Contemporary Implant Dentistry

Contemporary Implant Dentistry

Editor: Patricia Baker

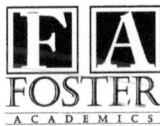

FA
FOSTER
ACADEMICS

www.fosteracademics.com

www.fosteracademics.com

FA
FOSTER
ACADEMICS

Cataloging-in-Publication Data

Contemporary implant dentistry / edited by Patricia Baker.
    p. cm.
Includes bibliographical references and index.
ISBN 978-1-63242-610-9
1. Dental implants. 2. Dentures. 3. Dentistry. I. Baker, Patricia.
RK667.I45 C66 2019
617.693--dc23

Foster Academics,
118-35 Queens Blvd., Suite 400,
Forest Hills, NY 11375, USA

ISBN 978-1-63242-610-9 (Hardback)

Contents

Preface

The world is advancing at a fast pace like never before. Therefore, the need is to keep up with the latest developments. This book was an idea that came to fruition when the specialists in the area realized the need to coordinate together and document essential themes in the subject. That's when I was requested to be the editor. Editing this book has been an honour as it brings together diverse authors researching on different streams of the field. The book collates essential materials contributed by veterans in the area which can be utilized by students and researchers alike.

A surgical component which serves as an orthodontic anchor between the bone of the jaw or skull and a dental prosthesis is called a dental implant. A dental prosthesis can range from a bridge, a denture to a facial prosthesis. Osseointegration is a biological process in which a material forms a bond with the bone. This process is the foundation of modern implant dentistry. Computed tomography along with CAM/CAD simulations and surgical guidelines are used to determine the position of implants with respect to the adjacent teeth. Temporary anchorage devices are a special type of small diameter dental implants which are used to assist the movement of the tooth. Root analog ceramic implants are currently the most technologically advanced form of dental implants. They are produced using CT or DVT scans and can be placed without any surgery after tooth extraction. In this book, the various advancements in implant dentistry are glanced at and their applications as well as ramifications are looked at in detail. For all readers who are interested in this field, the case studies included herein will serve as an excellent guide to develop a comprehensive understanding.

Each chapter is a sole-standing publication that reflects each author's interpretation. Thus, the book displays a multi-facetted picture of our current understanding of application, resources and aspects of the field. I would like to thank the contributors of this book and my family for their endless support.

Editor

Drug Delivery Systems in Bone Regeneration and Implant Dentistry

Sukumaran Anil, Asala F. Al-Sulaimani,
Ansar E. Beeran, Elna P. Chalisserry,
Harikrishna P.R. Varma and Mohammad D. Al Amri

1. Introduction

Bone regeneration is a complex, well-orchestrated physiological process involving a number of cell types and intracellular and extracellular molecular signaling pathways [1]. Bone grafts provide a structural framework for clot development, maturation and remodeling that supports bone formation in osseous defects. These materials must possess biocompatibility and osteoconductivity, as well as the properties that support osteogenesis. The ideal characteristics of a bone graft are that it must be nontoxic, non-antigenic, resistant to infection, easily adaptable, readily and sufficiently available to stimulate new attachment and able to trigger osteogenesis [2].

Osseous defects in the oral cavity have been successfully managed with a variety of biological and synthetic materials, including autografts, allografts, xenografts and alloplastic materials. Although autografts are unequivocally accepted as the gold standard, donor site morbidity and limitations on the quantity of bone that can be harvested demand that clinicians seek alternatives [3]. In light of the immunological and disease transfer risks from allogeneic bone, research has focused extensively on developing alloplastic bone substitutes that are predominantly based on ceramics, such as calcium phosphates (CaP), calcium sulfates, and bioactive glasses [4]. In general, these ceramic materials are renowned for their osteoconductive and bioactive properties [5]. The most commonly used ceramics are the CaP-based ceramics hydroxyapatite (HA) and beta tricalcium phosphate [6].

Considering engineered grafts, the most important factor is to prepare a three-dimensional structure consisting of biodegradable material, generally called a scaffold [7]. The nature and structure of the scaffold should support cell proliferation and differentiation, accelerating the process of tissue regeneration. Furthermore, the growth factor providing a scaffold to an injury site should enhance progenitors, causing inflammatory cells to migrate and activate the healing process [8, 9]. However, among the basic challenges for scaffold implantation is to control infection due to bacterial load, which can create immune problems and finally result in implant rejection. To overcome implant-related infection and bacterial load on the scaffold, antibiotic drug incorporation and its controlled release have been suggested as a promising strategy [10]. Bone is among the few tissues of the human body that has high endogenous healing capacity. Various concepts for local drug delivery to bone have been developed in recent decades to overcome such healing deficits.

Several methods are used for drug loading and release from scaffolds. However, the basic aim for drug release is to reduce infections and bacterial load to the site of implant, but if the drug is released too quickly, there could be a chance of infection because the entire drug has drained from the scaffold in the initial time itself. Similarly, if there is too much delay to drug release, infection can set in further, making it more difficult to manage the healing of wounds. Hence, better options for drug release would incorporate higher antibiotic release at the initial time and sustained release at an effective rate to inhibit the risk of infection from bacteria in the scaffold at an effective level [11]. Different techniques have been used for drug loading to the scaffold, and controlled release has been studied. One of the simplest strategies is the application of biodegradable polymer coatings loaded with specific drugs onto the scaffold structure. The other methods reported for coating the drug-loaded polymer have included solvent casting, thermally induced phase separation, evaporation, freeze drying and foam coating. Among these methods, an interesting approach for drug loading and release consists of combining drug-loaded microspheres with a macroporous scaffold `matrix' [12-15].

In a recent study, a biodegradable nanoporous bioceramic system was used as a highly bioresorbable matrix for drug delivery. This study emphasized the efficacy of hydroxyapatite-based material having interconnected nanoporosity as a vehicle for a therapeutic agent. An in vitro experiment was conducted with the goal of assessing this material and comparing it with commercially available gentamicin-loaded PMMA cement. It was found that the nanoporous bioceramic granules could act as antibiotic carriers, exhibiting a high initial burst effect followed by sustained low-level release for 3 weeks. It was very effective, confirming that the concentration of drug eluted was greater than that needed to maintain bactericidal levels [16].

In addition to the above-mentioned technique, magnetic nanoparticle-incorporated materials have also been used as a bone regeneration scaffold, and they are schematically represented in figure 3 [17]. To obtain homogenous dispersion of magnetic particle loading and surfactant, a porous structure generated by ceramic crystals, the in-situ method was followed. Further, it was made to a specific shape, and the specific drug was loaded via dip loading or other methods. The drug-loaded scaffold was placed at the defective site in the presence of a magnetic field (MF), which facilitated easy drug release from the scaffold, helping to protect it from bacterial colonization, and the MF stimulated the scaffold for cell proliferation. Recently released in vitro results support MF-induced bone regeneration [18-20].

Engineered biomaterials combined with growth factors, such as bone morphogenetic protein-2 (BMP-2), have been demonstrated to constitute an effective approach in bone tissue engineering because they can act both as a scaffold and as a drug delivery system to promote bone repair and regeneration. Despite the substantial progress made in developing porous materials as bone substitutes, the realization of synthetic structure able to harness fully bone's capability of regenerating and remodeling itself and to mimic the complicated physiochemical attributes of bone continues to present challenges.

In the following sections of this chapter, the materials and drug delivery techniques used to enhance bone regeneration and to control infection are discussed. The methods to enhance the surface of titanium implants to promote osseointegration are also detailed.

2. Bone regeneration materials

2.1. Calcium phosphate ceramics

The calcium phosphates have been widely studied due to their biocompatibility, tailorable bio-absorbability and bioactivity. Calcium phosphates have been used as novel delivery carriers for antibiotics, anti-inflammatory agents, analgesics, anticancer drugs, growth factors, proteins and genes [21, 22]. Furthermore, they can be synthesized using simple methods, and these drugs can easily be incorporated via different routes, such as wet chemical processes, solid state reactions, hydrothermal and micelle-mediated processes, etc. [23, 24]. Most of the polymeric systems show an acidic nature, and their degradation by-products can alter drug activity. The major advantages of CaPs, compared with other biodegradable polymeric systems, is that the degradation ions are Ca^{2+} and PO_4^{3-} ions, which already exist in the body in higher concentrations [25].

Nanotechnology-derived calcium phosphates have also successfully maintained a sustained and steady drug release over time. Calcium phosphate scaffolds not only provide initial structural integrity for bone cells but also direct their proliferation and differentiation and assist in the ultimate assembly of new tissue. Therefore, ceramic nanoscaffolds are usually 3-D and porous, although in some cases they consist of 2-D coatings or films. They mimic the in vivo environment of cells more completely than nanoparticles.

Therefore, most drug-eluted ceramic nanoscaffolds serve multiple functions, such as drug delivery, directing cell growth or tissue generation, and mechanical support. Indeed, the mechanical support provided by ceramic scaffolds far exceeds that provided by polymeric scaffolds. Studies have shown that drug-release kinetics could be further controlled by tailoring calcium phosphate nanoparticle grain size, surface area and calcium-to-phosphorus ratios [26]. Hollow silica nanospheres have been fabricated into well-controlled shapes and sizes using self-templating molecules [20]. For example, studies have shown that hollow silica nanospheres were capable of entrapping an eight-fold greater quantity of drug species than solid silica nanospheres. Time-delayed multiple-stage release profiles were also possible with these hollow silica nanospheres [27].

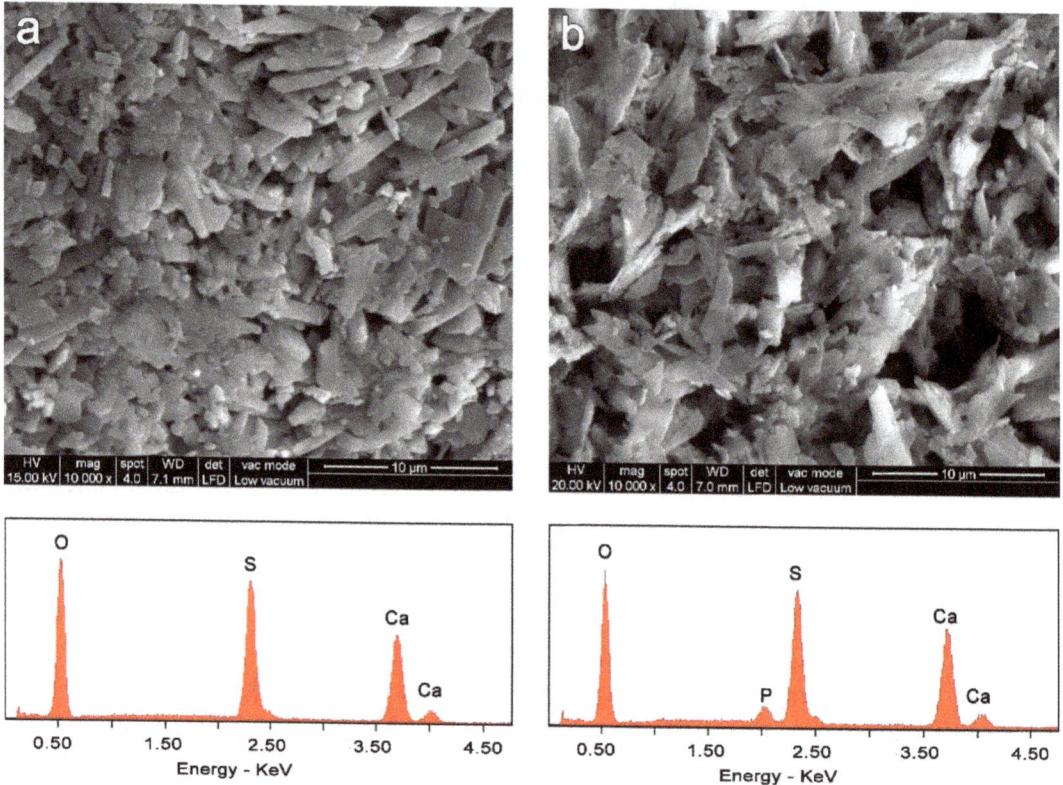

Figure 1. The micromorphology (SEM) of calcium sulfate-phosphate injectable cement. **a)** The set cement surface of unmodified low-dimensional medical grade calcium sulfate (crystal sizes less than 5 microns). **b)** The phosphate-containing material, which inhabits very small crystal formations grown into folding sheets. Energy dispersive (EDS) data, corresponding to the samples, are shown below each. The phosphorous content in the second sample is evident, whereas no separate phosphate phase appeared in XRD. The phosphate content resides as a substitution in the calcium sulfate crystals.

2.2. Porous spherical hydroxyapatite granules for drug delivery

Calcium phosphate-based bioceramics, such as hydroxyapatite (HA), are known for their excellent biocompatibility due to their similarity in composition to the apatite found in natural bone [28]. Various forms of HA bone grafts, such as dense and porous blocks, dense and porous granules, and powder forms, are available as bone substitutes [29]. The porous matrices enable cell migration and provide favorable conditions for nutrient transport, tissue infiltration, and vascularization [30, 31]. The spherically shaped particles are suitable for implantation as injectable bone cements, and the inter-granular space promotes cell migration and the growth of extracellular matrix [32, 33].

Porous HA is produced using methods such as ceramic slip foaming [34], positive replication of reticulated foam scaffolds [35], burnout of sacrificial porogens, such as polymer beads [3], and techniques that exploit naturally occurring porous calcium-based structures, such as the hydrothermal conversion of either coral or bone [36, 37]. Porous spherical HA granules can be used for drug delivery systems. The various pore and channel structures of spherical granules were obtained by adjusting the ratio of water to HA powder and the amount of sodium chloride (NaCl). Earlier studies focused on the use of anti-inflammatory or anti-bacterial drug release from HA, to control inflammation and infection at the site of implantation [38]. Currently, several drugs have been found to enhance bone formation, and the loading of HA with these drugs and agents could be a very effective method for enhancing bone formation at the site of implantation [39, 40]. Research is under way to control the drug release rate using the complex micro-channel structures of HA granules [41].

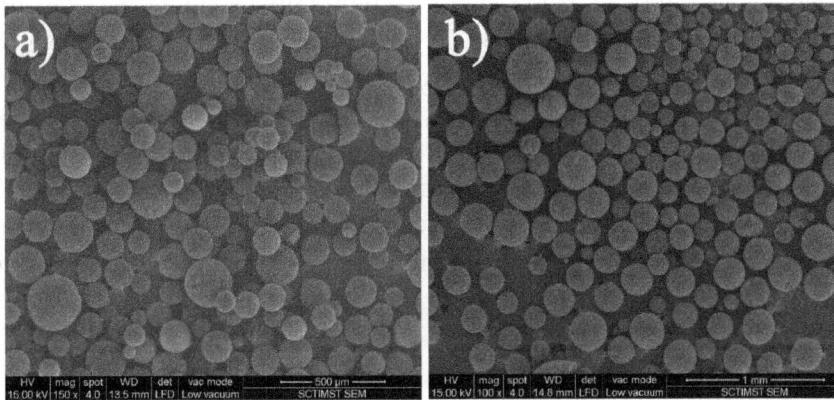

Figure 2. Scanning electron microscopic images of: a) polycaprolactone polymer microspheres; and b) magnetic hydroxyapatite-loaded polycaproctone polymer microspheres.

2.3. Demineralized bone matrix

Bone void fillers, such as demineralized bone matrix (DBM), offer a broad range of materials, structures and delivery systems to use in bone grafting procedures. Allogenic DBM possesses osteoinductive properties and could serve as an ideal drug delivery device for prophylactic treatment in a variety of different anatomical locations [42, 43]. The use of DBM would allow for the release of the entire quantity of antibiotic as the material is being remodeled.

2.4. Carriers and delivery systems for growth factors

Growth factors (GFs), such as bone morphogenetic protein, transforming growth factor-beta, fibroblast growth factor, platelet-derived growth factor, and insulin-like growth factor, are proteins secreted by cells that act on the appropriate target cell or cells to perform specific actions. A variety of so-called bone-graft substitutes, including demineralized bone matrix, calcium phosphate-containing preparations and Bioglass (BG), are also potential carriers for recombinant proteins [44]. Bioglass and calcium phosphate-based materials, such as hydroxyapatite, coralline hydroxyapatite, and tricalcium phosphate, have been shown to be biocompatible and to provide osteoconductive scaffolds that could potentially be combined with GFs to enhance bone repair [45].

Demineralized bone matrix preparations are particularly attractive as potential carriers for growth factors because they are osteoconductive and can have some osteoinductive potential as well. The disadvantages of these materials include poor handling characteristics and concerns about their overall bio-resorbability, as well as limited potential for remodeling and an unclear understanding of their effects on bone strength [46]. Recombinant bone morphogenetic protein (BMP) has been used to enhance the bone regeneration in graft and implant osseointegration in dentistry [47]. Recombinant human BMP-2 (rhBMP-2) has been shown to be effective in bone regeneration [48].

Among surface modification techniques, coating the implant surface with bone stimulating agents, such as GFs, is very promising. The most commonly used GFs include bone morphogenetic proteins (BMP-2), TGF-β1, platelet-derived growth factor, insulin-like growth factor and combinations [47, 49]. The actual mechanisms of GF combinations are not fully understood. From early reported studies, after implantation, both GFs (TGF-β and BMP) could directly increase the local pool of osteoprogenitor cells by stimulating their migration [50]. The circulation of pathways acts as a source of osteoprogenitor cells throughout ectopic BMP-induced bone regeneration. Similarly, the presence of both TGF-β1 and BMP-7 cooperatively interact to increase angiogenesis and vascular invasion after their co-administration increased vessel constitution [51]. The results demonstrated that the presence of GF associated with implant surfaces improved bone regeneration, vascular invasion and angiogenesis. Research is under way to optimize the carrier properties and the characteristics of the GF and its dose to maximize the regeneration potential.

2.5. Nanoscaffolds

The application of nanotechnology for drug delivery and the use of nanometer scale materials has helped to develop innovative approaches in this field. At this scale, materials display different physicochemical properties due to their small size, surface structure and high surface area. The nanoparticles based ceramic scaffolds have also demonstrated great potential for controlled drug delivery and is currently a fast growing research area. The ceramic nanoscaffolds have several advantages such as high porosity, high volume-to-area ratios, high surface area, high structural stability and long degradation times. These properties make them potent systems for controlled release of drugs. At the implantation sites drugs/chemical agents are applied for decreasing infection, reducing inflammation, and increasing bone growth on titanium surfaces. The nanotubular titania and calcium phosphate-based nanoscaffolds have showed good potential for drug and growth factor delivery.

2.6. Magnetic nanoparticles (FE-hydroxyapatite)

Superparamagnetic nanoparticles (MNPs) have been progressively explored for their potential in biomedical applications and in particular as contrast agents for diagnostic imaging, for magnetic drug delivery and, more recently, for tissue engineering applications [52-54]. MNPs have been used for biomedical applications, such as in hyperthermia [55], as a contrast agent for diagnostic imaging [56], for magnetic drug delivery [57, 58] [13], and for cell mechanosensitive receptor manipulation to induce cell differentiation [59].

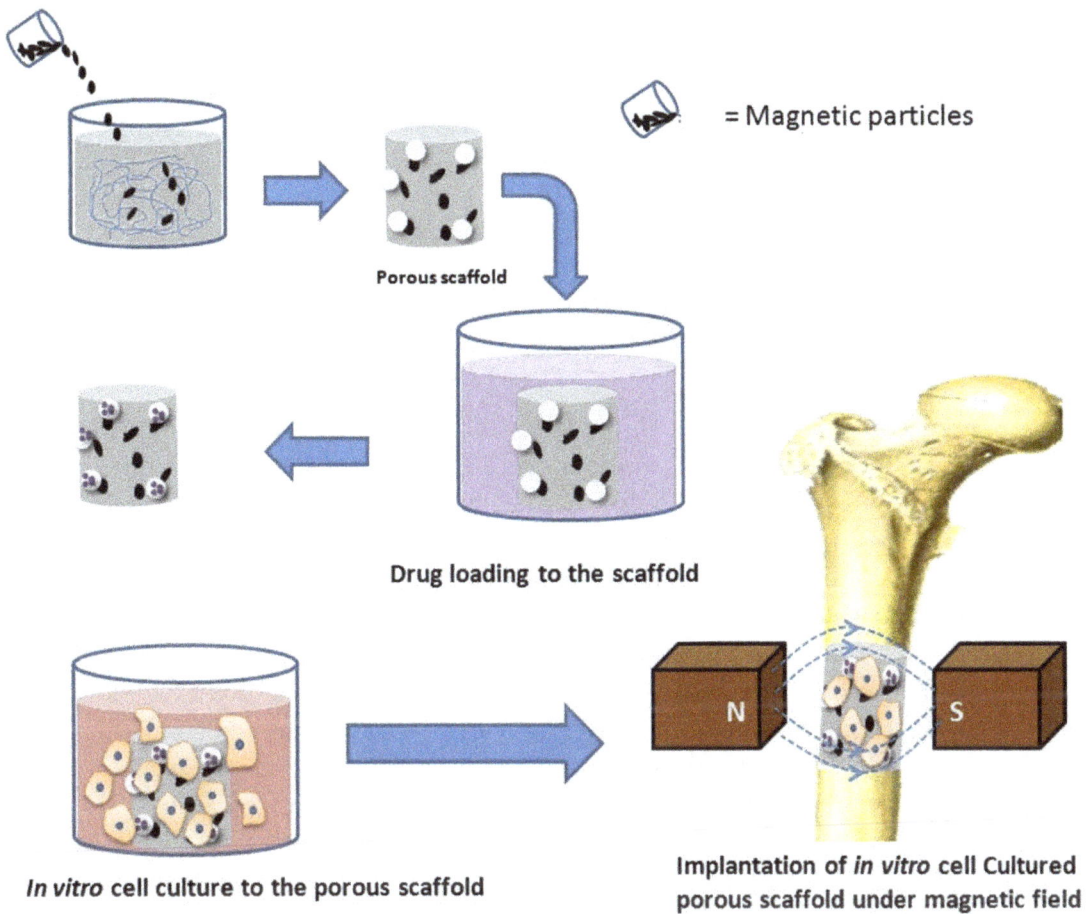

= Magnetic particles

Porous scaffold

Drug loading to the scaffold

In vitro cell culture to the porous scaffold

Implantation of *in vitro* cell Cultured porous scaffold under magnetic field

Figure 3. Schematic presentation of engineered magnetic scaffold preparation and implantation.

The most popular MNPs used in medicine and biotechnology are iron oxide-based phases, but their potential as a tissue engineering scaffold has not yet been fully assessed [60]. Although Fe is a vital element in the human body, its concentration within hard tissue is low, and its presence into the body scarcely affects bone remodeling [61]. In contrast, the biocompatibility and bioactivity of HA are already well established [62-64], and, in fact, more than 60% of the currently available bone graft substitutes involve calcium phosphate-based materials [65]. Hence, a Fe-HA phase endowed with superparamagnetic ability could be used as an active scaffold for bone and osteochondral regeneration or as a nontoxic, biodegradable, magnetic nanocarrier [17, 66, 67].

2.7. Chitosan hydroxy apatite

Chitosan is considered an appropriate functional material for biomedical applications because of its high biocompatibility, biodegradability, non-antigenicity and adsorption properties [68, 69]. The mechanical and biological properties of chitosan scaffolds could be improved by the incorporation of bioceramics, such as HA, β-tricalcium phosphate and calcium phosphate biomaterials, such as gelatin alginate, or inorganic material, such as wollastonite [70, 71]. Chitosan scaffolds are osteoconductive and can enhance bone formation both in vitro and in vivo [72]. Currently, the development of chitosan-nanohydroxyapatite (nHA) composites through in situ hybridization by ionic diffusion processes, freezing and lyophilization, stepwise co-precipitation, and mineralization via double diffusion are being undertaken successfully [73-75].

3. Surface functionalization of titanium implants

The long-term success of dental implants also depends on the complex **biointegration** of these alloplastic materials, determined by the responses of the different surrounding host tissues. The osteoinductivity of calcium phosphate coatings has attracted significant interest, using various coating techniques, including plasma spraying, magnetron sputtering, electrophoretic deposition, hot isostatic pressing, sol-gel deposition, pulsed laser deposition, ion beam dynamic mixing deposition, electrospray deposition, biomimetic deposition, and electrolytic deposition [76]. Non-ceramic implant coating is also used, allowing for drug incorporation during the coating process. The currently available techniques can be broadly divided into three categories, including hydrogel coatings, layer-by-layer coatings, and immobilization. Techniques such as 'dip-coating' methods and 'layer-by-layer' (LbL) coating techniques are used for the incorporation of BMP-2 and TGF-β1 to the implant surface [77].

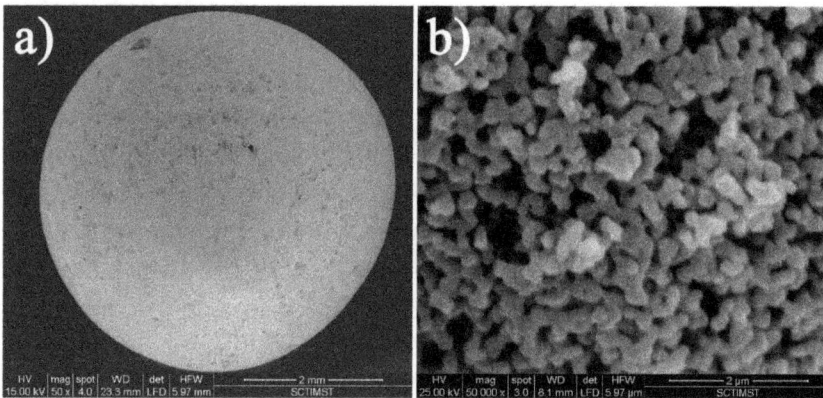

Figure 4. a) Scanning electron microscopic pictures of HAP microspheres; b) high-resolution SEM picture showing interconnected nanopores.

3.1. Nanotubular titanium surface

Nanotubular titania structures can be readily fabricated via direct anodization of titanium implants into an electrochemical cell that uses the titanium as an anode and platinum as a cathode in the presence of fluorine-based electrolytes [78, 79]. Penicillin-based antibiotics could be loaded to the nanotubular titania as a drug delivery platform by co-precipitating the drug and calcium phosphate crystals onto the nanostructures [80, 81].

Anodic oxidation has many advantages for surface modification, such as its ability to fabricate porous TiO_2 films through dielectric breakdown, the changeability of the crystalline structure and the chemical composition of the oxide film depending on the fabrication conditions, and it has been suggested to provide storage room for the delivery of GFs, such as rhBMP-2, to enhance osseointegration [82, 83]. In vitro studies have suggested that a dose response could be produced with appropriate period of delivery of the GF to the cells [84].

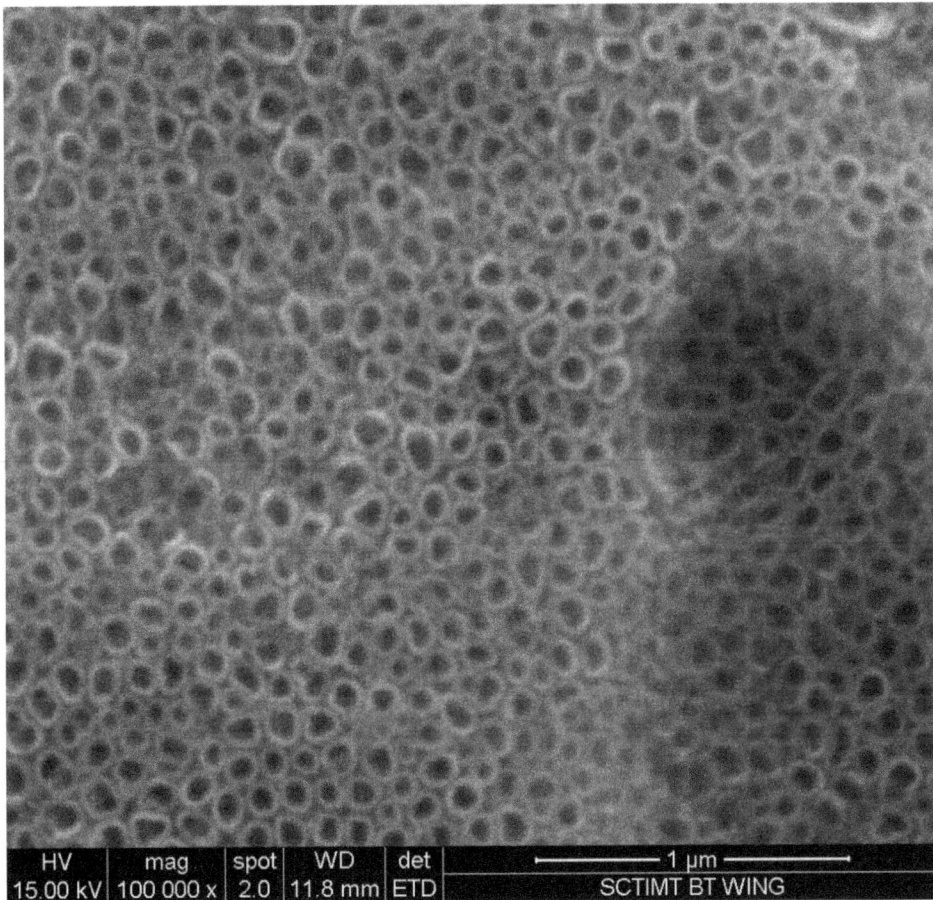

| HV | mag | spot | WD | det | 1 μm |
| 15.00 kV | 100 000 x | 2.0 | 11.8 mm | ETD | SCTIMT BT WING |

Figure 5. Scanning electron microscopic image of an anodized titanium implant surface showing uniform nano-tubules of titanium oxide throughout the surface.

3.2. Hydroxyapatite

Coating of titanium implant surfaces with HA has shown better integration with bone. HA can be coated to the surface by plasma spraying, sputtering, pulse laser deposition and electrostatic multilayer assemblies, fabricated using the layer-by-layer technique [85]. HA coatings enhance new bone formation on implant surfaces with a line-to-line fit, in areas with

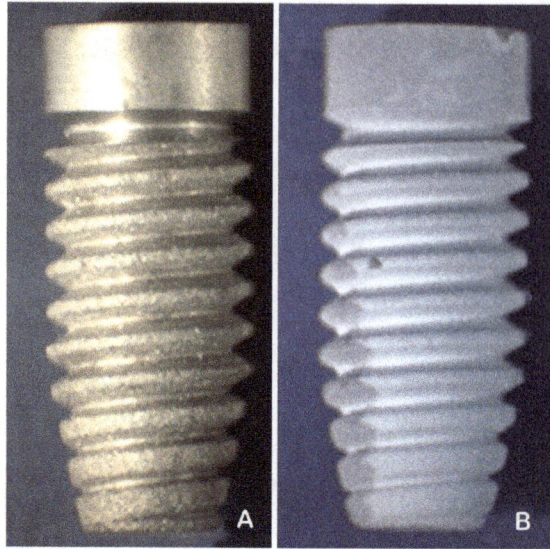

Figure 6. a) An anodized titanium implant; b) An anodized titanium implant coated with hydroxyapatite.

gaps of 1-2 mm between the coated implant and the surrounding bone. The coating also helps to prevent the formation of fibrous tissue that would normally result due to the micro-movements of an uncoated titanium implant [86].

HA coatings have been used as a method for the delivery of GFs, bioactive molecules, and DNA [85, 87, 88]. HA coatings augmented with bone morphogenetic protein-7 (BMP-7), placed on segmental femoral diaphyseal replacement prostheses, improved bone ingrowth in a canine extra-cortical bone-bridging model. Titanium alloy plasma-sprayed porous HA coatings, infiltrated with collagen, recombinant human bone morphogenetic protein (rhBMP-2) and RGD peptide, improved mesenchymal stem cell (MSC) adhesion, proliferation and differentiation in vitro and increased bone formation in ectopic muscle and intra-osseous locations in vivo [85].

Another group used hydroxyapatite nanoparticles complexed with chitosan into nanoscale non-degradable electrostatic multilayers, which were capped with a degradable poly(b-amino ester)-based film incorporating physiological amounts of rhBMP-2 [89]. Plasmid DNA, bound to calcium phosphate coatings deposited on poly-lactide-co-glycolide (PLG), was shown to be released in vitro according to the properties of the mineral and solution environment [87]. These methods of delivery of bioactive molecules extended the function of HA as a coating to enhance new bone formation around implants.

3.3. Antibiotics: Surface tethering of antibiotics

The initial adhesion and colonization of bacteria to an implant surface are considered to play key roles in the pathogenesis of infections related to biomaterials [90]. Two recent strategies are: (1) coating implants with antibiotics; and (2) covalently attaching antimicrobial molecules onto the implant surface. The objective of these bioactive surfaces is to disrupt the colonization

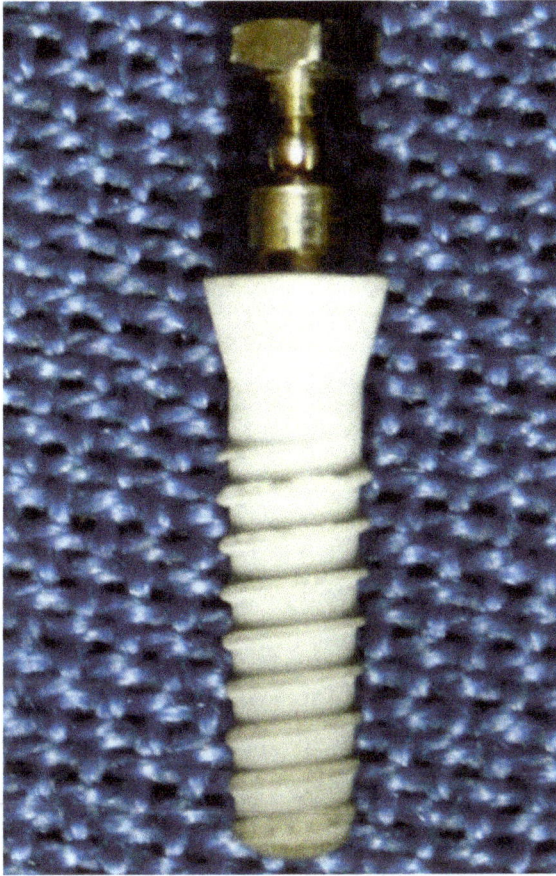

Figure 7. Hydroxyapatite-coated titanium implant.

of the microbes or to prevent bacterial adhesion to the implant and subsequent development of biofilm [91]. Hydrophilic surfaces have been shown to be less prone to become infected with microorganisms than hydrophobic surfaces [92]. The topical application of antibiotics on the implant surface might be more efficient because bacteria are killed locally directly upon binding, before the formation of biofilm. Local delivery of antibiotics has long been applied in bone cements used to repair orthopedic and dental implants [93].

Antibiotics such as gentamicin are incorporated into the cement, which slowly releases the drugs after setting *in situ*. Local delivery can prevent adhesion and growth of significant numbers of bacteria. HA coatings are frequently applied to dental implants to stimulate osseointegration and to accelerate bone formation. Antibiotics can be co-precipitated on titanium surfaces to obtain drug-releasing surface coatings. Studies have shown that antibiotics with optimal calcium-chelating properties had long lasting antimicrobial properties [94, 95]. Alt et al [96] demonstrated that both gentamicin-hydroxyapatite and gentamicin-RGD (arginine-glycineaspartate)-HA coatings could release antibiotics for up to twenty-four hours without inhibiting new bone formation. Erythromycin-impregnated strontium-doped calcium polyphosphate (SCPP) was found to inhibit bacterial growth completely for up to 14 days [97]

Nanoporous implants are suitable for the incorporation of antibiotics to obtain controlled release of drugs [98]. Nanostructured surfaces play a major role in advanced biomedical implant design because these surfaces have been studied for their enhanced bioactive properties, as well as their antagonistic behavior toward bacterial colonization. To maintain sustained drug elution properties and better bone bonding ability, significant efforts have been undertaken to develop bioactive hollow nanostructures on implant surfaces [99]. In this context, one of the implant titania nanotubular surfaces created via anodization showed enhanced bioactivity, conjugated with the capacity to store diverse compounds and control their elution. The anodization technique could create porous structures with controlled sizes of three-dimensional networks on metallic surfaces [100].

Anodization followed by HA coating was adopted as a surface modification technique to make drug-loadable Ti implants for dental applications. Self-organized titania nano-tubes were grown on titanium substrate as drug-carrying vehicles by coating HA ceramic using laser deposition. Nanostructured surfaces were achieved on titanium via anodization in a glycerol-NH_4F electrolyte system, followed by annealing. The nano-tubules were then capped with HA deposited with pulsed laser ablation. HA-coated polished titanium, nano-structured titanium and hydroxyapatite coated nano-structured titanium were analyzed for their drug-carrying capacity using gentamicin sulfate. The ceramic-coated anodized substrates were found to be most efficient among the aforementioned three compounds in controlled delivery for longer than 160 h, with drug content of 0.5 $\mu g/cm^2$, compared to the anodized substrate, which delivered the whole drug within 140 h. It was thus evident that laser deposition facilitated the controlled release of drug, compared to the anodized and bare substrates. This study proposed the application of laser deposition of bioceramics, such as HA, over nano-structured titanium for drug-eluting metallic implants [101].

3.4. Tan-Ag coatings

Due to the risk of the development of antibiotic resistance associated with antibiotic-loaded coatings, non-antibiotic agents in the coating have been used as alternatives. Among the various dopants, silver nanoparticles are among the most popular agents used due to their inhibition of bacterial adhesion, broad anti-bacterial spectrum, long lasting anti-bacterial effects, and propensity for being less prone to the development of resistance. Ag and Cu are known to be efficient antibacterial agents because of their specific antimicrobial activity and the nontoxicity of active Ag and Cu ions to human cells [102, 103]. Sputter coating of Ag, along with HA, resulted in an antibacterial-bioactive coating, which inhibited bacterial attachment without cytotoxic effects [104]. TaN-Ag nano-composite coating of titanium dental implants also showed significant antibacterial properties without any cytotoxic effects. Hence, it could be concluded that coating of titanium implants with materials having antimicrobial properties might be useful in preventing infection [105].

3.5. Bisphosphonate

Bisphosphonates (BPs) constitute a group of drugs that inhibit osteoclast action and the resorption of bone, and they are used to treat metabolic diseases such as osteoporosis, Paget's disease, hypercalcemia of malignancy and multiple myeloma [106]. The nitrogen-containing BPs are more potent, and they accumulate in maximum concentrations in the matrix and osteoclasts [107]. BPs have a high affinity for bone minerals and bind strongly to HA, resulting in selective uptake to the target organ and high local concentrations in bone, particularly at sites of active bone remodeling. The BPs have similar chemical structures to pyrophosphate, but their chemical stability is greater. In pyrophosphates, the phosphate group is bonded through phosphoanhydride bond (P-O-P), whereas in BP, P is bonded through a germinal carbon atom (P-C-P); hence, these bonds are resistant to hydrolysis under acidic conditions [108]. The affinity of BP to Ca^{2+} ions helps to target specific bony sites, and BP can be coupled with a gamma-emitting radioisotope, such as technetium, for simultaneous bone scanning [109]. BPs inhibit osteoclast differentiation, reduce their activity, and induce their apoptosis [110]. The nitrogen-containing BPs bind to and inhibit farnesyl pyrophosphate synthase (FPPS), a key enzyme of the mevalonate pathway, thereby preventing the prenylation and activation of small GTPases, which are essential for the bone-resorption activity and survival of osteoclasts [111].

Systemic and local delivery of BPs improved the osseointegration of dental implants in osteoporotic animal models [112-116]. Improved osseointegration and the mechanical stability of titanium implants were reported in ovariectomized rats supplemented with alendronate [112]. Kurth et al [113] showed enhanced integration of HA-coated titanium implants via the administration of ibandronate to osteoporotic rats. Similar observations of enhanced osseointegration have been reported in other studies via the local release of BPs (pamidronate and zoledronic acid) from the surface coatings of implants [115, 116]. An experimental study in an ovariectomized rabbit model showed that systemic zoledronic acid (ZA) administration improved the osseointegration of titanium implants [117].

3.6. Simvastatin

Statins are prescribed to decrease cholesterol biosynthesis by the liver, thereby reducing serum cholesterol concentrations and lowering the risk of heart attack. A liposoluble statin, simvastatin, could induce the expression of bone morphogenetic protein (BMP) 2 mRNA and, as a result, promote bone formation on the calvaria of mice following daily subcutaneous injections [118, 119]. Another study showed that the topical application of statins to alveolar bone increased bone formation and concurrently suppressed osteoclast activity at the bone healing sites [120]. Yang et al [119] demonstrated that simvastatin-loaded porous titanium surface potently increased ALP activity and the extracellular accumulation of proteins, such as osteocalcin and type I collagen, in mouse preosteoblast MC3T3-E1 cells. Du et al [121] demonstrated that administration of simvastatin resulted in significant improvement in the osseointegration of titanium implants in osteoporotic rats. This finding could be attributed to the increased expression of bone morphogenic protein 2, which stimulates osteoblast differentiation [118]. Statins are known to enhance the expression of VEGF (vascular endothelial growth factor), a bone anabolic factor, in osteoblasts and to regulate osteoblast function by increasing the expression of bone sialoprotein (BSP), osteocalcin (OCN), and type I collagen (COL-I), as well as suppressing the gene expression of collagenases, such as matrix metalloproteinase (MMP)-1 and MMP-13 [122, 123]. Thus the competitive inhibition of simvastatin interferes with the malevonate pathway, leading to decreased protein prenylation, which is necessary for normal osteoclast function [118].

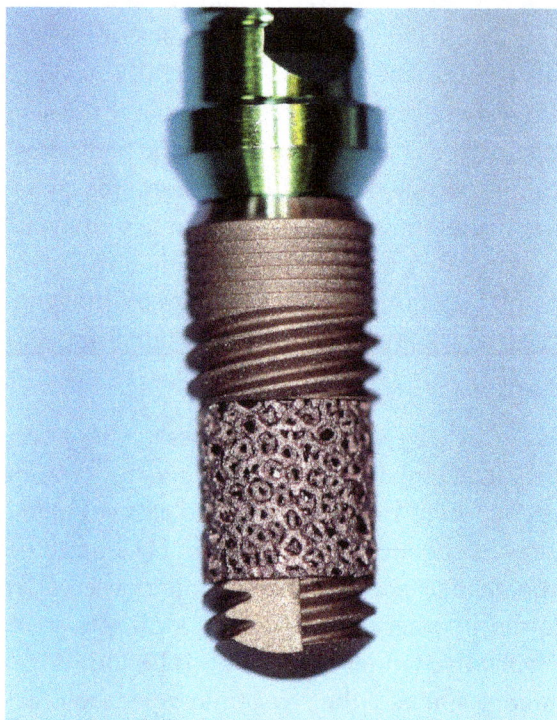

Figure 8. A trabecular implant that could be used to load drugs.

3.7. Calcitonin

Calcitonin (CT), produced by the C-cells of thyroid tissue, has been reported to stimulate hard tissue formation [124]. It acts on bone tissue via the suppression of osteolysis and the induction of Ca^{2+} release. It was reported that CT inhibited osteoclastic bone resorption by binding to specific cell surface receptors [125]. This hormone favors bone formation, inhibits osteoclastic activity and prevents osteopenia [126-128]. In vitro and in vivo studies have shown that this hormone stimulates the growth of bone tissue [40, 129, 130]. Calcitonin also showed increases in the amount and rate of bone formation, as observed in rat calvaria and extraction sockets in dogs [131].

3.8. Pantaprazole

A class of substituted benzimidazoles known as proton pump inhibitors (PPIs) have been shown to promote bone regeneration and peri-implant healing. Examples of these drugs include omeprazole and pantoprazole, which are employed clinically in the treatment of gastroesophageal reflux disorder (GERD). PPI-loaded calcium phosphate cements demonstrated not only inherent biocompatibility and osteoconductivity but also the ability to retard bone resorption through a drug delivery mechanism [132, 133]. Pantoprazole-loaded calcium phosphate cements inhibited osteoclastic resorption without interfering with the peri-implant bone resorption rate in a study performed rat femoral condyles [134]. Another advantage of the addition of omeprazole is that it inhibits osteoclastic acidification, which help to inhibit bone resorption and increases the lifespan of osteoclasts [135]. The drugs were dissolved in dimethyl sulfoxide to the desired concentration and were added to the liquid phase of the calcium phosphate.

4. Conclusions

Drug delivery systems (DDS) targeting specific organs and tissues and their bioavailability at specific sites have become critical issue in modern medicine. Local drug delivery systems in bone could be used to promote regeneration, prevent infection, or treat post-surgical pain. The quest for new bone scaffold materials to overcome the shortcomings of existing materials, such as ceramics and polymers, is undertaken to overcome the limited mechanical properties required for temporary bone substitutes. Mixing of polymers, natural or synthetic, and inorganic components, such as HA, TCP and BG, might help to develop better composite scaffolds that combine the advantages of both biodegradable polymers and bioactive ceramics [136].

If DDS are used in combination with implants, the coating strategies should allow for the choice of a drug or combination of drugs and their doses, localization and release due to intra-operative considerations. HA coatings on titanium implants themselves provide an osteoconductive and an osteoinductive approach for the enhancement of bone formation. These biological properties could be augmented further by adding growth factors and other molecules to produce a truly osteoinductive platform.

Proteins or glycosaminoglycans, such as collagen and chondroitin sulfate, provide a biomimetic coating on the surface of an implant, which can improve osseointegration [137]. Biomolecules such as GFs are also widely used for implant coatings, to modulate cellular functions, such as decreasing inflammation, enhancing stem cell differentiation, inducing blood vessel formation, or acting as chemoattractants for circulating osteoprogenitors [138, 139]. Although the implant materials available for the reconstruction of craniofacial bone defects have shown favorable results in most craniofacial and dental applications, the presence of complications related to infection and poor osseointegration still represent challenges in the biomedical field.

The current trend in the field of bone repair indicates that the tissue engineering field is moving toward the development of biomaterials with improved surfaces that will stimulate bone formation and avoid infections through the incorporation of surface modification techniques and antibacterial coatings and agents, as well as the incorporation of GFs, stem cells and other pharmacological drugs.

Author details

Sukumaran Anil[1*], Asala F. Al-Sulaimani[2], Ansar E. Beeran[3], Elna P. Chalisserry[4], Harikrishna P.R. Varma[3] and Mohammad D. Al Amri[5]

*Address all correspondence to: drsanil@gmail.com

1 Department of Periodontics and Community Dentistry, College of Dentistry, King Saud University, Riyadh, Saudi Arabia

2 King Saud University, Riyadh, Saudi Arabia

3 Biomedical Technology Wing, Sree Chitra Tirunal Institute for Medical Sciences & Technology, Poojappura, India

4 College of Dentistry, King Saud University, Riyadh, Saudi Arabia

5 Department of Prosthetic Dental Sciences, College of Dentistry, King Saud University, Riyadh, Saudi Arabia

References

[1] Kempene DH, Creemers LB, Alblas J, Lu L, Verbout AJ, Yaszemski MJ, Dhert WJ. Growth factor interactions in bone regeneration. Tissue engineering Part B, Reviews 2010; 16(6):551-566.

[2] Romagnoli C, D'Asta F, Brandi ML. Drug delivery using composite scaffolds in the context of bone tissue engineering. Clinical Cases in Mineral and Bone Metabolism 2013; 10(3):155.

[3] Moy PK, Lundgren S, Holmes RE. Maxillary sinus augmentation: histomorphometric analysis of graft materials for maxillary sinus floor augmentation. Journal of oral and maxillofacial surgery : official journal of the American Association of Oral and Maxillofacial Surgeons 1993; 51(8):857-862.

[4] Zamet JS, Darbar UR, Griffiths GS, Bulman JS, Bragger U, Burgin W, Newman HN. Particulate bioglass as a grafting material in the treatment of periodontal intrabony defects. Journal of clinical periodontology 1997; 24(6):410-418.

[5] Ignatius AA, Ohnmacht M, Claes LE, Kreidler J, Palm F. A composite polymer/tricalcium phosphate membrane for guided bone regeneration in maxillofacial surgery. Journal of biomedical materials research 2001; 58(5):564-569.

[6] Knabe C, Driessens FC, Planell JA, Gildenhaar R, Berger G, Reif D, Fitzner R, Radlanski RJ, Gross U. Evaluation of calcium phosphates and experimental calcium phos-

phate bone cements using osteogenic cultures. Journal of biomedical materials research 2000; 52(3):498-508.

[7]   Langer R, Vacanti JP. Tissue engineering. Science 1993; 260(5110):920-926.

[8]   Furth ME, Atala A, Van Dyke ME. Smart biomaterials design for tissue engineering and regenerative medicine. Biomaterials 2007; 28(34):5068-5073.

[9]   Lee SH, Shin H. Matrices and scaffolds for delivery of bioactive molecules in bone and cartilage tissue engineering. Advanced drug delivery reviews 2007; 59(4-5): 339-359.

[10] Sussman C, Bates-Jensen BM: Wound care: a collaborative practice manual: Lippincott Williams & Wilkins; 2007.

[11] Adams CS, Antoci V, Jr., Harrison G, Patal P, Freeman TA, Shapiro IM, Parvizi J, Hickok NJ, Radin S, Ducheyne P. Controlled release of vancomycin from thin sol-gel films on implant surfaces successfully controls osteomyelitis. Journal of orthopaedic research : official publication of the Orthopaedic Research Society 2009; 27(6):701-709.

[12] Maquet V, Jerome R: Design of macroporous biodegradable polymer scaffolds for cell transplantation. In Materials Science Forum: 1997. Trans Tech Publ; 1997:15-42.

[13] Thomson RC, Yaszemski MJ, Powers JM, Mikos AG. Hydroxyapatite fiber reinforced poly(alpha-hydroxy ester) foams for bone regeneration. Biomaterials 1998; 19(21): 1935-1943.

[14] Zhang Y, Zhang M. Calcium phosphate/chitosan composite scaffolds for controlled in vitro antibiotic drug release. Journal of biomedical materials research 2002; 62(3): 378-386.

[15] Cabanas MV, Pena J, Roman J, Vallet-Regi M. Tailoring vancomycin release from beta-TCP/agarose scaffolds. European journal of pharmaceutical sciences : official journal of the European Federation for Pharmaceutical Sciences 2009; 37(3-4):249-256.

[16] Simon D, Manuel S, Varma H. Novel nanoporous bioceramic spheres for drug delivery application: a preliminary in vitro investigation. Oral surgery, oral medicine, oral pathology and oral radiology 2013; 115(3):e7-14.

[17] Panseri S, Cunha C, D'Alessandro T, Sandri M, Giavaresi G, Marcacci M, Hung CT, Tampieri A. Intrinsically superparamagnetic Fe-hydroxyapatite nanoparticles positively influence osteoblast-like cell behaviour. Journal of nanobiotechnology 2012; 10:32.

[18] Panseri S, Cunha C, D'Alessandro T, Sandri M, Russo A, Giavaresi G, Marcacci M, Hung CT, Tampieri A. Magnetic hydroxyapatite bone substitutes to enhance tissue regeneration: evaluation in vitro using osteoblast-like cells and in vivo in a bone defect. PloS one 2012; 7(6):e38710.

[19] Singh RK, Patel KD, Lee JH, Lee EJ, Kim JH, Kim TH, Kim HW. Potential of magnetic nanofiber scaffolds with mechanical and biological properties applicable for bone regeneration. PloS one 2014; 9(4):e91584.

[20] Yang L, Sheldon BW, Webster TJ. Nanophase Ceramics for Improved Drug Delivery: Current Opportunities and Challenges. American Ceramic Society Bulletin 2010; 89(2):24-31.

[21] Ginebra M, Traykova T, Planell J. Calcium phosphate cements as bone drug delivery systems: a review. Journal of Controlled Release 2006; 113(2):102-110.

[22] Kim K, Fisher JP. Nanoparticle technology in bone tissue engineering. J Drug Target 2007; 15(4):241-252.

[23] Barth BM, Sharma R, Altinoglu EI, Morgan TT, Shanmugavelandy SS, Kaiser JM, McGovern C, Matters GL, Smith JP, Kester M et al. Bioconjugation of calcium phosphosilicate composite nanoparticles for selective targeting of human breast and pancreatic cancers in vivo. ACS nano 2010; 4(3):1279-1287.

[24] Cheng X, Kuhn L. Chemotherapy drug delivery from calcium phosphate nanoparticles. International journal of nanomedicine 2007; 2(4):667-674.

[25] Wang S, McDonnell EH, Sedor FA, Toffaletti JG. pH effects on measurements of ionized calcium and ionized magnesium in blood. Archives of pathology & laboratory medicine 2002; 126(8):947-950.

[26] Melville AJ, Rodriguez-Lorenzo LM, Forsythe JS. Effects of calcination temperature on the drug delivery behaviour of Ibuprofen from hydroxyapatite powders. Journal of materials science Materials in medicine 2008; 19(3):1187-1195.

[27] Chen JF, Ding HM, Wang JX, Shao L. Preparation and characterization of porous hollow silica nanoparticles for drug delivery application. Biomaterials 2004; 25(4): 723-727.

[28] Suchanek W, Yoshimura M. Processing and properties of hydroxyapatite-based biomaterials for use as hard tissue replacement implants. Journal of Materials Research 2011; 13(01):94-117.

[29] Paul W, Sharma CP. Development of porous spherical hydroxyapatite granules: application towards protein delivery. Journal of materials science Materials in medicine 1999; 10(7):383-388.

[30] Jones AC, Milthorpe B, Averdunk H, Limaye A, Senden TJ, Sakellariou A, Sheppard AP, Sok RM, Knackstedt MA, Brandwood A et al. Analysis of 3D bone ingrowth into polymer scaffolds via micro-computed tomography imaging. Biomaterials 2004; 25(20):4947-4954.

[31] Karageorgiou V, Kaplan D. Porosity of 3D biomaterial scaffolds and osteogenesis. Biomaterials 2005; 26(27):5474-5491.

[32] Ribeiro CC, Barrias CC, Barbosa MA. Preparation and characterisation of calcium-phosphate porous microspheres with a uniform size for biomedical applications. Journal of materials science Materials in medicine 2006; 17(5):455-463.

[33] Zyman Z, Glushko V, Filippenko V, Radchenko V, Mezentsev V. Nonstoichiometric hydroxyapatite granules for orthopaedic applications. Journal of materials science Materials in medicine 2004; 15(5):551-558.

[34] Akao M, Aoki H, Kato K. Mechanical properties of sintered hydroxyapatite for prosthetic applications. Journal of Materials Science 1981; 16(3):809-812.

[35] Slosarczyk A. Highly Porous Hydroxyapatite Material. Powder Metall Int 1989; 21(4): 24-25.

[36] Roy DM, Linnehan SK. Hydroxyapatite formed from coral skeletal carbonate by hydrothermal exchange. Nature 1974; 247(5438):220-222.

[37] Dard M, Bauer A, Liebendorger A, Wahlig H, Dingeldein E. Preparation physio-chemical and biological evaluation of a hydroxyapatite ceramic from bovine spongiosa. Act Odonto Stom 1994; 185:61-69.

[38] Schlapp M, Friess W. Collagen/PLGA microparticle composites for local controlled delivery of gentamicin. J Pharm Sci 2003; 92(11):2145-2151.

[39] Kim JH, Park YB, Li Z, Shim JS, Moon HS, Jung HS, Chung MK. Effect of alendronate on healing of extraction sockets and healing around implants. Oral diseases 2011; 17(7):705-711.

[40] Doğan H, Ozcelik B, Senel S. The effect of calcitonin on osseous healing in guinea pig mandible. Journal of endodontics 2001; 27(3):160-163.

[41] Hong MH, Son JS, Kim KM, Han M, Oh DS, Lee YK. Drug-loaded porous spherical hydroxyapatite granules for bone regeneration. Journal of materials science Materials in medicine 2011; 22(2):349-355.

[42] Sassard WR, Eidman DK, Gray PM, Block JE, Russo R, Russell JL, Taboada EM. Augmenting local bone with Grafton demineralized bone matrix for posterolateral lumbar spine fusion: avoiding second site autologous bone harvest. Orthopedics 2000; 23(10):1059-1064; discussion 1064-1055.

[43] Lewis CS, Supronowicz PR, Zhukauskas RM, Gill E, Cobb RR. Local antibiotic delivery with demineralized bone matrix. Cell Tissue Bank 2012; 13(1):119-127.

[44] Schmitt JM, Hwang K, Winn SR, Hollinger JO. Bone morphogenetic proteins: an update on basic biology and clinical relevance. Journal of orthopaedic research : official publication of the Orthopaedic Research Society 1999; 17(2):269-278.

[45] Lieberman JR, Daluiski A, Einhorn TA. The role of growth factors in the repair of bone. Biology and clinical applications. The Journal of bone and joint surgery American volume 2002; 84-A(6):1032-1044.

[46] Cornell CN. Osteoconductive Materials and Their Role as Substitutes for Autogenous Bone Grafts. Orthopedic Clinics of North America 1999; 30(4):591-598.

[47] Tatakis DN, Koh A, Jin L, Wozney JM, Rohrer MD, Wikesjo UM. Peri-implant bone regeneration using recombinant human bone morphogenetic protein-2 in a canine model: a dose-response study. Journal of periodontal research 2002; 37(2):93-100.

[48] Wikesjö UM, Sorensen RG, Wozney JM. Augmentation of Alveolar Bone and Dental Implant Osseointegration: Clinical Implications of Studies with rhBMP-2 A Comprehensive Review. The Journal of Bone & Joint Surgery 2001; 83(1_suppl_2):S136-S145.

[49] Bessho K, Carnes DL, Cavin R, Chen HY, Ong JL. BMP stimulation of bone response adjacent to titanium implants in vivo. Clinical oral implants research 1999; 10(3): 212-218.

[50] Janssens K, ten Dijke P, Janssens S, Van Hul W. Transforming growth factor-beta1 to the bone. Endocrine reviews 2005; 26(6):743-774.

[51] Duneas N, Crooks J, Ripamonti U. Transforming growth factor-beta 1: induction of bone morphogenetic protein genes expression during endochondral bone formation in the baboon, and synergistic interaction with osteogenic protein-1 (BMP-7). Growth factors 1998; 15(4):259-277.

[52] Jain TK, Reddy MK, Morales MA, Leslie-Pelecky DL, Labhasetwar V. Biodistribution, clearance, and biocompatibility of iron oxide magnetic nanoparticles in rats. Mol Pharm 2008; 5(2):316-327.

[53] Prijic S, Scancar J, Cemazar M, Bregar VB, Znidarsic A, Sersa G. Increased cellular uptake of biocompatible superparamagnetic iron oxide nanoparticles into malignant cells by an external magnetic field. The Journal of membrane biology 2010; 236(1): 167-179.

[54] Sun C, Du K, Fang C, Bhattarai N, Veiseh O, Kievit F, Stephen Z, Lee D, Ellenbogen RG, Ratner B. PEG-mediated synthesis of highly dispersive multifunctional superparamagnetic nanoparticles: their physicochemical properties and function in vivo. ACS nano 2010; 4(4):2402-2410.

[55] Amirfazli A. Nanomedicine: magnetic nanoparticles hit the target. Nat Nanotechnol 2007; 2(8):467-468.

[56] Glossop JR, Cartmell SH. Tensile strain and magnetic particle force application do not induce MAP3K8 and IL-1B differential gene expression in a similar manner to fluid shear stress in human mesenchymal stem cells. Journal of tissue engineering and regenerative medicine 2010; 4(7):577-579.

[57] Gupta AK, Gupta M. Synthesis and surface engineering of iron oxide nanoparticles for biomedical applications. Biomaterials 2005; 26(18):3995-4021.

[58] Arruebo M, Fernández-Pacheco R, Ibarra MR, Santamaría J. Magnetic nanoparticles for drug delivery. Nano Today 2007; 2(3):22-32.

[59] Kanczler JM, Sura HS, Magnay J, Green D, Oreffo RO, Dobson JP, El Haj AJ. Controlled differentiation of human bone marrow stromal cells using magnetic nanoparticle technology. Tissue engineering Part A 2010; 16(10):3241-3250.

[60] Singh N, Jenkins GJ, Asadi R, Doak SH. Potential toxicity of superparamagnetic iron oxide nanoparticles (SPION). Nano Rev 2010; 1.

[61] Morrissey R, Rodriguez-Lorenzo LM, Gross KA. Influence of ferrous iron incorporation on the structure of hydroxyapatite. Journal of materials science Materials in medicine 2005; 16(5):387-392.

[62] Landi E, Celotti G, Logroscino G, Tampieri A. Carbonated hydroxyapatite as bone substitute. Journal of the European Ceramic Society 2003; 23(15):2931-2937.

[63] Landi E, Tampieri A, Celotti G, Sprio S, Sandri M, Logroscino G. Sr-substituted hydroxyapatites for osteoporotic bone replacement. Acta biomaterialia 2007; 3(6): 961-969.

[64] Landi E, Tampieri A, Mattioli-Belmonte M, Celotti G, Sandri M, Gigante A, Fava P, Biagini G. Biomimetic Mg-and Mg, CO< sub> 3</sub>-substituted hydroxyapatites: synthesis characterization and in vitro behaviour. Journal of the European Ceramic Society 2006; 26(13):2593-2601.

[65] Laurencin C, Khan Y, El-Amin SF. Bone graft substitutes. Expert review of medical devices 2006; 3(1):49-57.

[66] Tampieri A, D'Alessandro T, Sandri M, Sprio S, Landi E, Bertinetti L, Panseri S, Pepponi G, Goettlicher J, Banobre-Lopez M et al. Intrinsic magnetism and hyperthermia in bioactive Fe-doped hydroxyapatite. Acta biomaterialia 2012; 8(2):843-851.

[67] Xu H-Y, Gu N. Magnetic responsive scaffolds and magnetic fields in bone repair and regeneration. Frontiers of Materials Science 2014; 8(1):20-31.

[68] Thein-Han WW, Misra RD. Biomimetic chitosan-nanohydroxyapatite composite scaffolds for bone tissue engineering. Acta biomaterialia 2009; 5(4):1182-1197.

[69] Muzzarelli R, Baldassarre V, Conti F, Ferrara P, Biagini G, Gazzanelli G, Vasi V. Biological activity of chitosan: ultrastructural study. Biomaterials 1988; 9(3):247-252.

[70] George M, Abraham TE. Polyionic hydrocolloids for the intestinal delivery of protein drugs: alginate and chitosan--a review. Journal of controlled release : official journal of the Controlled Release Society 2006; 114(1):1-14.

[71] Li Z, Ramay HR, Hauch KD, Xiao D, Zhang M. Chitosan-alginate hybrid scaffolds for bone tissue engineering. Biomaterials 2005; 26(18):3919-3928.

[72] Muzzarelli RA, Mattioli-Belmonte M, Tietz C, Biagini R, Ferioli G, Brunelli MA, Fini M, Giardino R, Ilari P, Biagini G. Stimulatory effect on bone formation exerted by a modified chitosan. Biomaterials 1994; 15(13):1075-1081.

[73] Hu Q. Preparation and characterization of biodegradable chitosan/hydroxyapatite nanocomposite rods via in situ hybridization: a potential material as internal fixation of bone fracture. Biomaterials 2004; 25(5):779-785.

[74] Manjubala I, Scheler S, Bossert J, Jandt KD. Mineralisation of chitosan scaffolds with nano-apatite formation by double diffusion technique. Acta biomaterialia 2006; 2(1): 75-84.

[75] Kong L, Gao Y, Cao W, Gong Y, Zhao N, Zhang X. Preparation and characterization of nano-hydroxyapatite/chitosan composite scaffolds. J Biomed Mater Res A 2005; 75(2):275-282.

[76] de Jonge LT, Leeuwenburgh SC, Wolke JG, Jansen JA. Organic-inorganic surface modifications for titanium implant surfaces. Pharmaceutical research 2008; 25(10): 2357-2369.

[77] Wildemann B, Bamdad P, Holmer C, Haas NP, Raschke M, Schmidmaier G. Local delivery of growth factors from coated titanium plates increases osteotomy healing in rats. Bone 2004; 34(5):862-868.

[78] Kim K-H, Kwon T-Y, Kim S-Y, Kang I-K, Kim S, Yang Y, Ong JL. Preparation and characterization of anodized titanium surfaces and their effect on osteoblast responses. Journal of Oral Implantology 2006; 32(1):8-13.

[79] Yao C, Webster TJ. Anodization: a promising nano-modification technique of titanium implants for orthopedic applications. J Nanosci Nanotechnol 2006; 6(9-10): 2682-2692.

[80] Yao C, Webster TJ. Prolonged antibiotic delivery from anodized nanotubular titanium using a co-precipitation drug loading method. Journal of Biomedical Materials Research Part B: Applied Biomaterials 2009; 91(2):587-595.

[81] Jia H, Kerr LL. Sustained ibuprofen release using composite poly (lactic-co-glycolic acid)/titanium dioxide nanotubes from Ti implant surface. Journal of pharmaceutical sciences 2013; 102(7):2341-2348.

[82] Kim HS, Yang Y, Koh JT, Lee KK, Lee DJ, Lee KM, Park SW. Fabrication and characterization of functionally graded nano-micro porous titanium surface by anodizing.ooJournal of biomedical materials research Part B, Applied biomaterials 2009; 88(2):427-435.

[83] Bae IH, Yun KD, Kim HS, Jeong BC, Lim HP, Park SW, Lee KM, Lim YC, Lee KK, Yang Y et al. Anodic oxidized nanotubular titanium implants enhance bone morphogenetic protein-2 delivery. Journal of biomedical materials research Part B, Applied biomaterials 2010; 93(2):484-491.

[84] Puleo DA, Huh WW, Duggirala SS, DeLuca PP. In vitro cellular responses to bioerodible particles loaded with recombinant human bone morphogenetic protein-2. Journal of biomedical materials research 1998; 41(1):104-110.

[85] He J, Huang T, Gan L, Zhou Z, Jiang B, Wu Y, Wu F, Gu Z. Collagen-infiltrated porous hydroxyapatite coating and its osteogenic properties: in vitro and in vivo study. J Biomed Mater Res A 2012; 100(7):1706-1715.

[86] Soballe K, Hansen ES, Brockstedt-Rasmussen H, Bunger C. Hydroxyapatite coating converts fibrous tissue to bone around loaded implants. The Journal of bone and joint surgery British volume 1993; 75(2):270-278.

[87] Choi S, Murphy WL. Sustained plasmid DNA release from dissolving mineral coatings. Acta biomaterialia 2010; 6(9):3426-3435.

[88] Saran N, Zhang R, Turcotte RE. Osteogenic protein-1 delivered by hydroxyapatite-coated implants improves bone ingrowth in extracortical bone bridging. Clinical orthopaedics and related research 2011; 469(5):1470-1478.

[89] Shah NJ, Hong J, Hyder MN, Hammond PT. Osteophilic multilayer coatings for accelerated bone tissue growth. Advanced materials 2012; 24(11):1445-1450.

[90] Ribeiro M, Monteiro FJ, Ferraz MP. Infection of orthopedic implants with emphasis on bacterial adhesion process and techniques used in studying bacterial-material interactions. Biomatter 2012; 2(4):176-194.

[91] Ketonis C, Parvizi J, Jones LC. Evolving strategies to prevent implant-associated infections. The Journal of the American Academy of Orthopaedic Surgeons 2012; 20(7): 478-480.

[92] Pavithra D, Doble M. Biofilm formation, bacterial adhesion and host response on polymeric implants—issues and prevention. Biomedical Materials 2008; 3(3):034003.

[93] Webb JC, Spencer RF. The role of polymethylmethacrylate bone cement in modern orthopaedic surgery. The Journal of bone and joint surgery British volume 2007; 89(7):851-857.

[94] Oosterbos CJ, Vogely H, Nijhof MW, Fleer A, Verbout AJ, Tonino AJ, Dhert WJ. Osseointegration of hydroxyapatite-coated and noncoated Ti6Al4V implants in the presence of local infection: a comparative histomorphometrical study in rabbits. Journal of biomedical materials research 2002; 60(3):339-347.

[95] Stigter M, Bezemer J, De Groot K, Layrolle P. Incorporation of different antibiotics into carbonated hydroxyapatite coatings on titanium implants, release and antibiotic efficacy. Journal of controlled release 2004; 99(1):127-137.

[96] Alt V, Bitschnau A, Bohner F, Heerich KE, Magesin E, Sewing A, Pavlidis T, Szalay G, Heiss C, Thormann U et al. Effects of gentamicin and gentamicin-RGD coatings on

bone ingrowth and biocompatibility of cementless joint prostheses: an experimental study in rabbits. Acta biomaterialia 2011; 7(3):1274-1280.

[97] Ren WP, Song W, Esquivel AO, Jackson NM, Nelson M, Flynn JC, Markel DC. Effect of erythromycin-doped calcium polyphosphate scaffold composite in a mouse pouch infection model. Journal of biomedical materials research Part B, Applied biomaterials 2014; 102(6):1140-1147.

[98] Zilberman M: Active Implants and Scaffolds for Tissue Regeneration. In Studies in Mechanobiology, Tissue Engineering and Biomaterials. Volume 8. Springer 2011:XII, 516

[99] Tovar N, Jimbo R, Witek L, Anchieta R, Yoo D, Manne L, Machado L, Gangolli R, Coelho PG. The physicochemical characterization and in vivo response of micro/nanoporous bioactive ceramic particulate bone graft materials. Materials science & engineering C, Materials for biological applications 2014; 43:472-480.

[100] Gultepe E, Nagesha D, Sridhar S, Amiji M. Nanoporous inorganic membranes or coatings for sustained drug delivery in implantable devices. Advanced drug delivery reviews 2010; 62(3):305-315.

[101] Rajesh P, Mohan N, Yokogawa Y, Varma H. Pulsed laser deposition of hydroxyapatite on nanostructured titanium towards drug eluting implants. Materials science & engineering C, Materials for biological applications 2013; 33(5):2899-2904.

[102] Zhang W, Chu PK. Enhancement of antibacterial properties and biocompatibility of polyethylene by silver and copper plasma immersion ion implantation. Surface and Coatings Technology 2008; 203(5-7):909-912.

[103] Huang H-L, Chang Y-Y, Lai M-C, Lin C-R, Lai C-H, Shieh T-M. Antibacterial TaN-Ag coatings on titanium dental implants. Surface and Coatings Technology 2010; 205(5):1636-1641.

[104] Chen W, Liu Y, Courtney HS, Bettenga M, Agrawal CM, Bumgardner JD, Ong JL. In vitro anti-bacterial and biological properties of magnetron co-sputtered silver-containing hydroxyapatite coating. Biomaterials 2006; 27(32):5512-5517.

[105] Chen Y, Zheng X, Xie Y, Ji H, Ding C, Li H, Dai K. Silver release from silver-containing hydroxyapatite coatings. Surface and Coatings Technology 2010; 205(7): 1892-1896.

[106] Cotte FE, Fardellone P, Mercier F, Gaudin AF, Roux C. Adherence to monthly and weekly oral bisphosphonates in women with osteoporosis. Osteoporosis international : a journal established as result of cooperation between the European Foundation for Osteoporosis and the National Osteoporosis Foundation of the USA 2010; 21(1): 145-155.

[107] Russell RG, Watts NB, Ebetino FH, Rogers MJ. Mechanisms of action of bisphosphonates: similarities and differences and their potential influence on clinical efficacy.

Osteoporosis international : a journal established as result of cooperation between the European Foundation for Osteoporosis and the National Osteoporosis Foundation of the USA 2008; 19(6):733-759.

[108] Russell RG. Bisphosphonates: mode of action and pharmacology. Pediatrics 2007; 119 Suppl 2:S150-162.

[109] Bisaz S, Jung A, Fleisch H. Uptake by bone of pyrophosphate, diphosphonates and their technetium derivatives. Clinical science and molecular medicine 1978; 54(3): 265-272.

[110] Drake MT, Clarke BL, Khosla S. Bisphosphonates: mechanism of action and role in clinical practice. Mayo Clinic proceedings Mayo Clinic 2008; 83(9):1032-1045.

[111] Schindeler A, Little DG. Bisphosphonate action: revelations and deceptions from in vitro studies. J Pharm Sci 2007; 96(8):1872-1878.

[112] Narai S, Nagahata S. Effects of alendronate on the removal torque of implants in rats with induced osteoporosis. Int J Oral Maxillofac Implants 2003; 18(2):218-223.

[113] Kurth AH, Eberhardt C, Muller S, Steinacker M, Schwarz M, Bauss F. The bisphosphonate ibandronate improves implant integration in osteopenic ovariectomized rats. Bone 2005; 37(2):204-210.

[114] Giro G, Sakakura CE, Goncalves D, Pereira RM, Marcantonio E, Jr., Orrico SR. Effect of 17beta-estradiol and alendronate on the removal torque of osseointegrated titanium implants in ovariectomized rats. J Periodontol 2007; 78(7):1316-1321.

[115] Yoshinari M, Oda Y, Inoue T, Matsuzaka K, Shimono M. Bone response to calcium phosphate-coated and bisphosphonate-immobilized titanium implants. Biomaterials 2002; 23(14):2879-2885.

[116] Peter B, Pioletti DP, Laib S, Bujoli B, Pilet P, Janvier P, Guicheux J, Zambelli PY, Bouler JM, Gauthier O. Calcium phosphate drug delivery system: influence of local zoledronate release on bone implant osteointegration. Bone 2005; 36(1):52-60.

[117] Yildiz A, Esen E, Kurkcu M, Damlar I, Daglioglu K, Akova T. Effect of zoledronic acid on osseointegration of titanium implants: an experimental study in an ovariectomized rabbit model. Journal of oral and maxillofacial surgery : official journal of the American Association of Oral and Maxillofacial Surgeons 2010; 68(3):515-523.

[118] Mundy G, Garrett R, Harris S, Chan J, Chen D, Rossini G, Boyce B, Zhao M, Gutierrez G. Stimulation of bone formation in vitro and in rodents by statins. Science 1999; 286(5446):1946-1949.

[119] Yang F, Zhao SF, Zhang F, He FM, Yang GL. Simvastatin-loaded porous implant surfaces stimulate preosteoblasts differentiation: an in vitro study. Oral surgery, oral medicine, oral pathology, oral radiology, and endodontics 2011; 111(5):551-556.

[120] Ayukawa Y, Yasukawa E, Moriyama Y, Ogino Y, Wada H, Atsuta I, Koyano K. Local application of statin promotes bone repair through the suppression of osteoclasts and

the enhancement of osteoblasts at bone-healing sites in rats. Oral surgery, oral medicine, oral pathology, oral radiology, and endodontics 2009; 107(3):336-342.

[121] Du Z, Chen J, Yan F, Xiao Y. Effects of Simvastatin on bone healing around titanium implants in osteoporotic rats. Clinical oral implants research 2009; 20(2):145-150.

[122] Maeda T, Kawane T, Horiuchi N. Statins augment vascular endothelial growth factor expression in osteoblastic cells via inhibition of protein prenylation. Endocrinology 2003; 144(2):681-692.

[123] Maeda T, Matsunuma A, Kurahashi I, Yanagawa T, Yoshida H, Horiuchi N. Induction of osteoblast differentiation indices by statins in MC3T3-E1 cells. Journal of cellular biochemistry 2004; 92(3):458-471.

[124] Ubios AM, Jares Furno G, Guglielmotti MB. Effect of calcitonin on alveolar wound healing. Journal of oral pathology & medicine : official publication of the International Association of Oral Pathologists and the American Academy of Oral Pathology 1991; 20(7):322-324.

[125] Rao LG, Heersche JN, Marchuk LL, Sturtridge W. Immunohistochemical demonstration of calcitonin binding to specific cell types in fixed rat bone tissue. Endocrinology 1981; 108(5):1972-1978.

[126] Dahlin C, Linde A, Gottlow J, Nyman S. Healing of bone defects by guided tissue regeneration. Plastic and reconstructive surgery 1988; 81(5):672-676.

[127] Ichikawa M, Nakamuta H, Hoshino T, Ogawa Y, Koida M. Anti-osteopenic effect of nasal salmon calcitonin in type 1 osteoporotic rats: comparison with subcutaneous dosing. Biological & pharmaceutical bulletin 1994; 17(7):911-913.

[128] Arisawa EA, Brandao AA, Almeida JD, da Rocha RF. Calcitonin in bone-guided regeneration of mandibles in ovariectomized rats: densitometric, histologic and histomorphometric analysis. International journal of oral and maxillofacial surgery 2008; 37(1):47-53.

[129] Reginster JY, Azria M, Gaspar S, Bleicher M, Franchimont N, Behhar M, Albert A, Franchimont P. Endogenous production of specific antibodies does not decrease hypocalcemic response to calcitonin in young rabbits. Calcified tissue international 1992; 50(6):518-520.

[130] Almeida JD, Arisawa EA, da Rocha RF, Carvalho YR. Effect of calcitonin on bone regeneration in male rats: a histomorphometric analysis. International journal of oral and maxillofacial surgery 2007; 36(5):435-440.

[131] Foster SC, Kronman JH. The effects of topical thyrocalcitonin on the extraction sites in the jaws of dogs. Oral surgery, oral medicine, and oral pathology 1974; 38(6): 866-873.

[132] Costa-Rodrigues J, Reis S, Teixeira S, Lopes S, Fernandes MH. Dose-dependent inhibitory effects of proton pump inhibitors on human osteoclastic and osteoblastic cell activity. The FEBS journal 2013; 280(20):5052-5064.

[133] Rzeszutek K, Sarraf F, Davies JE. Proton pump inhibitors control osteoclastic resorption of calcium phosphate implants and stimulate increased local reparative bone growth. The Journal of craniofacial surgery 2003; 14(3):301-307.

[134] Sheraly A, Lickorish D, Sarraf F, Davies J. Use of gastrointestinal proton pump inhibitors to regulate osteoclast-mediated resorption of calcium phosphate cements in vivo. Current drug delivery 2009; 6(2):192-198.

[135] Väänänen HK, Zhao H. Osteoclast function: biology and mechanisms. Principles of Bone Biology, 3rd ed Academic Press, San Diego, USA 2008:193-209.

[136] Porter JR, Ruckh TT, Popat KC. Bone tissue engineering: a review in bone biomimetics and drug delivery strategies. Biotechnology progress 2009; 25(6):1539-1560.

[137] Rammelt S, Illert T, Bierbaum S, Scharnweber D, Zwipp H, Schneiders W. Coating of titanium implants with collagen, RGD peptide and chondroitin sulfate. Biomaterials 2006; 27(32):5561-5571.

[138] Liu Y, de Groot K, Hunziker EB. BMP-2 liberated from biomimetic implant coatings induces and sustains direct ossification in an ectopic rat model. Bone 2005; 36(5): 745-757.

[139] Goodman SB, Yao Z, Keeney M, Yang F. The future of biologic coatings for orthopaedic implants. Biomaterials 2013; 34(13):3174-3183.

2

Immediate Loading in Implant Dentistry

Ilser Turkyilmaz and Ashley Brooke Hoders

1. Introduction

Planning for immediate implant placement requires an accurate diagnosis and specific case selection [1-3]. Adequate planning can be accomplished using the various technologies that are available to us today, and it is important to remember that any alteration to position in relationship to the prosthesis used during planning can compromise the final result with alteration of occlusion, esthetics and biomechanics resulting. In order to accurately plan, a thorough clinical evaluation will be necessary and should include assessment of smile line, gingival morphology, the inter-arch relationship, condition and gingival margin positions of adjacent teeth, as well as supporting tissue conditions [4-6].

If the presenting conditions are deemed unfavorable, it is important that corrections be made via reconstruction of soft tissue, bone, and tooth positioning. An adequate amount of bone is important because a deficiency can jeopardize stability and lead to recession, loss of papilla and inadequate positioning; an inadequate amount of soft tissue will lead to a poor esthetic outcome [7-9]. Therefore, when bone quality and quantity are not sufficient, you must use regeneration techniques during the initial phase of treatment such as guided bone regeneration, orthodontics, and/or grafting. Other important things to be considered for immediate loading include the implant having primary stability [10,11]. Things that would contraindicate immediate loading include lack of primary stability, parafunction, pathology in the region of implant placement, and systemic alterations such as severe periodontal disease, poor oral hygiene, and smoking. Careful evaluation must be completed before immediate placement and loading be considered.

2. Immediate loading

2.1. Concepts and protocols

Ever since dental implants were first successfully employed in restoring completely edentulous mandibles in 1951, implant supported dental rehabilitations of various designs and complexity have been shown to be a reliable and predictable treatment option for both partially and fully edentulous patients [12-14]. The original Branemark protocol dictated that the initial phase of implant integration be at least 4 to 6 months before any restoration was placed [15]. "Conventional loading", as it is now known, is a reliable, safe, predictable, and accepted treatment modality that has been used as a point of comparison for other dental implant loading protocols.

Within the last decade, clinicians have increasingly begun to explore the possibilities of decreasing treatment time by early placement of the implant-supported restoration, or by placing implants in extraction sockets at the time of extraction [16-18]. Investigators are now increasingly reporting protocols designed to promote shortened treatment periods for implant-supported prostheses.

The concept of implant immediate loading includes all of the advantages of a one stage surgical approach. Also, during the osseointegration process, the patient does not have to use a removable denture, which increases function, speech, stability, comfort and improves certain psychological factors [19]. Splinted implants can decrease the risk of overload to each implant because of the greater surface area and improved biomechanical distribution [20,21].

The primary goal for immediate loading is establishment of direct bone implant contact. The terminology when it comes to immediate loading can sometimes be ambiguous and there many classifications in the literature, so it is important to understand the different techniques that can be used [22]:

2.1.1. Terminology for the timing of implant loading

Immediate loading: The placement of implants and insertion of restorations are completed in the same day.

Early loading: The restoration is connected to the implants at a second procedure but earlier than the conventional healing period of 3 to 6 months; time of loading should be considered in days/weeks.

Delayed loading: The restoration is connected at a second procedure after a conventional healing period of 3 to 6 months.

2.1.2. Terminology for implant loading

Occlusal loading: The crown/bridge is in contact with opposing dentition in centric occlusion.

Nonocclusal loading: The crown/bridge is not in contact in centric occlusion with opposing dentition in centric occlusion.

The concept of an immediate restoration includes a nonsubmerged first stage surgery and also implies that the occlusal surfaces and implants are loaded with a provisional of definitive restoration [23-25]. A delayed or staged loading refers to an implant prosthesis with occlusal load after more than 3 months (mandible) or 6 months (maxilla) post-implant insertion. Using a delayed approach allows you to use a 2 stage surgical procedure that covers implants with tissue or one stage approach that exposes a portion of the implant at the initial surgery.

2.2. Factors affecting time of loading

Some of the variables that can impact your ability to immediately load include surgical trauma, bone loading trauma, and treatment plans related to implant number. Alveolar and residual bone has a cortical and trabecular component that can be modified by modeling and remodeling. Remodeling allows the bone to respond to its local environment or allows bone repair after traumatic situation [26]. The bone is generally lamellar bone but woven bone might occur during the repair process. Typically, lamellar bone and woven bone are the primary bone tissue types observed around a dental implant. Lamellar bone and woven bone are the primary bone tissue types found around a dental implant. Lamellar bone is organized, highly mineralized and is the strongest bone type. Woven bone is unorganized, less mature, less mineralized and has lower strength and is more flexible [26]. Woven bone can form at a rate of 60μm (micrometers) per day, whereas lamellar bone forms at a rate of up to 10μm per day.

The rationale behind immediate loading is not only to reduce the risk of fibrous tissue formation but also to promote lamellar bone maturation to sustain a continued occlusal load. So when compared to the 2 stage approach, the repair of the implant is separated from the early loading response by 3-6 months. The process of osteotomy preparation and implant insertion causes a regional acceleratory phenomenon of bone repair around the implant interface [26]. Therefore, the organized lamellar bone in the preparation site becomes woven and unorganized next to the implant and at 4 months the bone is still only 60% mineralized lamellar bone- this is sufficient in most bone types and situation for implant loading.

The concept of immediate loading challenges the conventional load-free healing time of 3-6 months before the insertion of restoration. The bone in the thread design is stronger on the day of implant placement as opposed to 3 months later as more mature lamellar bone exists in the implant threads. However, the cellular connection between the implant surface and bone cells does not exist yet [26,27]. On the day of implant placement, there is residual cortical and trabecular bone around the implant and the implant has some contact with this prepared bone. Surgical trauma triggers early cellular repair and increased vascularization to stimulate repair process to injured bone [26,27]. Woven bone formation by appositional growth may start to form as early as the second week after implant placement at a rate of 30-50μm per day. Approximately 3-5 weeks after implant placement, the implant bone interface is weakest and at highest risk of overload since the implant-bone interface is least mineralized and unorganized during this time.

2.3. Risk factors for immediate loading

It has been found that immediate loaded failure occurred between 3-5weeks post-operative from mobility without infection [28-29]. The risk of immediate occlusal overload can be decreased by utilizing some techniques such as having more vital bone in contact with the implant interface, minimizing the surgical trauma at implant placement, including thermal injury and mechanical trauma that may result in microfracture of bone during implant placement. In addition, the microfracture of bone may lead to osteonecrosis and possible fibrous and granulation tissue encapsulation around the implant. Death of osteoblasts has been reported to occur at 40 °C [30-31].

Sharawy et al. [32], reported that heat generated in bone next to implant drills depends on design and revolutions of the drill. It was found that the drill rpm of 2500 generated less heat than 2000 rpm and 1250 rpm caused the highest heat and the longest recovery period regardless of drill design. Some other factors that need to be entertained to keep heat minimum may include the drill sharpness, the depth of the osteotomy, the amount of bone prepared, the variation in cortical thickness and the temperature and solution chemistry of the irrigant.

When the implant is substantially compressed against the bone, the interface between implant and bone has a greater area of repair. Self-tapping via implant itself, meaning the implant cuts the bone during placement, can result in greater bone remodeling/woven bone around the implant in initial healing compared to bone tapping before implant placement. The implant should not have any mobility on insertion; excess strain within the bone from torque and space filling may also increase risk of microdamage at the interface [33-35].

The recommended protocol for immediate load is to insert the implant with a torque of 45-60 Ncm [36-37]. This stability helps to ensure that the implant has a relatively rigid fixation in good quality bone. Additional torque may result in pressure necrosis and increase the strain magnitude at the interface and increase amount of damage and remodeling which could decrease strength of bone implant interface.

An alternate approach is to use a reverse torque test of 20Ncm to evaluate the quality of the bone and the interface at initial fixation for evaluating delayed healing. If the implant does not unthread at 20Ncm the resistance indicates that the bone is sufficient density to consider immediate loading.

Once the bone begins to receive occlusal loads by the implant restoration, the interface begins to remodel again. However, the trigger is strain transfer from occlusal function rather than trauma of implant placement. *Repair bone* is woven bone from surface trauma but *reactive woven bone is* woven bone formed from mechanical or loading response. The remodeling from mechanical strain can be called *bone turnover* and not only repairs damaged bone but also allows the implant interface to adapt to its biomechanical situation. The *interface remodeling rate* is the period of time for bone at the implant interface to be replaced with new bone [26].

Strain is the change in length of material/original length measured as % change [26]. The loaded bone next to an implant changes its shape, which is measured as strain. Micro-strain conditions 100 times less than the ultimate strength of bone may trigger a cellular response. Bone fractures at strain levels of 1-2% but bone begins to disappear or form fibrous tissue, which is named the *pathologic overload zone* when strain levels of 20-40%. There-fore, the mechanical load is too severe, fibrous tissue may form at the implant interface rather than bone. Fibrous tissue at an implant interface may cause clinical mobility instead of rigid connection called osseointegration.

The ideal microstrain level for bone is the *adapted zone* and is called *ideal load bearing zone* [26]. The remodeling rate of bone in the jaws is in the physiologic zone of 40% of each year; the bone can remodel and remain an organized, mineralized, lamellar structure at these levels. The intermediate level of microstrain with the ideal load bearing zone and pathologic overload is called the *mild overload zone* [26]. In this strain region, bone begins its healing process to repair microfractures and the bone that is in a fatigue risk of failure. Bone in this range is reactive woven bone. Microstrain from overload or trauma causing accelerated bone repair causes less mineralized bone to form and less organized bone that is weaker [26].

Localized overload and possible implant failure might be possible due to excess stresses along the implant interface. However, immediate loading does not cause excessive stresses necessarily [26]. Initial response of bone at the implant interface has been evaluated on immediately loaded implants: direct bone-implant-contact with favorable bone quality around the implant has been reported. Brunski showed that a direct bone-implant interface may develop as long as the implant moves less than 100 μm and micromotion beyond 150 resulted in fibrous tissue encapsulation instead of a osseointegration [38]. Studies have shown that immediate loading of an implant interface did not increase risk of fibrous tissue formation. Long term results suggest that loaded implants have less marrow spaces and more compact bone. Greater direct bone contact was noted at the interface, suggesting that early occlusal loading may enhance bone remodeling and further increase bone density compared with unloaded implants [38].

Canullo et al., reported that the extension of bone remodeling was less extensive in cases of immediate placement (1.7mm) rather than delayed placement (3.0mm) [39]. Despite this limit in the healing zone, it has been shown that bone can fill osseous defects around implants if they are 3-walled in nature and <1.5-2.0mm wide. Other interventions such as autogenous bone grafts have been shown to be more osteogenic when used in conjunction with immediately placed implants. However, immediate placement does present some disadvantages. These can include unpredictable site morphology, a potentially limited amount of soft tissue, and risk of failure due to residual periosteal infection. Despite these potential disadvantages, immediate implant placement and immediate implant loading have shown to be favorable in maintaining or increasing bone heights around implants [1-4].

2.4. Biomechanical considerations

Any treatment plans involving immediate loading should have the goal to minimize the occlusal overload risk and its resultant increase in the remodeling rate of bone. The regional acceleratory phenomenon may replace the bone interface without the additional risk of biomechanical overload. The lower the stress applied to the bone, the lower the microstrain in the bone [26]. This provides conditions that increase the functional surface area to the implant bone interface. The surface area of load may be increased by variables including implant number, implant size, implant design, and body surface conditions. Force applied to the implant bone interface is related to the strain observed and some other factors such as patient conditions, implant position and direction of occlusal load.

Two approaches for immediate occlusal loading with edentulous patient include: over-engineering by placing more implants than the usual treatment plan for the conventional healing period; using selected implants around the arch (3+) to immediately restore with a transitional fixed prosthesis. In this approach, enough number of implants, which are needed to support a fixed prosthesis, are left submerged for the healing period. So, even if all immediately loaded implants fail, a fixed restoration can still be provided to the patient. If any immediately loaded implants survive, then they are also used in the final restoration [40]. This technique can be used where moderate to abundant bone is present in the posterior and anterior to the mental foramen. A study by Scortecci, involved loading all implants initially and splinting all for increased area of load transfer which could decrease stresses along the developing multiple interfaces and increases the stability, retention, and strength of transitional prosthesis during initial healing phase [41]. This technique allows you to use additional implants.

The functional surface area of occlusal load transfer along implant interface may be increased by increasing the implant number, especially when the devices are splinted through bridgework. The biomechanical approach loads additional implants when immediate loading is planned. The lowest percentage of survival for a full arch restoration corresponded to a fewer number of loaded implants.

A rule in traditional prosthetics is that 3 pontics in the posterior of the mouth are contraindicated for a fixed prosthesis because of the amount of force and the flexibility and fatigue strength of the restoration [27]. When only 3 are used to support an immediate restoration there are often 3-4 pontics cantilevered. It has been suggested that additional implants should be placed with the staged healing approach in case one or more fails during the initial loading period. They can then be used in the final restoration to decrease the number of pontics and increase retention of final restoration

An increased number of implants reduces the risk of overload due to the increased implant surface area but also increases the retention of the restoration and decreases the number of pontics [27]. If fracture to a prosthesis or partially unretained restorations occur, the portion that is retained may act as a lever and overload the implants. The increased retention minimizes the occurrence of partially unretained restorations during healing which would be another source of overload to the implants supporting the restoration [27]. Decreases in pontic number also reduce the risk of fracture of the transitional restoration that could be a source of additional load to the remaining implants supporting the prosthesis. As a general rule, more implants should be inserted in maxilla to compensate for less dense bone and increased directions of force often found in the upper arch [27].

The most common number of implants used for a mandibular overdenture is 4-6 splinted in anterior mandible [5,24,42]. In a partially edentulous patient missing multiple teeth, ideally 1 implant should be placed for each missing tooth. For missing single teeth, the implant size, design or surface may be more important. Load may be reduced by reducing occlusal the contact and having a nonfunctional scheme.

The greater the benefit:risk ratio or the lower the risk, the more immediate loading should be considered. For example, a completely edentulous mandible restored with an overdenture supported by 4+ implants is a very low risk condition. If the patient can not tolerate a mandibular denture and does not wear it, the immediate load protocol would be a high benefit. An example of a high risk for immediate load would be posterior single tooth implant- the implant number can not be increased and you can not engage cortical bone; this would be of low benefit when out of the esthetic zone. Additional studies to evaluate risks especially in maxilla are expected [43].

2.5. Factors related to implant type/design

The area of load may also be increased by considering implant size, design, and surface. You can decrease stress by decreasing force applied to the prosthesis. These forces are influenced by patient factors, implant position, cantilever forces, occlusal load direction, occlusal contact positions, and diet.

Implant diameter and length are often emphasized in reports as these values give insight into the bone-to-implant surface area that an implant will provide. Avila et al., described that larger implants provided greater bone-to-implant contact and less susceptibility to cantilever forces following restoration [44]. More importantly, thread design and dimensions dictate the functional bone-to-implant surface area that will resist forces when a given implant is loaded along a given functional axis. Tapered implants offer a conical shape that is consistent with a natural root form but have less surface area which in turn results in increased crestal bone stresses and less primary stability.

For each 3mm increase in length beyond 10mm, you can increase the surface area by more than 20% for a cylinder implant design. Most stresses to an implant bone interface are concentrated at crestal bone. Therefore, increased implant length does little to decrease stress that occurs at the transosteal region around implant. But because immediately restored implant loads the interface before the establishment of a cellular connection, the implant length is more relevant especially in softer bone.

Benefits of increased length are found in the initial stability of the bone implant interface. Remodeling of the interface does not occur uniformly around implant- one region of interface remodels and other remains stable. Added length may allow remodeling in one region while other can stabilize implant. Added length can also allow implant to engage opposing cortical plate which can increase initial stability. Cortical bone has a lower remodeling rate and ensures stable condition during early loading. When trying to evaluate what length implant should be placed, it is important to consider that the survival rate of 10mm or less implants drops to less than 85% in traditional healing; Schnitman et al., found a 50% failure rate in immediately loaded implants with length of 10mm or less [45]. However, recent literature suggests that a high degree of survivability can be reproduced with implants that are at least 3mm in diameter and 8mm in length when splinted with other implants [46,47]. These findings, along with the innovations in implant design, suggest that these values should be revisited.

The functional surface area of each implant support system is related to the width and shape of the implant. Wider root form implants of the same length provide greater bone contact than narrower implants. Occlusal stresses are greatest in concentration at the crest of the ridge after the implant has integrated, so the width may be more important to the length of the implant to decrease the risk of crestal bone overload. Overload can cause early crestal bone loss in immediately loaded implants. The diameter of the implant increases in the molar area for immediate loading, especially when the density is less or the forces are greater. Increasing the width of the implant in molar sites or adding additional implants to increase the surface area in the posterior region can help alleviate overload that may result in crestal bone loss.

The implant body design needs to be more specific for immediate load because maximum stability is needed at the time of placement. After placement, bone has not had time to grow into the recesses or undercuts in the implant body or attach to the conditioned surface before occlusal load is applied. A threaded implant body and insertion process provides a better chance of stabilization. The implant design has a greater impact on the functional surface area than the implant size. The functional surface area is greater during immediate load, and a threaded implant presents many advantages over a pressfit type of implant for immediate load because the design features do not require integration to resist loads and have a greater surface area to resist occlusal forces [48].

The number, spacing, and orientation of the threads affect the amount of area available to resist the forces during immediate loading [49,50]. A greater number of threads means a greater functional surface area at the time of immediate load. The smaller the distance between threads, the greater the thread number corresponds to the surface area. Thread depth is also a variable to consider. Greater depth means a greater functional surf area for immediate load application. Functional surface area is more important when the number of implants cannot increase (less than 4 adjacent teeth are being replaced).

Thread geometry can affect the strength of early osseointegration and bone implant interface. A V- shaped thread design withstands a 10x greater shear force applied to bone compared to a square thread shape. Bone is strongest in compression and weakest in shear loading. Compressive force transfer would decrease microstrain to bone as compared to shear force. Therefore, a square thread design may provide a benefit in immediate load protocols.

The higher the remodeling rate of a loaded interface creates a higher woven bone ratio and weaker bone interface. A square threaded implant design with deeper threads has a 10x reduction in resorption rate. When considering a tapered implant design for immediate load, consider that this type of design allows for a less overall surface area compared to a straight design of the same length, width, and thread number. A tapered design will also have less thread depth near the apical portion of the implant, which reduces the surface area but decreases initial fixation. Thread depth and a tapered body can combine to improve initial stability, and may be a good option in lower density bone when less than 4 teeth are replaced and implant position and number can not be manipulated. Implant number, position and patient factors are more relevant to success and there have been few trials that compare immediate load with different implant thread designs and tapered implant bodies in the edentulous patient [50,51].

When the implant surface is modified with a roughened texture, this increases the bone to implant contact [52,53]. The shear strength of an implant with a roughened texture has been shown to be 5x greater than implants with smooth surface. The surface condition also affects the rate and percentage of bone contact, and lamellar bone formation. Surface coatings and conditions of the implant have been shown to be most beneficial during the initial healing and early loading conditions. For immediate loading, the most desirable surface is one that will allow the greatest percent of bone formation, has the highest bone-implant contact percentage with the highest mineralization rate, and the fastest lamellar bone formation.

A rough surface will initially increase stability; a machined surface is less successful to do so, especially in low density bone. A hydroxyapatite (HA) coating has been shown to decrease resorption rates during occlusal loading, which can increase the percentage of lamellar bone formation at the interface. If the bone is not an ideal density for immediate loading, the surface condition of the implant body may decrease the risk of occlusal overload. In summary, a rough surface provides a better condition than a machine surface; and in good quality bone, the types of surface condition is less relative to the overall implant survival [54].

Strain placed on the bone is influenced by the stress directed to the implant interface [26]. Ways that stress can be reduced include increasing the surface area that supports the occlusal load or by decreasing the force that is applied to the prosthesis. It has been recommended to not remove the prosthesis once it is delivered within first 2 weeks, and that resorbable sutures may be beneficial.

3. General considerations for treatment planning

Patient factors such as bruxism and clenching parafunction are forces that are high in magnitude, extensive in duration, and generate primarily horizontal forces to the implant. Parafunction presents a considerable risk and potential contraindication for immediate load due to this resulting in the poorest implant survival data [55]. There is an increased risk of abutment screw loosening, unretained prostheses, fracture of the transitional restoration used in immediate loading when a lever forms and increasing the risk of occlusal overload.

Implant position is an important factor for the edentulous patient. In the partially edentulous patient it is important to eliminate cantilevers on two implants supporting 3 teeth rather than position the implants next to each other with a cantilever. There will be less stress directed towards the implant interface when implants are not in a straight line in an edentulous site [24,36]. Cross-arch splinting is a very effective way to reduce stress within the entire implant support system, especially when there is an antero-posterior (AP) distance between the splinted implants. The splinted arch concept for the completely edentulous patient is advantageous for the immediate load transitional restoration. A line is drawn from the distal of each posterior implant. The distance from this line to the center of the most anterior implant is called the *anteroposterior distance* (A-P spread). The greater the A-P spread is between the center of the most anterior implant or implants and the most distal aspect of the posterior implants, the smaller is the resultant loads on the implant system from cantilevered forces because of the stabilizing effect of the A-P distance [27].

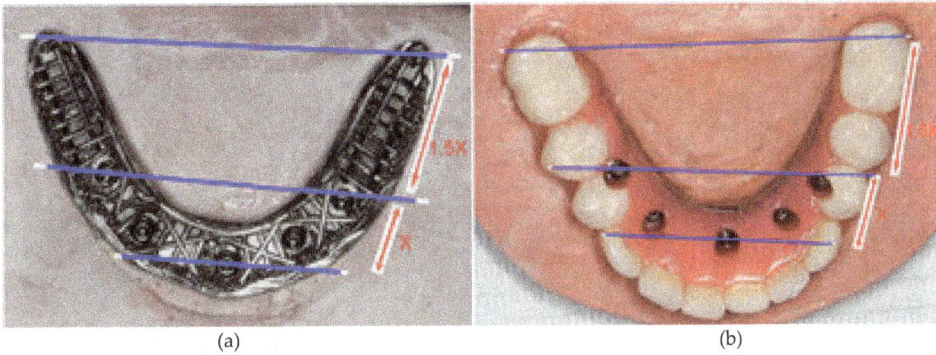

Figure 1. A-P spread and length of cantilever for framework (a) and final restoration (b).

A square arch form involves smaller A-P spreads between splinted implants and should have shorter-length cantilevers. A tapered arch form has the largest distance between anterior and posterior implants and may have the longest cantilever design [27].

3.1. Treatment planning of mandible

The mandible should be divided into three sections when planning for implant placement: canine to canine; bilateral posterior. This is different from the maxilla, which needs more implant support because the bone is less dense and the direction of force is outside of the arch in all excursive movements; here you must consider the maxilla in at least 4 sections depending on the magnitude of force and the shape of the arch. These sections include the bilateral canine area and the bilateral posterior areas; at least 1 implant should be inserted into each [6] section and splinted during immediate load for the completely edentulous patient.

Concerns about medial mandibular flexure with cross-arch splinting suggests that the final restoration should be fabricated in at least 2 sections when implants are placed in both posterior quadrants and fewer than 3 adjacent pontics are present [56]. The following photos show the restoration of an mandible with a 2-piece implant-supported fixed restoration.

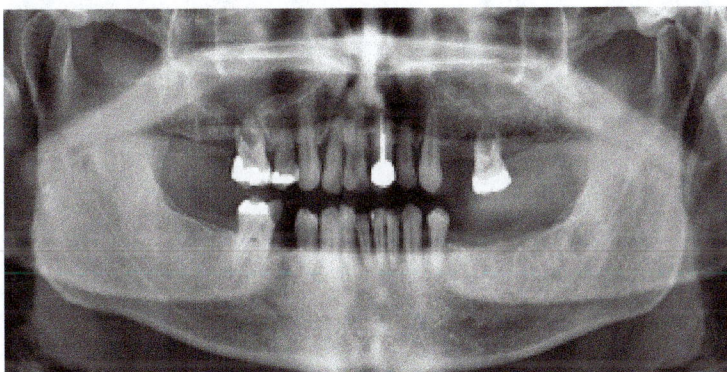

Figure 2. Panoramic radiograph of patient before treatment.

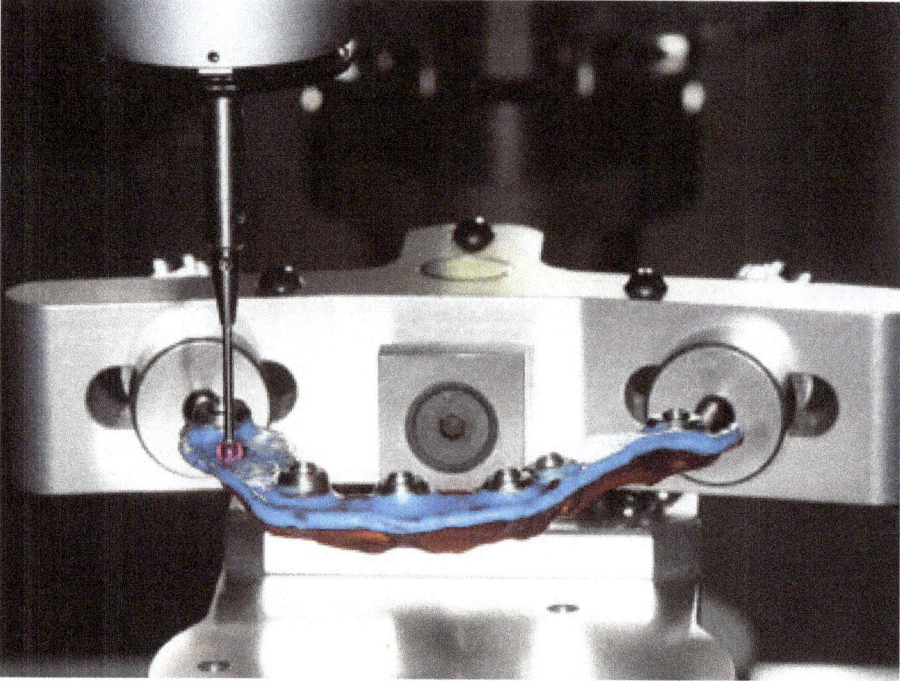

Figure 3. Scanning of tissue surface of mandibular wax pattern by using CAD/CAM.

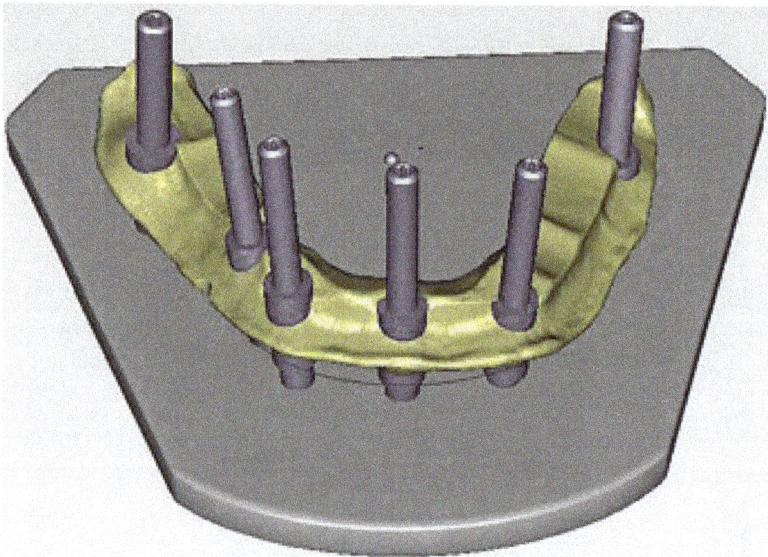

Figure 4. Final design of mandibular framework.

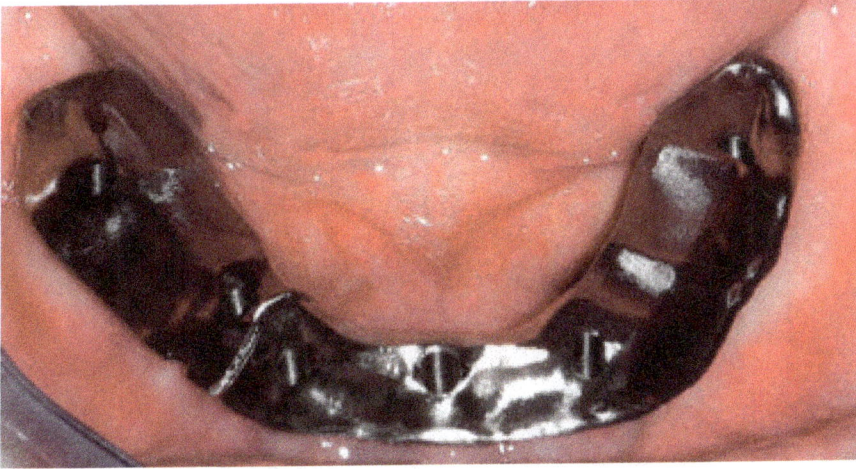

Figure 5. Clinical fit of mandibular framework verified after it was sectioned in two pieces.

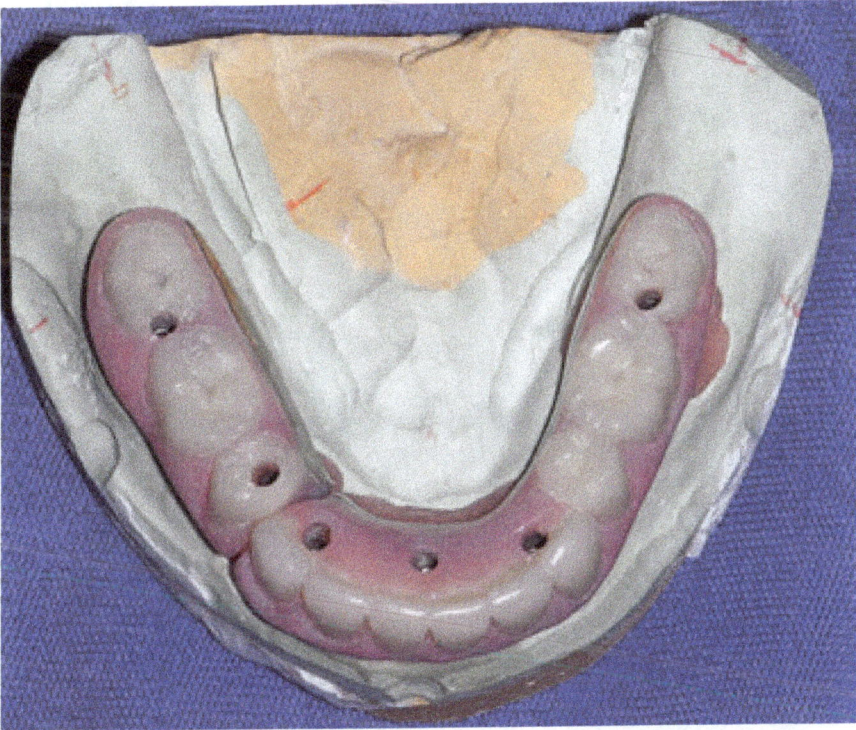

Figure 6. Implant-supported screw-retained fixed dental prosthesis, in two pieces, was fabricated in the laboratory.

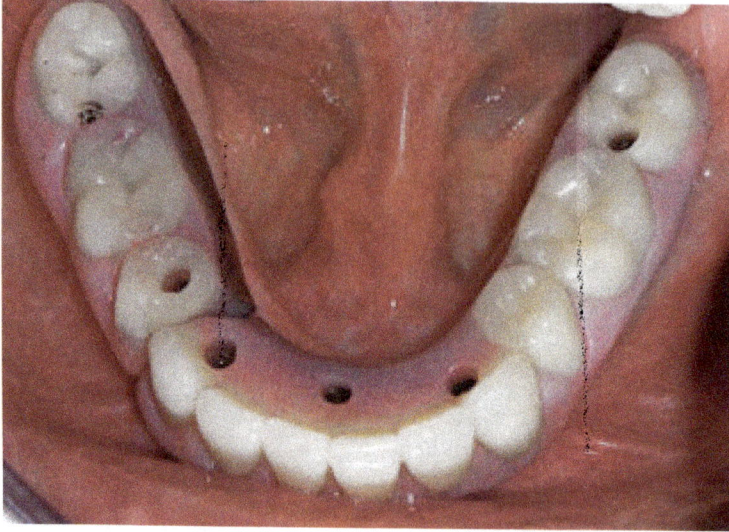

Figure 7. Occlusal view of mandibular implant- supported screw-retained fixed dental prosthesis at delivery.

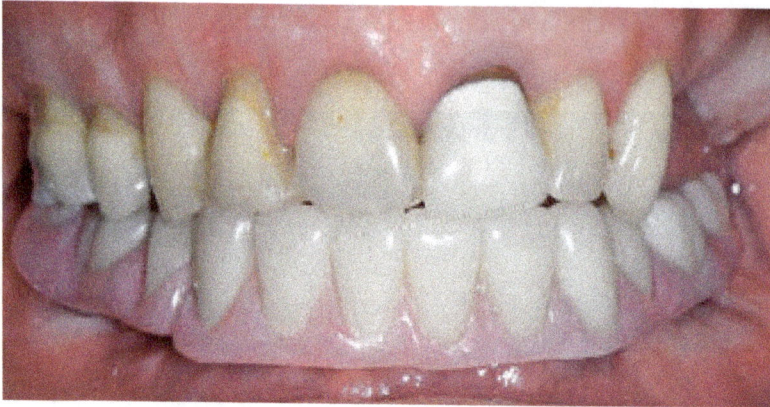

Figure 8. Intra-oral view after inserting mandibular restoration.

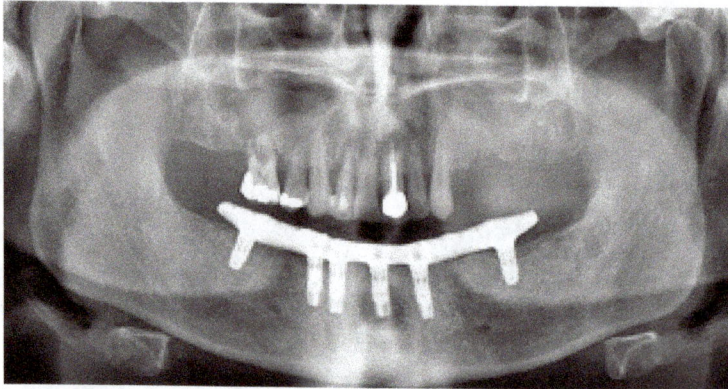

Figure 9. Panoramic radiograph at delivery.

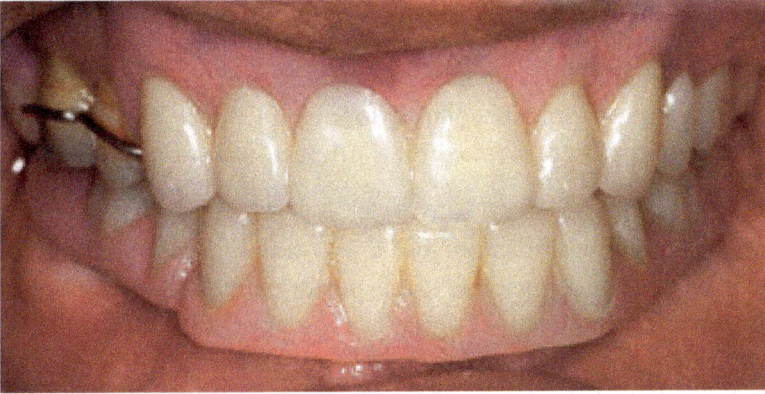

Figure 10. Intra-oral view after inserting interim maxillary removable partial denture.

3.2. Factors influencing restorative plans

Cantilevers increase moment loads to implant bone interface and can increase the amount of crestal bone loss observed, increase abutment screw loosening, increased implant body fracture, and increase the risk of implant failure. The immediate load transitional should not have a posterior cantilever -not in esthetic zone- and bite forces are greater posteriorly; especially in the partially edentulous patients without a cross-arch support system. Partially uncemented restorations may result in a cantilever along the remaining implants; considering a definitive cement for transitional restoration to decrease the risk of partially retained restorations can be considered.

An occusal load direction along the implant interface may affect the resorption rate. Axial load has been shown to maintain the lamellar bone and has a lower resorption rate. The crown height can also serve as a vertical cantilever when angled forces or cantilevers placed. Flat occlusal planes in the posterior decrease risk of angled loads. The amount of force can be decreased by modifying the occlusal contacts so as to decrease or eliminate contact on the restoration. In the completely edentulous patient, parafunction may be eliminated by restoring with an immediate load overdenture and having the patient remove it at night. Having a stress relief attachment to implants can decrease the force transferred while the prosthesis is in function.

The patient's diet should also be a factor to consider and can lead to the fracture or loosening of the transitional due to overload. The patient should be instructed to eat only soft foods during the immediate loading period. The mechanical properties of bone should be considered as a less dense bone type has a lower strength. The bone-implant contact decreases for less dense bone, and the strength of the bone is directly related to its density, with the less dense bone type being weaker. The rate of resorption of dense cortical bone is slower than trabecular resorption rates; cortical bone is more likely to remain lamellar during the immediate load process than trabecular bone.

In summary, the greater number of implants, the greater length and width of implants, rough surfaces that provide greater surface area; placement of implants to maximize antero-posterior spread and decrease cantilevers should be considered in lower density bone types when planning for immediate load. The bone in the anterior is cortical bone at the crestal and apical areas; root forms implants should be placed to engage the opposing cortical plate when immediate load is contemplated to maximize primary stability and optimize mechanical conditions.

The posterior maxilla has a thin sinus floor and the mandibular canal location does not always allow engagement of the opposing cortex; the posterior maxilla is the area that caries the highest risk of implant failure when a 2 stage healing approach is used [57,58]. The implant number, width, and design are methods to decrease stresses to the interface in these regions. Use of conventional healing for type 3 or 4 bone quality when less than 10mm height exists. Bone grafting depends on many factors to be predictable: blood supply and lack of micro-movement [57-60]. Developing woven bone is at more risk of overload, and grafting is more predictable when soft tissue covers the graft and membranes are used. Immediately loaded implants should be placed in an existing bone volume that is adequate for both early load and that has the proper prosthetic design. Bone grafting before implant placement and then implant insertion and immediate loading after graft maturation is suggested when inadequate bone volume is present for proper reconstructive procedures.

3.3. Restoratively-driven treatment planning

Implant rehabilitation should always be prosthodontically driven [6]. This philosophy promotes a reduction in implant micromovement through appropriately positioned and loaded restorations. If restorations are inappropriately designed, a loss of osseointegration and/or prosthetic failure is more likely to occur. Axial implant loading is a desirable treatment goal since lateral forces greater than 30Ncm have been shown to produce micromotions greater than 100μm. Non-axial loading can also contribute to the loosening of abutment screws, a major cause of prosthodontic failure. Nordin et al., described that a high precision and passively fitting prosthesis reduced stresses and strains that could be detrimental to a healing implant [61]. In their study, they utilized the "Cresco Precision Method" to allow a high precision passive fit, intended to reduce stress and strain on the implant-bone interface during prosthetic fixation. Some researchers have implemented splinting and cross-arch stabilization on implants that are not loaded along their long axis. In an effort to avoid the maxillary sinus, Bevilacqua et al., placed distal implants in an angulated manner [62]. This technique has shown bone loss around the distal implants that is similar to more conventionally placed implants. Others have demonstrated 100% survivability using a similar concept called V-II-V, where 6 implants are placed into the maxilla at 30-45 degree angulations to the occlusal plane in the posterior maxilla to avoid the maxillary sinus.

Some researchers have reported that a similar prognosis could be expected whether or not the splinting of implants was utilized [63,64]. Especially when evaluating implant treatment in the maxilla, it is more common to find reports supporting reductions in micromovement and increases in overall survivability and success when splinting and cross-arch stabilization are used. Various combinations of prosthodontic materials are available, including: all-resin, metal reinforced resins and ceramics and all-ceramics. Literature describing the ability of each type of restoration to adequately splint immediately loaded implants to permit osseointegration suggests that stability, rather than the material used, is the critical factor. However, Collaert and De Bruyn reported resin fractures leading to prosthodontic failure and they subsequently altered their protocol to utilize metal reinforced fixed prostheses [65]. Nordin et al., reported failures of distal implants supporting all resin full-arch prostheses [61]. This failure is consistent with both Ibanez et al. [66], who reported that stability from splinting is the primary concern for success rather than other factors such as implant length, and Bergkvist et al.[67], who described impaired healing of implants under a removable prosthesis. Nordin et al., subsequently cited material thinness as the likely cause of inadequate rigidity, suggesting that if adequately thick, an all-resin fixed prosthesis would provide adequate splinting and cross-arch stabilization. Since implants are susceptible to overload with excessive micromotion and since they do not possess a periodontal ligament, pathologic bone strain and fibrotic healing are more likely to occur with poor occlusal management. An occlusal scheme that is perpendicular to the long axis of the implant, has freedom in centric relation, avoids cantilever forces, does not have interferences during excursive or protrusive movements and is in group function where possible also reduces non-axial forces on the implant and screw fixation components.

4. Conclusion

The more current reports suggest that the prevalence of implant survivability has increased and that previous recommendations may not reflect the survivability that current treatment planning and delivery options afford. Careful surgical preparation and performance, considerations in restoration design and maintenance, a regular recall regimen and good oral hygiene can predictably and consistently yield successful results. This has been proven continuously in the literature for the mandible. Although the maxilla has yet to prove itself in long term evidence based studies, the interim results of various investigations suggests that by carefully following guidelines and respecting the biology of the "softer" maxillary alveolar bone and the anatomic limitations of the upper jaw, clinicians may achieve long term success rates similar to those consistently realized in the mandible.

Author details

Ilser Turkyilmaz* and Ashley Brooke Hoders

*Address all correspondence to: ilserturkyilmaz@yahoo.com

Department of Comprehensive Dentistry, University of Texas Health Science Center at San Antonio, Texas, USA

References

[1] Mijiritsky E, Mardinger O, Mazor Z, Chaushu G. Immediate provisionalization of single-tooth implants in fresh-extraction sites at the maxillary esthetic zone: up to 6 years of follow-up. Implant Dentistry. 2009;18(4):326-33.

[2] Turkyilmaz I, Shapiro V. Immediate provisional restoration of an implant placed in a fresh primary maxillary canine extraction socket: a case report. General Dentistry. 2011;59(3):e105-9.

[3] D'Amato S, Redemagni M. Immediate postextraction implantation with provisionalization of two primary canines and related impacted permanent canines: a case report. The International Journal of Periodontics and Restorative Dentistry. 2014;34(2): 251-6.

[4] Kourkouta S. Implant therapy in the esthetic zone: smile line assessment. The International Journal of Periodontics and Restorative Dentistry. 2011;31(2):195-201.

[5] Turkyilmaz I. Prosthetic rehabilitation of an edentulous maxilla with microstomia, limited interarch space, and malaligned implants: a clinical report. Texas Dental Journal. 2012;129(4):389-95.

[6] Katsoulis J, Pazera P, Mericske-Stern R. Prosthetically driven, computer-guided implant planning for the edentulous maxilla: a model study. Clinical Implant Dentistry and Related Research. 2009;11(3):238-45.

[7] Butler B, Kinzer GA. Managing esthetic implant complications. Compendium of Continuing Education in Dentistry. 2012;33(7):514-8, 520-2.

[8] Chow YC, Wang HL. Factors and techniques influencing peri-implant papillae. Implant Dentistry. 2010;19(3):208-19.

[9] Pinho T, Neves M, Alves C. Multidisciplinary management including periodontics, orthodontics, implants, and prosthetics for an adult. American Journal of Orthodontics and Dentofacial Orthopedics. 2012;142(2):235-45.

[10] Turkyilmaz I, McGlumphy EA. Influence of bone density on implant stability parameters and implant success: a retrospective clinical study. BMC Oral Health. 2008 24;8:32.

[11] Pan CY, Chou ST, Tseng YC, Yang YH, Wu CY, Lan TH, Liu PH, Chang HP. Influence of different implant materials on the primary stability of orthodontic mini-implants. The Kaohsiung Journal of Medical Sciences. 2012;28(12):673-8.

[12] Turkyilmaz I. 26-year follow-up of screw-retained fixed dental prostheses supported by machined-surface Branemark implants: a case report. Texas Dental Journal. 2011;128(1):15-9.

[13] Grandi T, Guazzi P, Samarani R, Grandi G. Immediate loading of four (all-on-4) postextractive implants supporting mandibular cross-arch fixed prostheses: 18-month

follow-up from a multicentre prospective cohort study. European Journal of Oral Implantology. 2012;5(3):277-85.

[14] Turkyilmaz I, Tozum TF, Fuhrmann DM, Tumer C. Seven-year follow-up results of TiUnite implants supporting mandibular overdentures: early versus delayed loading. Clinical Implant Dentistry and Related Research. 2012;14 Suppl 1:e83-90.

[15] Branemark PI, Hansson BO, Adell R, Breine U, Lindstrom J, Hallen O, Ohman A. Osseointegrated implants in the treatment of the edentulous jaw. Experience from a 10-year period. Scandinavian Journal of Plastic and Reconstructive Surgery. 1977;16:1-132.

[16] Johansson B, Friberg B, Nilson H. Digitally planned, immediately loaded dental implants with prefabricated prostheses in the reconstruction of edentulous maxillae: a 1-year prospective, multicenter study. Clinical Implant Dentistry and Related Research. 2009;11(3):194-200.

[17] Rungcharassaeng K, Kan JY, Yoshino S, Morimoto T, Zimmerman G. Immediate implant placement and provisionalization with and without a connective tissue graft: an analysis of facial gingival tissue thickness. The International Journal of Periodontics and Restorative Dentistry. 2012;32(6):657-63.

[18] Singh A, Gupta A, Yadav A, Chaturvedi TP, Bhatnagar A, Singh BP. Immediate placement of implant in fresh extraction socket with early loading. Contemporary Clinical Dentistry. 2012;3(Suppl 2):S219-22.

[19] Turkyilmaz I, Suarez JC, Company AM. Immediate implant placement and provisional crown fabrication after a minimally invasive extraction of a peg-shaped maxillary lateral incisor: a clinical report. The Journal of Contemporary Dental Practice. 2009;10(5):e73-80.

[20] Hauchard E, Fournier BP, Jacq R, Bouton A, Pierrisnard L, Naveau A. Splinting effect on posterior implants under various loading modes: a 3D finite element analysis. The European Journal of Prosthodontics and Restorative Dentistry. 2011;19(3):117-22.

[21] Wang TM, Leu LJ, Wang J, Lin LD. Effects of prosthesis materials and prosthesis splinting on peri-implant bone stress around implants in poor-quality bone: a numeric analysis. International Journal of Oral and Maxillofacial Implants. 2002;17(2): 231-7.

[22] Aparicio C, Rangert B, Sennerby L. Immediate/early loading of dental implants: a report from the Sociedad Española de Implantes World Congress consensus meeting in Barcelona, Spain, 2002. Clinical Implant Dentistry and Related Research. 2003;5(1): 57-60.

[23] Lindeboom JA, Frenken JW, Dubois L, Frank M, Abbink I, Kroon FH. Immediate loading versus immediate provisionalization of maxillary single-tooth replacements:

a prospective randomized study with BioComp implants. Journal of Oral and Maxillofacial Surgery. 2006;64(6):936-42.

[24] Turkyilmaz I. Alternative method to fabricating an immediately loaded mandibular hybrid prosthesis without impressions: a clinical report. The International Journal of Periodontics and Restorative Dentistry. 2012;32(3):339-45.

[25] Abboud M, Wahl G, Guirado JL, Orentlicher G. Application and success of two stereolithographic surgical guide systems for implant placement with immediate loading. International Journal of Oral and Maxillofacial Implants. 2012;27(3):634-43.

[26] Misch CE. Bone Density: A Key Determinant for Treatment Planning. In: Contemporary Implant Dentistry, (Misch CE) 3rd ed. Mosby Elsevier, St. Louis, Missouri;2008. pp. 130-146.

[27] Bidez MW, Misch CE. Clinical Biomechanics in Implant dentistry. In: Contemporary Implant Dentistry, (Misch CE) 3rd ed. Mosby Elsevier, St. Louis, Missouri;2008. pp. 543-556.

[28] Buchs AU, Hahn J, Vassos DM. Efficacy of threaded hydroxyapatite-coated implants in the anterior mandible supporting overdentures. Implant Dentistry. 1996;5(3): 188-92.

[29] Sakka S, Baroudi K, Nassani MZ. Factors associated with early and late failure of dental implants. Journal of Investigative and Clinical Dentistry. 2012;3(4):258-61.

[30] Eriksson AR, Albrektsson T, Albrektsson B. Heat caused by drilling cortical bone. Temperature measured in vivo in patients and animals. Acta Orthopaedica Scandinavica. 1984;55(6):629-31.

[31] Albrektsson T, Eriksson A. Thermally induced bone necrosis in rabbits: relation to implant failure in humans. Clinical Orthopaedics and Related Research. 1985;(195): 311-2.

[32] Sharawy M, Misch CE, Weller N, Tehemar S. Heat generation during implant drilling: the significance of motor speed. Journal of Oral and Maxillofacial Surgery. 2002;60(10):1160-9.

[33] Turkyilmaz I, Aksoy U, McGlumphy EA. Two alternative surgical techniques for enhancing primary implant stability in the posterior maxilla: a clinical study including bone density, insertion torque, and resonance frequency analysis data. Clinical Implant Dentistry and Related Research. 2008;10(4):231-7

[34] Menicucci G, Pachie E, Lorenzetti M, Migliaretti G, Carossa S. Comparison of primary stability of straight-walled and tapered implants using an insertion torque device. The International Journal of Prosthodontics. 2012;25(5):465-71.

[35] Trisi P, Perfetti G, Baldoni E, Berardi D, Colagiovanni M, Scogna G. Implant micromotion is related to peak insertion torque and bone density. Clinical Oral Implants Research. 2009;20(5):467-71

[36] Turkyilmaz I. Use of reciprocating saw for alveolar ridge reduction in the anterior mandible for immediate load implant-supported hybrid dentures. Journal of Oral and Maxillofacial Surgery. 2010;68(6):1334-7.

[37] Javed F, Romanos GE. The role of primary stability for successful immediate loading of dental implants. A literature review. Journal of Dentistry. 2010;38(8):612-20

[38] Brunski JB. In vivo bone response to biomechanical loading at the bone/dental-implant interface. Advances in Dental Research. 1999;13:99-119

[39] Canullo L, Rasperini G. Preservation of peri-implant soft and hard tissues using platform switching of implants placed in immediate extraction sockets: a proof-of-concept study with 12- to 36-month follow-up. International Journal of Oral and Maxillofacial Implants. 2007;22(6):995-1000.

[40] Schnitman PA, Wohrle PS, Rubenstein JE. Immediate fixed interim prostheses supported by two-stage threaded implants: methodology and results. The Journal of Oral Implantology. 1990;16(2):96-105.

[41] Scortecci G. Immediate function of cortically anchored disk-design implants without bone augmentation in moderately to severely resorbed completely edentulous maxillae. The Journal of Oral Implantology. 1999;25(2):70-9.

[42] Grandi T, Guazzi P, Samarani R, Grandi G. Immediate loading of four (all-on-4) post-extractive implants supporting mandibular cross-arch fixed prostheses: 18-month follow-up from a multicentre prospective cohort study. European Journal of Oral Implantology. 2012;5(3):277-85.

[43] Rocci A, Rocci M, Scoccia A, Martignoni M, Gottlow J, Sennerby L. Immediate loading of maxillary prostheses using flapless surgery, implant placement in predetermined positions, and prefabricated provisional restorations. Part 2: a retrospective 10-year clinical study. International Journal of Oral and Maxillofacial Implants. 2012;27(5):1199-204.

[44] Avila G, Galindo P, Rios H, Wang HL. Immediate implant loading: current status from available literature. Implant Dentistry. 2007;16(3):235-45.

[45] Schnitman PA, Wohrle PS, Rubenstein JE, DaSilva JD, Wang NH. Ten-year results for Brånemark implants immediately loaded with fixed prostheses at implant placement. International Journal of Oral and Maxillofacial Implants. 1997;12(4):495-503.

[46] [46]. Mertens C, Meyer-Baumer A, Kappel H, Hoffmann J, Steveling HG. Use of 8-mm and 9-mm Implants in Atrophic Alveolar Ridges: 10-Year Results. International Journal of Oral and Maxillofacial Implants. 2012;27(6):1501-8.

[47] Atieh MA, Zadeh H, Stanford CM, Cooper LF. Survival of short dental implants for treatment of posterior partial edentulism: a systematic review. International Journal of Oral and Maxillofacial Implants. 2012;27(6):1323-31.

[48] Arnhart C, Kielbassa AM, Martinez-de Fuentes R, Goldstein M, Jackowski J, Lorenzoni M, Maiorana C, Mericske-Stern R, Pozzi A, Rompen E, Sanz M, Strub JR. Comparison of variable-thread tapered implant designs to a standard tapered implant design after immediate loading. A 3-year multicentre randomised controlled trial. European Journal of Oral Implantology. 2012;5(2):123-36.

[49] Chong L, Khocht A, Suzuki JB, Gaughan J. Effect of implant design on initial stability of tapered implants. The Journal of Oral Implantology. 2009;35(3):130-5.

[50] Sadowsky SJ. Immediate load on the edentulous mandible: treatment planning considerations. Journal of Prosthodontics. 2010;19(8):647-53.

[51] Schiroli G. Immediate tooth extraction, placement of a Tapered Screw-Vent implant, and provisionalization in the esthetic zone: a case report. Implant Dentistry. 2003;12(2):123-31.

[52] Yang GL, Song LN, Jiang QH, Wang XX, Zhao SF, He FM. Effect of strontium-substituted nanohydroxyapatite coating of porous implant surfaces on implant osseointegration in a rabbit model. International Journal of Oral and Maxillofacial Implants. 2012;27(6):1332-9.

[53] Cheng Z, Guo C, Dong W, He FM, Zhao SF, Yang GL. Effect of thin nano-hydroxyapatite coating on implant osseointegration in ovariectomized rats. Oral Surgery, Oral Medicine, Oral Pathology and Oral Radiology. 2012;113(3):e48-53.

[54] [54]. Nicu EA, Van Assche N, Coucke W, Teughels W, Quirynen M. RCT comparing implants with turned and anodically oxidized surfaces: a pilot study, a 3-year follow-up. Journal of Clinical Periodontology. 2012;39(12):1183-90.

[55] Goodacre CJ, Bernal G, Rungcharassaeng K, Kan JY. Clinical complications with implants and implant prostheses. The Journal of Prosthetic Dentistry. 2003;90(2):121-32.

[56] Flanagan D. An overview of complete artificial fixed dentition supported by endosseous implants. Artificial Organs. 2005;29(1):73-81.

[57] Sesma N, Pannuti C, Cardaropoli G. Retrospective clinical study of 988 dual acid-etched implants placed in grafted and native bone for single-tooth replacement. International Journal of Oral and Maxillofacial Implants. 2012;27(5):1243-8.

[58] Turkyilmaz I, McGlumphy EA. Influence of bone density on implant stability parameters and implant success: a retrospective clinical study. BMC Oral Health. 2008;8:32.

[59] Wagner W, Wiltfang J, Pistner H, Yildirim M, Ploder B, Chapman M, Schiestl N, Hantak E. Bone formation with a biphasic calcium phosphate combined with fibrin

sealant in maxillary sinus floor elevation for delayed dental implant. Clinical Oral Implants Research. 2012;23(9):1112-7.

[60] Clementini M, Boniello R, Gasparini G, Moro A, Pelo S. Surgical treatment of severe athropic maxilla by means of multiple extraoral harvesting. Oral Implantology (Rome). 2009;2(3):4-10.

[61] Nordin T, Graf J, Frykholm A, Hellden L. Early functional loading of sand-blasted and acid-etched (SLA) Straumann implants following immediate placement in maxillary extraction sockets. Clinical and radiographic result. Clinical Oral Implants Research. 2007;18(4):441-51

[62] Bevilacqua M, Tealdo T, Menini M, Pera F, Mossolov A, Drago C, Pera P. The influence of cantilever length and implant inclination on stress distribution in maxillary implant-supported fixed dentures. The Journal of Prosthetic Dentistry. 2011;105(1): 5-13.

[63] Al-Ansari A. No difference between splinted and unsplinted implants to support overdentures. Evidence Based Dentistry. 2012;13(2):54-5.

[64] Stoumpis C, Kohal RJ. To splint or not to splint oral implants in the implant-supported overdenture therapy? A systematic literature review. Journal of Oral Rehabilitation. 2011;38(11):857-69.

[65] Collaert B, De Bruyn H. Early loading of four or five Astra Tech fixtures with a fixed cross-arch restoration in the mandible. Clinical Implant Dentistry and Related Research. 2002;4(3):133-5.

[66] Ibanez JC, Tahhan MJ, Zamar JA, Menendez AB, Juaneda AM, Zamar NJ, Monqaut JL. Immediate occlusal loading of double acid-etched surface titanium implants in 41 consecutive full-arch cases in the mandible and maxilla: 6- to 74-month results. Journal of Periodontology. 2005;76(11):1972-81.

[67] Bergkvist G. Immediate loading of implants in the edentulous maxilla. Swedish Dental Journal Supplement. 2008;(196):10-75.

3

Miniscrew Applications in Orthodontics

Fatma Deniz Uzuner and Belma Işık Aslan

1. Introduction

Anchorage control during tooth movement is one of the main factors for ensuring successful orthodontic treatment. Anchorage can be defined as the resistance that a tooth or a group of teeth offer when they are subjected to a force [1]. The aim of orthodontic treatment is to maintain sufficient anchorage control to create appropriate force systems that provide the desired treatment effects.

Recently, implants have been used as skeletal anchorage devices for orthodontic purposes [2-5]. Temporary anchorage devices (TADs) [1,9,10], including miniplates, implants and miniscrews, have been used for skeletal anchorage [6-8]. TADs are inserted into the bone and aim to enhance orthodontic anchorage either by supporting the anchoring teeth or by being an independent anchorage unit eliminating the need for supporting teeth; they are removed once their function has been completed. They can be fixed into the bone either biomechanically (osseointegration) [11] or mechanically (cortical stabilization) [8]. Clinicians can better control anchorage by using TADs in orthodontic treatment, thereby achieving more satisfactory treatment results than could be achieved with conventional mechanics [6,12].

Currently, clinicians mostly prefer to use miniscrews for combined orthodontic treatment [13]. Despite the high success rate of miniplates, their invasive placement procedures require an oral surgeon and the associated high costs of such a procedure overshadow their use in terms of anchorage [1]. The use of osseointegrated mini-implants has also been limited because of the long waiting period for osseointegration, their large size and high cost [14,15]. Miniscrews, however, are available in favorable sizes, have relatively lower costs and are simple to insert and remove; therefore, they can be easily placed by an orthodontist with minimal tissue invasion [13]. Miniscrews obtain their stability mainly from mechanical retention in the bone [1,9], so they can be loaded immediately after placement [16]. In the literature, there is no general agreement about the terminology used [17,18]; this varies between 'miniscrews', 'microscrews', 'miniscrew implants'. and 'mini-implants' [13,19-21]. In this chapter, we refer to them as miniscrews. Miniscrews are now accepted as a simple and effective tool in daily orthodontic practice and orthodontists commonly use them in a variety of clinical situations [20-25].

This chapter focuses on the principles of application for miniscrews including screw sizes, application sites and fundamental placement methods. Management of complications, the use of miniscrews in specific orthodontic situations and appliance design are also discussed.

2. General considerations

2.1. Location and dimensions of the miniscrew

The stability of miniscrews immediately following their placement (primary stability) and during orthodontic treatment is important for clinicians in terms of achieving their desired treatment results. The primary factors for stability are the quality and quantity of the bone [26-28], as well as the thickness, type and health of the soft tissue [29].

Cortical bone with a thickness of less than 0.5 mm is not suitable for miniscrew placement. Higher success rates have been reported with cortical bone at least 1.0 mm thick [27].

To maximize stability, it is better to place miniscrews in the attached gingiva (keratinized gingiva), which is more resistant to inflammation and less likely to develop soft-tissue hypertrophy [26, 29]. However, if the miniscrew has to be placed in non-keratinized mucosa, a 3-mm vertical stab incision should be used to prevent the soft tissue from surrounding the miniscrew, as this small incision requires no sutures [1].

Placement site is another important factor in the success of miniscrews [30]. Miniscrews can be placed in the inter-radicular space between tooth roots, either buccally or lingually; in the hard palate (midpalatal/parapalatal region); below the anterior nasal spine; and in the infrazygomatic crest, maxillary tuberosity, edentulous areas, chin and retromolar areas [8,30].

Conflicting reports exist regarding success rates for miniscrews in the mandible and maxilla. Park et al. [31], found that the maxilla had a higher success rate than the mandible, while others [16, 30] reported that placement of the miniscrews in the maxilla or mandible was not associated with the success rate. Moon et al. [30] found that the area between the first and second premolars in the maxilla and mandible of both young and adult patients had the highest success rate.

In the maxilla, the buccal and palatal aspects of the posterior region have been defined as safe areas for miniscrew placement, while the maxillary tuberosity is not suitable because of the minimal bone thickness in the area [32]. Ishii et al. [33], and Poggio [32] reported that the safest region for placement is the inter-alveolar septum between the maxillary first molar and second premolar, 6–8 mm apical to the alveolar crest on the palatal side. The inter-radicular distance is greater on the palatal side; however, the thickness of the palatal mucosa renders this region less favorable. This problem could be alleviated by using a miniscrew with a longer head.

However, the midpalatal suture region is the most favorable placement site for miniscrews in terms of both bone and soft-tissue characteristics. This region, with its high density of cortical bone and thin keratinized soft tissue ensures the biomechanical stability of the miniscrews [23,34] and has been shown to have a higher success rate (90%) than the parapalatal suture region (84%) [35]. However, the parapalatal area is the most suitable region for miniscrew placement in adolescents for preventing developmental disturbances of the midpalatal suture, as the transverse growth of the midpalatal suture continues up until the late teens [36].

In the mandible, the safest region is either between the second premolar and first molar, or between the first and second molars, owing to the adequate bone thickness [22,32]. The thinnest bone was found between the first premolar and the canine. If a miniscrew has to be implanted into this region, it should be placed 11 mm below the alveolar crest [32]. Although the area between the second premolar and the first molar has thicker cortical bone than the area between the first and second premolars in the mandible, the success rate in this area is significantly lower [30]. These results suggest that other factors beyond bone quality, such as soft-tissue thickness [37], oral hygiene [38] and root proximity [39,40] might also affect the success rate of miniscrews.

Miniscrews are available in a variety of materials, shapes, head designs, length and diameter, being 5–12 mm long and having a diameter from 1.2 to 2.3 mm [6,11,20,41-43]. In general, 1.2–1.6 mm miniscrews are used. Because of its low success rate, the 1.0-mm diameter miniscrew is not suitable for clinical use [16]. However, the 1.2-, 1.3-and 1.5-mm diameter miniscrews have had similar or higher success rates than the 1.6-mm miniscrew [16,38]. The design of the miniscrew also affects primary stability, with a conical thread design achieving superior primary stability when compared with a cylindrical design [42].

Selection of the correct diameter and length depends on the region in which the miniscrew will be placed. If it is placed in the inter-radicular region, a miniscrew with a smaller diameter will be preferred, as it will decrease the risk of root damage [30]. The recommended diameter is 1.3 mm in the maxilla, 1.4 mm in the mandible and 1.5 or 1.6 mm in the midpalatal area [12].

Determining the length of the miniscrew primarily depends on the quality of the bone, the screw angulation, the soft-tissue thickness and the adjacent anatomic structures [8,38,44]. In regions with adequate cortical density, small miniscrews are preferred, while longer minis-crews are preferred if stability is required in trabecular bone.

The screw should be embedded into the bone at least 5–6 mm [45,46], yet deeper placements have been recommended when bone quality is low [47,48]. Minimal depth of placement is at least 6 mm for the maxilla and 4 mm for the mandible [12]. In maxillary buccal alveolar bone, 7–8 mm miniscrews are recommended, while 5–6 mm long miniscrews are suitable in the mandibular buccal bone [12]. Short screws can become dislodged when they are placed in the palatal region owing to the thick palatal soft tissue [44,49]. Long miniscrews (10–12 mm) are preferred in the palatal region to compensate for the thick palatal soft tissue and to keep 6-mm miniscrews embedded in the bone [48,49]. Because the midpalatal region has dense cortical bone, a long miniscrew may not be needed for stability.

2.2. Placement of the miniscrew

Before placing the miniscrews, clinicians should radiographically assess their position relative to the roots. Panaromic or periapical radiographs, however, may not provide adequate information for optimizing the placement of a miniscrew. Computed tomography (CT) or cone-beam CT can allow clinicians to make an accurate and reliable evaluation of bone thickness and the adjacent anatomic structures, and therefore improves the success rate and ensures safe placement of the screws [33,50,51].

The patient is instructed to rinse with a chlorhexidine solution; then, infiltrative anesthesia is applied. Light local anesthesia is preferred so that the nerve fibers in the periodontal ligament remain sensitive [12], and the patient is aware if the miniscrew touches the root of the tooth, allowing the clinician to change the insertion direction.

There are two different placement methods: self-tapping and self-drilling.

Self-tapping method: Before placing the miniscrew, a hole is drilled in the cortical bone and a miniscrew is screwed through this hole with a hand driver. The diameter of the pilot drill should be slightly smaller (0.2–0.3 mm) than the inner (or core) diameter of the miniscrew [46]. Care must be taken to keep the axis of the drill stable so as not to enlarge the hole. To reduce heat generation while drilling, clinicians should not apply too much pressure and should irrigate the bone with coolants [52,53].

Self-drilling method: Self-drilling is a simpler method for placing the miniscrew than self-tapping. The miniscrew is inserted into the bone without drilling and screwed in with the hand driver [12] or motor driver [54]. Using a motor driver is helpful for gaining a higher placement success rate [54]. Self-drilling screws are reported to have better stability, with more bone to metal contact than self-tapping screws [55,56].

An incision may be made in the soft tissue before drilling [54,57]. Miyawaki et al. [16], reported that the flapless (non-incision) group had a higher success rate than the flap surgery (incision) group. By contrast, Moon et al. [30], found no difference between non-incision and incision groups in their study.

Generally, miniscrews are inserted in the buccal or lingual cortical plates; this is defined as monocortical placement. Occasionally, the miniscrew can be placed across the entire width of the alveolus (bicortical placement). Although bicortical placement provides superior force resistance and stability compared with monocortical placement, more care has to be taken during placement. Bicortical placement may be preferred when increased orthodontic loading is needed or in cases where there is insufficient cortical bone thickness [58-60].

It is usually recommended that miniscrews are placed perpendicular (at an angle of 90°) to the bone surface [45]. However, this might not always be clinically achievable, and an angular approach might be needed. If the buccal alveolar bone volume is sufficient relative to the long axis of the teeth, the miniscrew can be placed at an angle of 30–40° for the upper jaw and 20–60° for the lower jaw [12]. This angular placement minimizes root contact, as there is relatively more space [50] and the surface area of cortical bone in contact with the miniscrew is increased, allowing placement of longer miniscrews and improved stability [12]. When placing a miniscrew at an angle into dense cortical bone using the self-drilling method, clinicians can damage the cortical bone; in such cases, the self-tapping method would be a better option [12].

Clinicians should apply slow and gentle force during insertion to avoid fracture of the miniscrew. The recommended insertion torque value is 5–10 N cm [61]. Insertion torque values are associated with the success of the procedure. The success rate of the miniscrew also depends on the clinician's experience and the type of the placement: whether self-tapping or self-drilling. If the self-tapping method is used, the following factors also affect the success rate: flap or flapless surgery, sterilization, pilot hole preparation depth and diameter, cooling technique, drill speed and pressure, direction of placement and placement procedure (steady or wiggling) [6,8,16,18,27,30,43,47].

The stability of the miniscrew should be checked after placement. If any mobility is detected, the implant needs to be removed. If primary stability is not achieved upon insertion, the miniscrew implant may loosen during orthodontic treatment [26].

Patients should be informed that they might have pain for 1–2 days and that they can take anti-inflammatory agents if required. Most patients do not have noticeable discomfort or inflammation. Patients need to be instructed in oral hygiene techniques [35] and should be advised that they can brush their teeth as usual. A compressed water spray such as Waterpik [12] and daily use of mouth rinses will be useful. Caution should be taken not to apply excessive force to the miniscrew while brushing and during mastication.

2.3. Timing of loading, force magnitude and direction

The timing of loading depends largely on the miniscrew type [62-65]. For osseointegrated miniscrews, loading can commence 2–3 months after placement. Miyawaki et al. [16], observed no significant difference between loading at 1–2 months and at 3 months after placement. However, miniscrews that do not require osseointegration are often used, and they can be loaded immediately [61].

The maximum force-load that a miniscrew can withstand remains controversial [66]. Dalstra et al. [67], recommended 50 g of immediate loaded force for miniscrews placed into thin cortical bone and fine trabeculae. Many studies have reported miniscrew stability with loading forces of 300 g or less [68,69]. In their study, Buchter et al. [69], evaluated the transverse loading of miniscrews placed in dense mandibular bone and reported that immediate loads of up to 900 centinewtons per millimetre [cN/mm] remained clinically stable. Kim et al. [70], investigated whether the specific directions of the force vectors were associated with the stability of miniscrews. The results indicated that miniscrews were fixed evenly in three dimensions and were not more resistant to any particular direction of load. Park [12] recommends loading immediately after placement and keeping the force minimal (< 70 g) until 2 months after placement, and then increasing the force up to 150–200 g.

Cortical thickness, miniscrew characteristics, force magnitude, direction and loading period are reported to be factors related to miniscrew stability [16,64-66,71]. However, one study found that the duration of loading did not influence the success rate of the miniscrews [70]. To prevent the miniscrew from loosening, the moments created during force application that may tend to unscrew the miniscrew have to be taken into consideration. To control these moments, clinicians have to carefully evaluate the force system applied to the miniscrew. If the application of such undesirable moments to the screw cannot be avoided, indirect anchorage is recommended [1,8].

Although the miniscrews may initially be stable, they may not remain stationary when subjected to orthodontic forces [72,73]. Liou et al. [72], placed miniscrews in the zygomatic buttress for direct anchorage and reported that when the screw was subjected to orthodontic force, extrusion and 0.4-mm tipping were observed at the level of the head of the screw. Liu et al. [73], evaluated the displacement of miniscrews placed in inter-radicular areas of the maxilla as anchorage for the en masse retraction of anterior teeth using three-dimensional CT registration evaluations. The researchers observed that both the molars and the miniscrews were displaced in the direction of force application and drifted mesially, but not by the same amount. The molars drifted mesially 0.91 mm and the miniscrews moved 0.23 mm on average. This result implied that the miniscrews might have come into contact with the roots following treatment. The different mesial-drift ratios of the molars and the miniscrews may be a critical factor in the loosening of miniscrews [74]. As a precaution, the researchers [73] advised placing the miniscrews mesially for long-term stability.

The conventional periodontal pressure–tension theory cannot explain the miniscrew displacement process. The Frost mechanostat theory instead identifies complex bone biomechanics [75,76]. The bone remodelling process at the bone–screw interface and the mechanism of screw displacement are correlated to the stress–strain field in the surrounding bone as a result of dynamic loading [77,78].

3. Complications

Complications may be related to factors such as the clinician, the patient and the miniscrews themselves [79].

Clinician-related complications: Clinicians' skills and experience are critical to the success rate of the procedure [70]. Once clinicians become accustomed to using miniscrews, their success rates increase [12]. Operators need to develop their skills to avoid damaging adjacent anatomical structures and the root of the tooth while placing the miniscrew.

Patient-related complications: These result from factors such as systemic diseases, periodontal disease, osteoporosis, drugs, pharmacologic prescriptions such as bisphosphonates, poor oral hygiene, smoking and cortical thickness of the bone [31,63,80-82], all of which can affect the stability of the miniscrew. It may be better not to use miniscrews for patients with adverse risk factors; however, if miniscrews have to be used, longer healing periods should be allowed and specific loading protocols should be applied [81,82]. It is notable that in their animal study, Park et al. [83], found that the presence of diabetes and variation in the placement system (self-drilling or self-tapping) did not affect the initial stability of orthodontic mini-implants.

Miniscrew-related complications: Anticipated complications with miniscrews include [6,72,79]:

1.   Pain and discomfort, irritation to tongue or cheek

2.   Inflammation around miniscrews

3.   Soft-tissue impingement

4.   Damage to surrounding anatomical structures

5.   Root injury

6.   Miniscrew mobility or failure

7.   Fracture of miniscrews

1.   Pain and discomfort, irritation to tongue or cheek

Generally, patients do not experience pain and discomfort following miniscrew placement [6,16,58,35]. If pain is present, it may last 1–2 days [58,47]. Kuroda et al. [38], analyzed patients' pain duration and intensity during the first 2 weeks after placement. One hour after placement, 95% of patients reported pain in the group in which miniscrews were placed after raising a mucoperiosteal flap, whereas in the group who had undergone a flapless approach, only 50% of patients reported pain. After 2 weeks, the values were 10% and 0% for the respective techniques.

Cheek irritation was generally not observed when miniscrews were placed in the buccal alveolar bone; however, when placed in the palatal area, tongue irritation primarily occurred. Bonding resin or a periodontal wound dressing can be applied to the head of the miniscrew to smooth its surface and to minimize soft-tissue irritation [1,84].

2.   Inflammation around miniscrews

Peri-implantitis is the most commonly observed complication, and is considered to be the major factor in implant failure [43]. The localization of the miniscrew, its relationship with the soft tissue and the hygiene habits of the patient are the main factors that affect inflammation [30]. Takaki et al. [35], reported that inflammation frequency depended on the degree of mucosal penetration and stated that chronic inflammation mostly occurred when miniscrews were placed in the anterior alveolar region of the maxilla. When the miniscrew was placed in the attached gingiva or in the palatal mucosa, less inflammation was observed [12]. By contrast, when miniscrews were placed in the oral mucosa, deep in the vestibule or near a frenulum, persistent inflammation occurred [29,31]. If miniscrews are placed 1 mm below the mucogingival junction, they do not produce serious inflammation. To prevent inflammation, the screws need to be thoroughly cleaned. Mild infections can be controlled by using antiseptic mouthwash and by brushing [35]. Taking a different view, Kim et al. [70], emphasized that unlike inflammation from poor oral hygiene, inflammation caused by mobile miniscrews was not controlled with improved oral hygiene. Therefore, inflammation or swelling around a miniscrew might be the result of it loosening, rather than the cause. When taking this view, primary stability becomes increasingly important.

3.   Soft-tissue impingement

In conditions where the miniscrew is placed deep in the vestibule, into the free gingiva or the retromolar area, the head of the miniscrews may become embedded in the overgrowth of surrounding soft tissue [85]. Placing miniscrews into attached gingiva can avoid soft-tissue impingement over the head of the screw. Additionally, the elastic chain, arch wire or coils may impinge on the gingiva and may cause inflammation, as well as gingival recession. Clinicians should be careful, as bending of the arch wire can eliminate impingement. Thin soft-tissue impingement overlying the miniscrew can be exposed with light finger pressure without having to apply a local anesthetic [85]. Soft-tissue impingement may be minimized by placing a wax pellet or an elastic separator over the miniscrew. Additionally, patients may be instructed to use chlorhexidine mouthwash. Rather than acting as an antibacterial agent and minimizing tissue inflammation, chlorhexidine reduces probable soft-tissue overgrowth by slowing down epithelialization [85,86].

4.   Damage to surrounding anatomical structures

While placing the miniscrew, the clinician needs to be careful not to cause damage to adjacent structures, nerves, arteries and the roots of the teeth. In the mandible, as the inferior alveolar nerve runs lingual and inferior to the molar roots and moves buccally at the premolar area, the miniscrews will be placed far above the inferior alveolar nerve and will not cause any damage. When placing the miniscrew in the palatal alveolar bone, angular placement near the apex of the roots of the maxillary molars will reduce the risk of making contact with the greater palatine nerve and artery, which are situated higher in the palate [12].

5.   Root injury

Iatrogenic root injury may occur while placing the miniscrew in a narrow inter-radicular space [87]. Clinicians need to evaluate the distance between the roots using periapical or panoramic radiographs to avoid root contact during placement. A safety clearance of 2 mm is recommended in interdental areas [64]. When this space is insufficient, the interdental space should be widened before placement during the alignment of the teeth.

Caution must be taken while placing the miniscrew. A small amount of local anesthesia is preferred to keep the nerve fibers in the periodontal ligament sensitive [12], so that the patients can feel it if the miniscrew touches the root. Clinicians can also sense contact with the root. During insertion of the miniscrew, cortical bone resistance may at the outset be quite strong; however, after penetrating the cortical bone, resistance remains minimal until the miniscrew is fully placed. If any strong resistance is felt, it should be used as an indicator of possible root contact [88]. Should this occur, the clinician should remove the miniscrew and change the insertion angulation. Angular placement of the miniscrew may minimize root contact. Placing the miniscrew slightly mesial to the contact point of teeth is also recommended. It has been shown that the distance from the outer bone surface to the buccal surface of the root is larger at the second premolars than that at the first molars [50].

Potential complications of root damage include root resorption, devitalization, dentoalveolar ankylosis and osteosclerosis [79, 89]. Researchers have determined that close proximity or contact between a miniscrew and a root can be a major risk factor for failure of the procedure [39, 40, 90]. This view is supported by Lee et al. [91], who reported that the incidence of root resorption increased when the distance between the miniscrew and the root was less than 0.6 mm, and that the incidence of bone resorption and ankylosis was increased when the miniscrew came close to the root surface, even without root contact.

Asscherickx et al. [89], reported that if damage occurs, recovery time is relatively quick. If trauma to the root does not involve the pulp and is limited to the cementum or the dentin of the tooth, the prognosis will not be heavily influenced and healing will take place [85,88]. After removal of the miniscrew, the damaged root will be repaired in 12–18 weeks [85]. In their animal studies, Kim and Kim [92] observed that when a miniscrew was left touching the root, the normal healing response did not occur; the root surface was mostly resorbed and partial repair began at 8 weeks.

During orthodontic treatment, contact between the root and the miniscrew may occur as the tooth moves. The tooth will then stop moving and the miniscrew may become mobile. If further tooth movement is required, the miniscrew must be removed and placed elsewhere.

6.   Miniscrew mobility or failure

Miniscrew dislodgement and mobility mostly occur in the first 1–2 months and more than 90% of the failures occur within the first 4 months [30]. When a miniscrew has resisted more than a 4-month period of force application, it can be considered successful and stable [30].

When mobility occurs, the clinician can tighten the miniscrew and leave it for 1–2 months with no loading, or light loading if necessary [1]. Supporting this recommendation, researchers reported that non-infected dental implants may reintegrate after tightening [93]; even when accidentally avulsed, an implant can become stable after reimplantation and immediate loading [94]. If stability cannot be regained, the miniscrew needs to be removed and replaced.

Miniscrew mobility and failure is mostly the result of low bone density owing to inadequate cortical thickness [85]. The health, thickness and type of soft tissue are other important factors in this context.

According to Moon et al. [30], sex, age, jaw (maxilla/mandible), soft-tissue management (incision/no incision) and placement side (left/right) are not related to the success rate of the miniscrew. By contrast, others have stated that miniscrews placed in the maxilla show a higher success rate than those placed in the mandible [10,31,35,43,54]. Occlusal stress and food impaction force may be factors causing mobility and failure of miniscrews in the mandible [35], while failure of miniscrews placed in the midpalatal area may be the result of tongue pressure [85].

There are conflicting reports about the relationship between success rate and the patient's age. Success rate tends to be lower in younger patients (< 20 years old) compared with older patients (> 20 years old) [54]. This may be because of the thinner cortical bone and poorer bone quality in younger patients. However, in another study, Park [95] reported that against expectations, the success rate was higher for the below 20 years age group compared with the over 20 years age group, which might be explained by the higher rate of metabolism in the young adult group. Contrarily, Miyawaki et al. [16], stated that there was no significant difference in the success rates of the below 20 years age group, the 20–30 years age group and the over 30 years age group.

Excessive stress at the screw–bone interface may cause miniscrew failure. Miniscrew geometry and the placement method (self-drilling/self-tapping) can have an effect on the stress distribution of the peri-screw bone. Self-drilling miniscrews have been reported to have greater screw–bone contact (mechanical grip) and holding strength compared with self-tapping screws [96,97], although the technique causes greater stress to the peri-screw bone. Placing a pilot hole before self-drilling may reduce this stress.

7. Fracture of miniscrews

Miniscrew fracture is a more serious clinical complication than root contact [87]. Fractures most commonly occur during the last turn of miniscrew insertion and the first turn of the removal phase [1,98]. Lima et al. [98], stated that excessive force and the inability of the implant to resist rotational forces during insertion were the main causes of fractures. Clinicians should apply slow and gentle force to avoid fracture of the miniscrew. If the insertion resistance reaches the fracture strength of the implant, it would be better to wait 1–2 min to relieve the internal stress accumulated in the miniscrew and the surrounding bone [1].

In their in vitro study, Choa et al. [87], evaluated the effects of insertion angle and implant thread type on the fracture properties of orthodontic miniscrews during insertion. They reported that maximum insertion torque increased with an increase in insertion angle. When a miniscrew contacts the artificial root at a critical contact angle, deformation or fracture of the miniscrew can occur at a lower insertion torque value than that of penetration.

The fracture of a miniscrew may also occur during the removal phase. Miniscrews can be easily removed by turning them in the opposite direction of placement. To eliminate the possibility of fracture, clinicians should apply gentle untightening pressure or use an ultrasonic scaler on the screw's head until the interface between the miniscrew and the bone breaks. If the removal torque approaches the fracture torque range, the clinician should wait 1–2 weeks before again attempting to remove it [1]. The greater the duration of the miniscrew in the bone and the older the patient, the greater the removal torque of the miniscrew [3]. Stress concentrates in the cervical part of the miniscrew during removal.

Fracture of miniscrews primarily depends on the screw size. Miniscrews with a smaller diameter are easier to place between the roots; however, a small decrease in this dimension results in a meaningful increase in the torsional strength and, therefore, in the risk of fracture [6,8,10]. Screws with a larger diameter demonstrate minimal fracturing. The core (inner) diameter affects fracturing more than the outer diameter. Clinicians may prefer to use a miniscrew with a larger diameter to reduce the risk of fracture; however, doing so will increase the fracture torque [22,99].

The material that the miniscrews are made of is also a factor that affects the likelihood of fracture. Pure titanium implants are preferred as they are more biocompatible than titanium alloy implants [1]; however, titanium alloys are stronger and provide more resistance to fracture [6].

4. Clinical applications

Planning of orthodontic treatment should consider the desired force system to act on the teeth that need to be moved, as well as any undesired effects on the anchorage unit of teeth. This will guide ideal placement of the miniscrew for the proper appliance design.

Clinicians also should be aware of any anatomical limitations for the placement of miniscrews. The location of the miniscrew will affect the appliance design and the force system. Therefore, clinicians should plan the placement area of the miniscrews in the buccal alveolar region and/ or in the palatal alveolar region or midpalatal area according to the required tooth movement. In conditions where miniscrews cannot be placed in the ideal position, the force direction should be adjusted depending on the changes in tooth movement during the treatment time.

Selection of the appropriate miniscrew design is crucial. Clinicians mostly prefer miniscrews with slotted heads, which are convenient for the attachment of different types of orthodontic wires (round, square or rectangular) and complex wire activations.

Many reports describe the application of miniscrew-supported orthodontic treatment for achieving a variety of orthodontic tooth movements, including intrusion [25,49,100], extrusion, space closure (distalization, mesialization) [24, 101], uprighting, eruption of impacted teeth [102] and the correction of canted occlusal planes [103]. In addition, miniscrews can be used in the application of dentofacial orthopedics such as rapid palatal expansion and Class II and III correction (Figure 1) [12,45,104,105]. This chapter does not cover the use of miniscrews for dentoskeletal orthopedics.

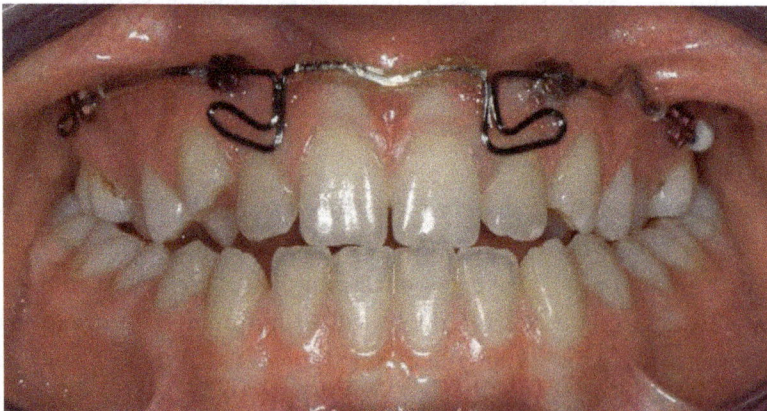

Figure 1. Miniscrews used in the application of dentofacial orthopedics with the placement of four miniscrews between the inter-radicular areas of the maxilla. Stainless steel arch wire (0.021 × 0.025 inch) was passively connected to the miniscrews, and two hook shapes were connected to the arch wire in the lateral root region for facemask elastics.

Miniscrews aim to strengthen orthodontic anchorage either by connecting to a tooth or a group of teeth to reinforce their anchorage (indirect anchorage) (Figure 2 and 3a) [105], or by acting as anchorage units themselves, eliminating the need for supporting teeth (direct anchorage) (Figures 3b and 4) [106].

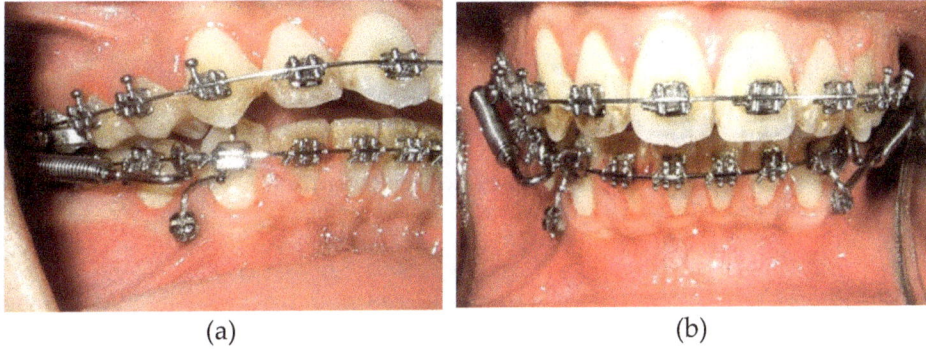

(a)   (b)

Figure 2. Miniscrew used as indirect anchorage to avoid buccal flaring of the anterior teeth with a forsus appliance.

Miniscrews are most often used for direct anchorage. Generally, direct forces are applied between the miniscrew and the target tooth by using elastic chain, elastic thread or a coil spring to move the tooth toward the miniscrew. If a miniscrew is used as a direct anchor, it is advantageous to place the miniscrew along the line of the desired tooth movement. If force applied between the tooth and the miniscrew causes undesirable moments, then the miniscrew should be used as indirect anchorage to support the anchorage teeth, rather than acting as a direct anchor [8].

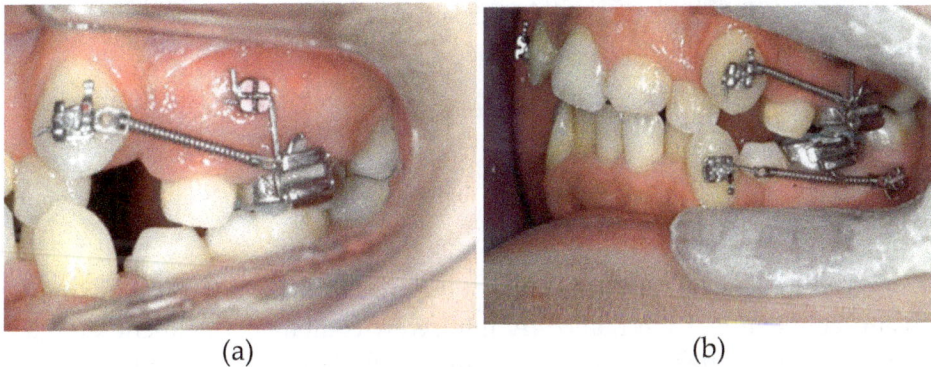

(a)   (b)

Figure 3. Canine distalization combined with miniscrew use as (a) indirect anchorage and (b) direct anchorage.

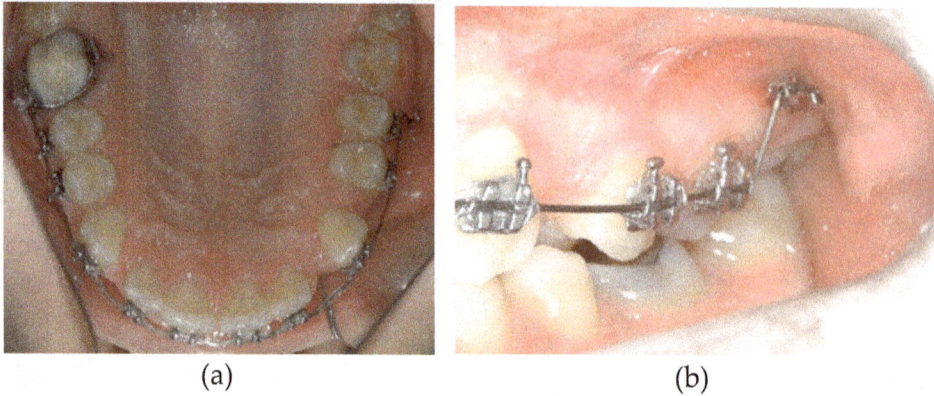

(a)   (b)

Figure 4. a and b: Use of a miniscrew for direct anchorage inserted between the second premolar and first molar where the molar could not be included in the arch wire because of incomplete eruption.

4.1. Intrusion

4.1.1. Intrusion of posterior teeth

Anterior open bites can be closed successfully through the intrusion of posterior teeth using various mechanical methods incorporating miniscrews (Figure 5).

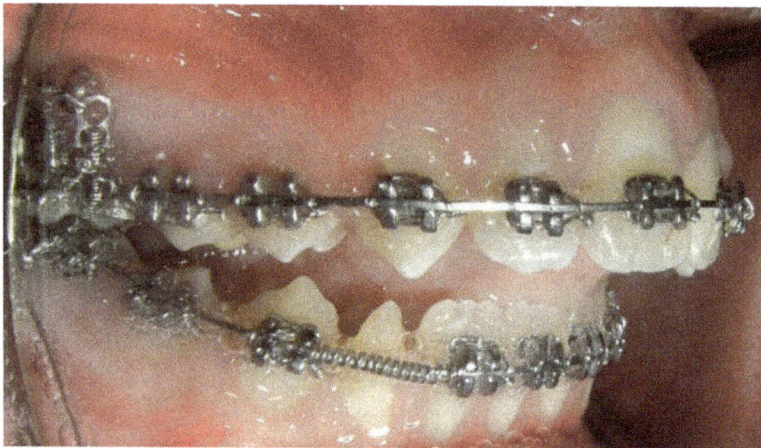

Figure 5. Miniscrew placed in the buccal vestibule apical to the maxillary molars, to be used for the intrusion of the posterior teeth to correct an anterior open bite.

Intrusion of posterior teeth is considered one of the most difficult types of tooth movement to achieve using conventional mechanics. A miniscrew-combined treatment may solve this problem. However, side effects such as buccal tipping have to be taken into consideration. As the intrusive force passes from the buccal to the centre of resistance, it will cause buccal tipping of the molars. When bilateral intrusion of posterior teeth is the goal, transpalatal arches can be used to avoid buccal tipping [20,21]. In unilateral intrusion, an additional miniscrew can be placed on the palatal side to apply a palatal intrusive force for achieving intrusion of the over-erupted molar without tipping (Figure 6a and b).

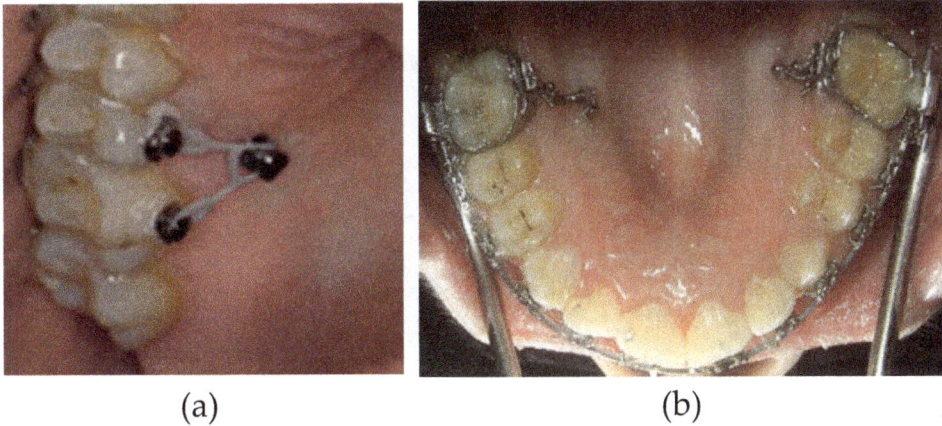

(a)　　　　　　　　　　　　　　　　(b)

Figure 6. a and b: Miniscrew in the palate to achieve intrusion of over-erupted posterior teeth.

4.1.2. Intrusion of anterior teeth

Miniscrews may be used to stabilize the molars during the incisor intrusion process, or can be placed anteriorly and used for direct application of the intrusive force to the incisors. The miniscrews should be placed as close to the midline of the anterior arch as possible. Alternately two miniscrews may be inserted into the lateral and canine interradicular area on both left and right sides.

4.2. Extrusion

While correcting an anterior open bite, activation of an extrusion arch results in mesial tipping and an intrusive force at the molars [107]. In such cases, miniscrews can be used to avoid these side effects.

In their case report, Roth et al. [108], treated an occlusal cant with miniscrew-supported mechanics by extruding the central incisors and the canine teeth. To avoid involving the other anterior teeth, a miniscrew was placed into the alveolus of the missing upper lateral incisor and an open coil was applied perpendicularly to an orthodontic wire connecting the central incisor and the canine.

4.3. Space closure

Generally, miniscrews are best suited to use as indirect anchorage during retraction of the anterior teeth or protraction of the posterior teeth [20]. In this way, the miniscrew is used to avoid undesirable movement of anchorage teeth, while conventional mechanics are used to close the space created (Figures 3a and 7).

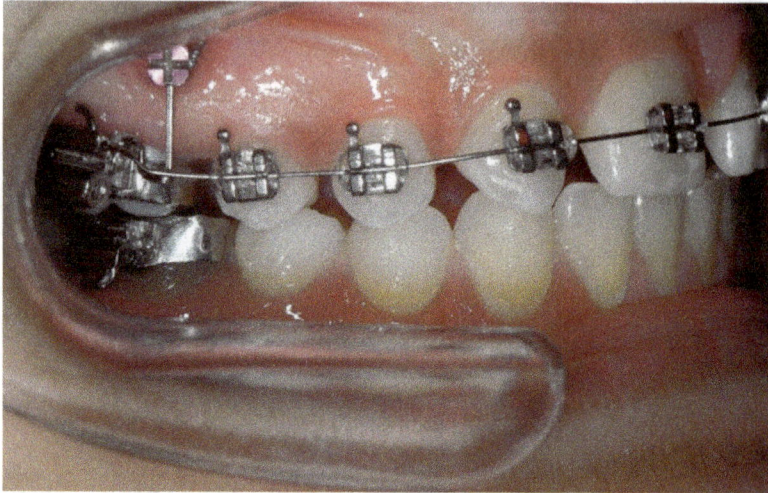

Figure 7. The use of a miniscrew as indirect anchorage during the distalization of the premolars and canine.

When direct anchorage is preferred for space closure, the direction and point of force application becomes crucial. Segmented arches may be preferred for canine distalization to provide a more appropriate force application point (Figure 8a and b). When the miniscrews are placed apically, a more favourable line of force direction passing closer to the centre of the resistance of the teeth can be achieved.

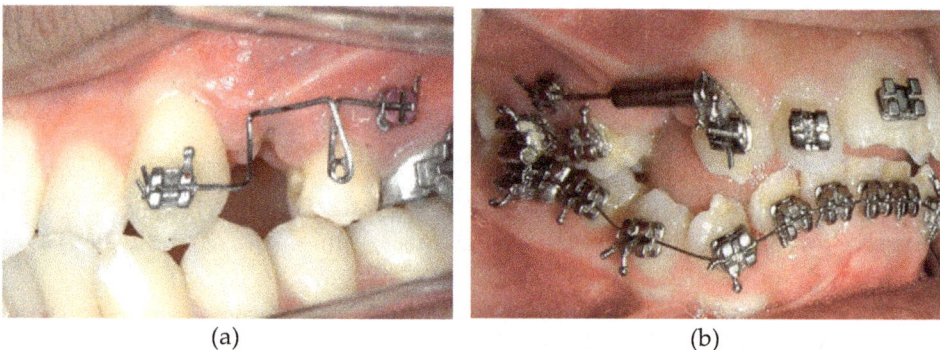

(a)   (b)

Figure 8. Miniscrews used as direct anchorage in canine distalization. Canine distalization with (a) a segmental arch and (b) a hybrid retraction arch.

Miniscrews can be used as direct anchorage when retracting the anterior teeth. Open coils/ elastic chains are applied directly between the miniscrew placed between the second premolar, the first molar and the hooks on the arch wire (Figure 9). Therefore, the point of force application is close to the centre of resistance of the anterior teeth, so that the anterior segment may slide bodily with minimal tipping; 150 g of force is used for retraction [109]. In some cases, miniscrews can be placed in the palatal region. Anchorage may be indirectly reinforced by connecting a transpalatal bar to a miniscrew in the palate [110].

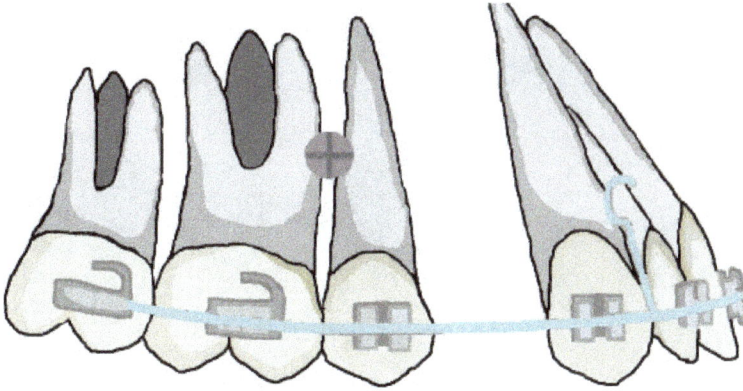

Figure 9. En mass retraction of the anterior teeth with miniscrew anchorage. Open coils/elastic chains can be applied directly between the miniscrew and the hooks on the arch wire.

4.4. Molar distalization

During molar distalization with conventional intraoral appliances, tipping and extrusion can occur in conjunction with the distal movement. In addition, reactive forces on the anterior anchoring teeth occur in the form of mesialization of upper anteriors/premolars and increased overjet. Many types and designs of appliances such as the pendulum [111,116], the Keles slide appliance [112], the distal-jet [113] and the compressed coil spring [116] can be combined with a miniscrew anchorage system (Figure 10).

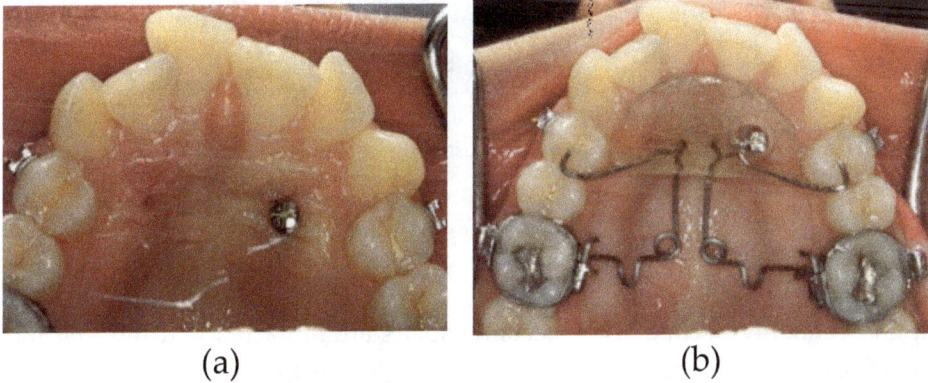

(a)   (b)

Figure 10. Miniscrew-supported pendulum application.

Miniscrew-supported molar distalization can only prevent undesired side effects on the anterior anchoring teeth; however, the side effects on the molars such as tipping, extrusion and rotation still remain. To avoid these undesired movements, miniscrew-supported mechanics can be designed (Figures 11 and 12). For bilateral molar distalization, rotation, tipping and extrusion can be controlled by placing the miniscrews in both the buccal and palatal region, and by using transpalatal arches [117].

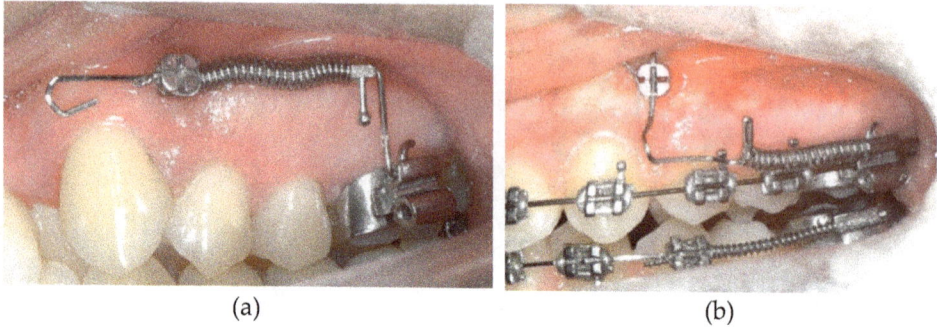

(a)   (b)

Figure 11. Design of the retraction unit may differ because of anatomic limitations, although the miniscrew is placed in the same region; (a) the distalizing force passes through the center of resistance of the first molar, which may provide parallel distalization rather than the system used in (b).

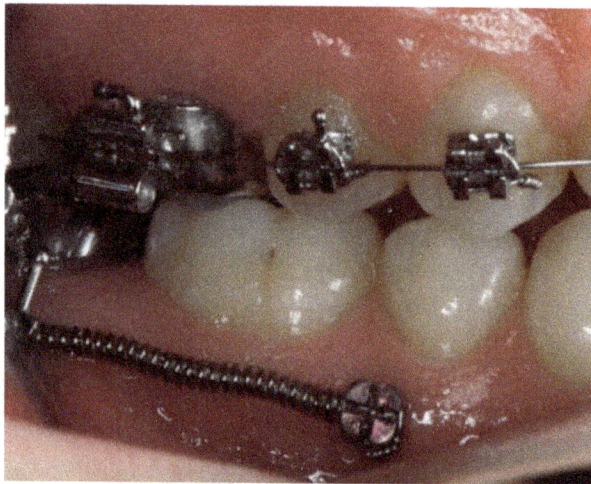

Figure 12. Mandibular second molar distalization with the use of direct miniscrew anchorage for the correction of mild Class III malocclusion.

4.5. Uprighting

Uprighting is generally needed when second molars are impacted and the first molar tips mesially because of early premolar extraction. Uprighting vectors with intrusion are very hard to accomplish; therefore, absolute anchorage is required. Miniscrews can be used as direct anchorage to prevent reactive forces on adjacent teeth that may result in negative side effects.

For second molar uprighting, a miniscrew can be placed in the buccal inter-radicular area of the second premolar and first molar. This area is the most reliable mandibular buccal cortical site.

For first molar uprighting, the miniscrew can be placed mesially in the area between the second and first premolars; 6-to 8-mm miniscrews are preferable and 0.17 × 0.25 inch TMA wires are preferred for preparing sectional arches with tip-back bending. Once the wire has been engaged by the miniscrew's head, intrusion and distalization forces are applied to the molar.

5. Conclusion

In dentistry today, it is becoming more difficult to cooperate with and satisfy patients. They have higher expectations for esthetics and comfort, yet they are impatient with longer treatment periods. Clinicians will continue to research alternative approaches to provide patients with their desired treatment outcomes over the shortest time possible. Because miniscrews provide an alternative to conventional mechanics for anchorage control, clinicians are showing increasing interest in this field. Desired treatment outcomes that are not possible with conventional mechanics may be achieved with miniscrew-supported orthodontic treatment. Miniscrews have recently become commonly accepted as a simple and effective tool in daily orthodontic practice.

With further studies and the development of new designs, appliances using miniscrews are expected to become more commonly used not only in orthodontic tooth movement, but also in the application of dentofacial orthopedics.

Acknowledgements

We thank Dr. Eren Korunmuş and Dr. Myumyun S. Myumyun for their valuable contributions in preparing this chapter.

Author details

Fatma Deniz Uzuner* and Belma Işık Aslan

*Address all correspondence to: fduzuner@yahoo.com.tr

Department of Orthodontics, Faculty of Dentistry, Gazi University, Emek Ankara, Turkey

References

[1] Lindauer SJ, Shroff B. Temporary anchorage devices: Biomechanical opportunities and challenges. In: R. Nanda and S. Kapila (ed.) Current therapy in orthodontics Mosby Inc. 2010; p278-290.

[2]   Gainsforth BL, Higley LB. A study of orthodontic anchorage possibilities in basal bone. American Journal of Orthodontics 1945;31: 406-417.

[3]   Linkow LI. Implant-orthodontics. Journal of Clinical Orthodontics 1970;4(12): 685-690.

[4]   Creekmore TD, Eklund MK. The possibility of skeletal anchorage. Journal of Clinical Orthodontics 1983;17(4): 266-269.

[5]   Costa A, Raffaini M, Melsen B. Miniscrews as orthodontic anchorage: a preliminary report. International Journal of Adult Orthodontics and Orthognathic Surgery 1998;13(3): 201-209.

[6]   Reynders R, Ronchi L, Bipat S. Mini-implants in orthodontics: a systematic review of the literature. American Journal of Orthodontics and Dentofacial Orthopedics 2009; 135(5): 564.e1-564.e19.

[7]   Huang LH, Shotwell IL, Wang HL. Dental implants for orthodontic anchorage. American Journal of Orthodontics and Dentofacial Orthopedics 2005; 127(6): 713-722.

[8]   Melsen B. Mini-implants: where are we? Journal of Clinical Orthodontics 2005;39(9) 539-547.

[9]   Mizrahi E, Mizrahi B. Mini-screw implants [temporary anchorage devices]: orthodontic and pre-prosthetic applications. Journal of Orthodontics 2007;34(2): 80-94.

[10] Chen CH, Chang CS, Hsieh CH, Tseng YC, Shen YS et al. The use of microimplants in orthodontic anchorage. Journal of Oral Maxillofacial Surgery 2006;64(8): 1209-1213.

[11] Roberts WE, Smith RK, Zilberman Y, Mozsary PG, Smith RS. Osseous adaptation to continuous loading of rigid endosseous implants. American Journal of Orthodontics and Dentofacial Orthopedics1984; 86(2): 95-111.

[12] Park HS. The usage of microimplants in orthodontics. In: R. Nanda and S. Kapila (ed.) Current therapy in orthodontics Mosby Inc. 2010; p291-300.

[13] Papadopoulos MA, Tarawneh F. The use of miniscrew implants for temporary anchorage in orthodontics: a comprehensive review. Oral Surg Oral Med Oral Pathol Oral Radiol Endod 2007;103 (5): e6-15.

[14] Higuchi KW and Slack JM. The use of titanium fixtures for intraoral anchorage to facilitate orthodontic tooth movement. International Journal of Oral Maxillofacial Implants 1991;6:338-344.

[15] Odman J, Lekholm U, Jemt T, Thilander B. Osseointegrated implants as orthodontic anchorage in the treatment of partially edentulous adult patients. European Journal of Orthodontics 1994;16(3): 187-201.

[16] Miyawaki S, Koyama I, Inoue M, Mishima K, Sugahara T et al. Factors associated with the stability of titanium screws placed in the posterior region for orthodontic

anchorage. American Journal of Orthodontics and Dentofacial Orthopedics 2003;124(4): 373-378.

[17] Cornelis MA, Scheffler NR, De Clerck HJ, Tulloch JF, Behets CN. Systematic review of experimental use of temporary skeletal anchorage devices in orthodontics. American Journal of Orthodontics and Dentofacial Orthopedics 2007;131(4): 52-58.

[18] Mah J, Bergstrand F. Temporary anchorage devices: a status report. Journal of Clinical Orthodontics 2005;39(3): 132-136.

[19] Heymann GC, Tulloch JF. Implantable devices as orthodontic anchorage: a review of current treatment modalities. Journal of Esthetic and Restorative Dentistry 2006;18(2): 68-80.

[20] Maino GB, Mura P, Bednar J. Miniscrew implants: the Spider Screw Anchorage System. Seminars in Orthodontics 2005;11(1): 40-46.

[21] Park HS, Kwon OW, Sung JH. Nonextraction treatment of an open bite with microscrew implant anchorage. American Journal of Orthodontics and Dentofacial Orthopedics 2006; 130(3): 391-402.

[22] Carano A, Velo S, Incorvati C, Poggio P. Clinical applications of the Mini-Screw-Anchorage-System (M.A.S.) in the maxillary alveolar bone. Progress in Orthodontics 2004;5:212-235.

[23] Kim YH, Yang SM, Kim S, Lee JY, Kim KE, Gianelly AA, Kyung SH. Midpalatal miniscrews for orthodontic anchorage. American Journal of Orthodontics and Dentofacial Orthopedics 2010;137(1): 66-72.

[24] Kyung SH, Hong SG, Park YC. Distalization of maxillary molars with a midpalatal miniscrews. Journal of Clinical Orthodontics 2003; 37(1) 22-26.

[25] Chang YJ, Lee HS, Chun YS. Microscrew anchorage for molar intrusion. Journal of Clinical Orthodontics 2004;38(6) 325-330.

[26] Wilmes B, Rademacher C, Olthoff G, Drescher D. Parameters affecting primary stability of orthodontic mini-implants. Journal of Orofacial Orthopedics 2006;67(3): 162-174.

[27] Motoyoshi M, Yoshida T, Ono A, Shimizu N. Effect of cortical bone thickness and implant placement torque on stability of orthodontic mini-implants. International Journal of Oral Maxillofacial Implants 2007;22(5): 779-784.

[28] Marquezana M, Mattosb CT, Sant'Annac EF, Gomes de Souzac MM, Maiac LC. Does cortical thickness influence the primary stability of miniscrews? A systematic review and meta-analysis. Angle Orthodontist 2014 Apr 2. [Epub ahead of print] DOI: 10.2319/093013-716.1

[29] Cheng SJ, Tseng IY, Lee JJ, Kok SH. A prospective study of the risk factors associated with failure of mini-implants used for orthodontic anchorage. International Journal of Oral Maxillofacial Implants 2004;19(1): 100-106.

[30] Moon CH, Lee DG, Lee HS, Im JS, Baek SH. Factors associated with the success rate of orthodontic miniscrews placed in the upper and lower posterior buccal region. Angle Orthodontist 2008;78(1): 101-106.

[31] Park HS, Jeong SH, Kwon OW. Factors affecting the clinical success of screw implants used as orthodontic anchorage. American Journal of Orthodontics and Dentofacial Orthopedics 2006;130(1): 18-25.

[32] Poggio PM, Incorvati C, Velo S, Carano A. "Safe zones": a guide for minis crew positioning in the maxillary and mandibular arch. Angle Orthodontist 2006;76(2): 191-197.

[33] Ishii T, Nojima K, Nishii Y, Takaki T, Yamaguchi H. Evaluation of the implantation position of mini-screws for orthodontic treatment in the maxillary molar area by a micro CT. The Bulletin of Tokyo Dental College 2004; 45(3): 165-172.

[34] Kang S, Lee SJ, Ahn SJ, Heo MS, Kim TW. Bone thickness of the palate for orthodontic mini-implant anchorage in adults. American Journal of Orthodontics and Dentofacial Orthopedics 2007;131(4):74-81.

[35] Takaki T, Tamura N, Yamamoto M, Takano N, Shibahara T et al. Clinical study of temporary anchorage devices for orthodontic treatment. Stability of micro/miniscrews and mini-plates: experience with 455 cases. Bulletin of Tokyo Dental College 2010;51(3): 151-163.

[36] Melsen B. Palatal growth studied on human autopsy material. A histologic microradiographic study. American Journal of Orthodontics 1975; 68(1): 42-54.

[37] Kim HJ, Yun HS, Park HD, Kim DH, Park YC. Soft-tissue and cortical-bone thickness at orthodontic implant sites. American Journal of Orthodontics and Dentofacial Orthopedics 2006;130(2): 177-82.

[38] Kuroda S, Sugawara Y, Deguchi T, Kyung HM, Takano-Yamamoto T. Clinical use of miniscrew implants as orthodontic anchorage: success rates and postoperative discomfort. American Journal of Orthodontics and Dentofacial Orthopedics 2007;131(1): 9-15.

[39] Asscherickx K, Vande Vannet B, Wehrbein H, Sabzevar MM. Success rate of miniscrews relative to their position to adjacent roots. European Journal of Orthodontics 2008;30(4): 330-335.

[40] Kuroda S, Yamada K, Deguchi T, Hashimoto T, Kyung HM, Takano-Yamamoto T. Root proximity is a major factor for screw failure in orthodontic anchorage. American Journal of Orthodontics and Dentofacial Orthopedics 2007;131(4): 68-73.

[41] Melsen B, Verna C. Miniscrew implants: the Aarhus anchorage system. Seminars in Orthodontics 2005;11(1): 24-31.

[42] Wilmes B, Ottenstreuer S, Su YY, Drescher D. Impact of implant design on primary stability of orthodontic mini-implants. Journal of Orofacial Orthopedics 2008;69(1): 42-50.

[43] Park HS, Jeong SH, Kwon OW. Factors affecting the clinical success of screw implants used as orthodontic anchorage. American Journal of Orthodontics and Dentofacial Orthopedics 2006;130(1): 18-25.

[44] Tseng YC, Hsieh CH, Chen CH, Shen YS, Huang IY, Chen CM. The application of mini-implants for orthodontic anchorage. International Journal of Oral and Maxillofacial Surgery 2006;35(8): 704-707.

[45] Lee J, Kim JY, Choic YJ, Kim KH, Chung CJ. Effects of placement angle and direction of orthopedic force application on the stability of orthodontic miniscrews. Angle Orthodontist 2013;83(4) 667-673.

[46] Oktenoglu BT, Ferrara LA, Andalkar N, Ozer AF, Sarioglu AC et al. Effects of hole preparation on screw pull out resistance and insertional torque: a biomechanical study. Journal of Neurosurgery 2001; 94(11): 91-96.

[47] Chaddad K, Ferreira AF, Geurs N, Reddy MS. Influence of surface characteristics on survival rates of mini-implants. Angle Orthodontist 2008;78(1): 107-113.

[48] Berens A, Wiechmann D, Dempf R. Mini-and micro-screws for temporary skeletal anchorage in orthodontic therapy. Journal of Orofacial Orthopedics 2006;67(6): 450-458.

[49] Park YC, Lee SY, Kim DH, Jee SH. Intrusion of posterior teeth using mini-screw implants. American Journal of Orthodontics and Dentofacial Orthopedics 2003;123(69 690-694.

[50] Park HS. An anatomical study using CT images for the implantation of micro-implants. Korean Journal of Orthodontics 2002;32(6): 435-441.

[51] Roze' J, Babu S, Saffazadeh A, Gayet-Delacroix M, Hoomaert A, Layrolle P. Correlating implant stability to bone structure. Clinical Oral Implants Research 2009;20(10): 1140-1145.

[52] Yacker MJ, Klein M. The effect of irrigation on osteotomy depth and bur diameter. International Journal of Oral Maxillofacial Implants 1996;11(5): 634-638.

[53] Matthews LS, Hirsch C. Temperatures measured in human cortical bone when drilling. Journal of Bone and Joint Surgery Am 1972;54(2): 297-308.

[54] Kim JS, Choi SH, Cha SK, Kim JH, Lee HJ et al. Comparison of success rates of orthodontic mini-screws by the insertion method. Korean Journal of Orthodontics 2012;42(5): 242-248.

[55] Kim JW, Ahn SJ, Chang YI. Histomorphometric and mechanical analyses of the drill-free screw as orthodontic anchorage. American Journal of Orthodontics and Dentofacial Orthopedics 2005;128(2): 190-194.

[56] Kim YH, Choi JH. The study about retention of miniscrews used for intraoral anchorage. Journal of the Korean Dental Association 2001;39: 684-687.

[57] Kim JW, Chang YI. Effect of drilling process in stability of micro-implants used for orthodontic anchorage. Korean Journal of Orthodontics 2002;32(2): 107-115.

[58] Freudenthaler JW, Haas R, Bantleon HP. Bicortical titanium screws for critical orthodontic anchorage in the mandible: a preliminary report on clinical applications. Clinical Oral Implants Research 2001;12(4): 358-363.

[59] Brettin BT, Grosland NM, Qian F, Southard KA, Stuntz TD, Morgan TA, Marshall SD, Southard TE. Bicortical vs monocortical orthodontic skeletal anchorage. American Journal of Orthodontics and Dentofacial Orthopedics 2008;134(5): 625-635.

[60] Holberg C, Winterhalder P, Rudzki-Janson I, Wichelhaus A Finite element analysis of mono-and bicortical mini-implant stability. European Journal of Orthodontics 2014;36(5): 550-556.

[61] Motoyoshi M, Hirabayashi M, Uemura M, Shimizu N. Recommended placement torque when tightening an orthodontic mini-implant. Clinical Oral Implants Research. 2006;17(1): 109-114.

[62] Luzi C, Verna C, Melsen B. A prospective clinical investigation of the failure rate of immediately loaded mini-implants used for orthodontic anchorage. Progress in Orthodontics 2007;8(1): 192-201.

[63] Gapski R,Wang HL, Mascarenhas P, Lang NP. Critical review of immediate implant loading. Clinical Oral Implants Research 2003;14(5): 515-527.

[64] Wang YC, Liou EJ. Comparison of the loading behavior of selfdrilling and predrilled miniscrews throughout orthodontic loading. American Journal of Orthodontics and Dentofacial Orthopedics 2008;133(1): 38-43.

[65] Yano S, Motoyoshi M, Uemura M, Ono A, Shimizu N. Tapered orthodontic miniscrews induce bone-screw cohesion following immediate loading. European Journal of Orthodontics 2006;28(6): 541-546.

[66] Motoyoshi M, Inaba M, Ono A, Ueno S, Shimizu N. The effect of cortical bone thickness on the stability of orthodontic miniimplants and on the stress distribution in surrounding bone. International Journal of Oral and Maxillofacial Surgery 2009;38(1): 13-18.

[67] Dalstra M, Cattaneo PM, Melson B. Load transfer of miniscrews for orthodontic anchorage. Orthodontics 2004; 1: 53-62.

[68] Kanomi R. Mini-implant for orthodontic anchorage. Journal of Clinical Orthodontics 1997;31(1): 763-767.

[69] Buchter A, Wiechmann D, Koerdt S, et al: Load-related implant reaction of mini-implants used for orthodontic anchorage. Clinical Oral Implants Research 2005;16(4): 473-479.

[70] Kim YH, Yang SM, Kim S, Lee JY, Kim KE, Gianelly AA, Kyung SH Midpalatal miniscrews for orthodontic anchorage: Factors affecting clinical success. American Journal of Orthodontics and Dentofacial Orthopedics 2010;137(1): 66-72.

[71] Park H, Lee Y, Jeong S, Kwon T. Density of the alveolar and basal bones of the maxilla and the mandible. American Journal of Orthodontics and Dentofacial Orthopedics 2008;133(1): 30-37.

[72] Liou EJ, Pai BC, Lin JC: Do miniscrews remain stationary under orthodontic forces? American Journal of Orthodontics and Dentofacial Orthopedics 2004;126(1): 42-47.

[73] Liu H, Lv T, Wang N, Zhao F, Wang K, Liud D. Drift characteristics of miniscrews and molars for anchorage under orthodontic force: 3-dimensional computed tomography registration evaluation. American Journal of Orthodontics and Dentofacial Orthopedics 2011;139(1): e83-e89.

[74] Park J, Cho HJ. Three-dimensional evaluation of interradicular spaces and cortical bone thickness for the placement and initial stability of microimplants in adults. American Journal of Orthodontics and Dentofacial Orthopedics 2009;136(3): 314.e1-12.

[75] Frost HM. Wolff's law and bone's structural adaptations to mechanical usage: an overview for clinicians. Angle Orthodontist1994; 64(3): 175-188.

[76] Frost HM. A 2003 update of bone physiology and Wolff's law for clinicians. Angle Orthodontist2004;74(1): 3-15.

[77] Zmudzki J, Walke W, Chladek W. Stresses present in bone surrounding dental implants in FEM model experiments. Journal of Achievements in Materials and Manufacturing Engineering 2008;27(1): 71-74.

[78] Lin D, Li Q, Li W, Swain M. Dental implant induced bone remodeling and associated algorithms. Journal of Mechanical Behavior of Biomedical Materials 2009; 2(5): 410-432.

[79] Kravitz ND, Kusnoto B. Risks and complications of orthodontic miniscrews. American Journal of Orthodontics and Dentofacial Orthopedics Orthop. 2007;131(4): 43-51.

[80] Chung KR, Kim SH, Kook YA. The C-orthodontic micro-implant. Journal of Clinical Orthodontics 2004;38(9): 478-486.

[81] Piesold JU, Al-Nawas B, Grotz KA. Osteonecrosis of the jaws by long-term therapy with bisphosphonates. Mund Kiefer und Gesichtschirurgie 2006;10(5): 287-300.

[82] Mengel R, Behle M, Flores-de-Jacoby L. Osseointegrated implants in subjects treated for generalized aggressive periodontitis: 10-year results of a prospective, long-term cohort study. Journal of Periodontology 2007;78(12): 2229-2237.

[83] Park JB, Kim EY, Paek J, Kook YA, Jeong DM et al. Primary stability of self-drilling and self-tapping mini-implant in tibia of diabetes-induced rabbits. International Journal of Dentistry Epub 2014 May 11; Article ID 429359 Doi: 10.1155/2014/429359

[84] Ludwig B, Glasl B, Lietz T, Bumann A, Bowman SJ. Techniques for attaching orthodontic wires to miniscrews. Journal of Clinical Orthodontics 2010;44(1): 36-40.

[85] Yamaguchi M, Inami T, Ito K, Kasai K, Tanimoto Y. Mini-Implants in the Anchorage Armamentarium: New Paradigms in the Orthodontics. International Journal of Biomaterials Epub 2012;Jun 5 Article ID 394121, 8 pages. Doi: 10.1155/2012/394121

[86] Othman S, Haugen E, Gjermo P. The effect of chlorhexidine supplementation in a periodontal dressing. Acta Odontologica Scandinavica 1989;47(6): 361-366.

[87] Choa IS, Kimb TW, Ahnc SJ, Yangd IH, Baekb SH. Effects of insertion angle and implant thread type on the fracture properties of orthodontic mini-implants during insertion. Angle Orthodontist 2013;83(4): 698-704.

[88] Brisceno CE, Rossouw PE, Carrillo R, Spears R, Buschang PH. Healing of the roots and surrounding structures after intentional damage with miniscrew implants. American Journal of Orthodontics and Dentofacial Orthopedics 2009;135(3): 292-301.

[89] Asscherickx K, Vannet BV, Wehrbein H, Sabzevar MM: Root repair after injury from mini-screw. Clinical Oral Implants Research 2005;16(5): 575-578.

[90] Chen YH, Chang HH, Chen YJ, Lee D, Chiang HH, Yao CC. Root contact during insertion of miniscrews for orthodontic anchorage increases the failure rate: an animal study. Clinical Oral implants Research 2008;19(1): 99-106.

[91] Lee YK, Kim JW, Baek SH, Kim TW, Chang YI. Root and bone response to the proximity of a mini-implant under orthodontic loading. Angle Orthodontist 2010;80(3): 452-458.

[92] Kim H, Kim TW. Histologic evaluation of root-surface healing after root contact or approximation during placement of miniimplants. American Journal of Orthodontics and Dentofacial Orthopedics 2011;139(6): 752-760.

[93] Ivanoff CJ, Sennerby L, Lekholm U. Reintegration of mobilized titanium implants: an experimental study in rabbit tibia. International Journal of Oral and Maxillofacial Surgery 1997;26(4): 310-315.

[94] Ogunsalu C. Reimplantation and immediate loading of an accidentally avulsed beaded implant: case report. Implant Dentistry 2004;13(1): 54-57.

[95] Park HS. Clinical study on success rate of microscrew implants for orthodontic anchorage. Korean Journal of Orthodontics 2003;33(3): 151-156.

[96] Heidemann W, Terheyden H, Gerlach KL. Analysis of the osseous/metal interface of drill free screws and self-tapping screws. Journal of Cranio-Maxillofacial Surgery 2001; 29(2): 69-74.

[97] Heidemann W, Terheyden H, Gerlach KL. In vivo studies of screw-bone contact of drill-free screws and conventional self-tapping screws. Mund-, Kiefer-und Gesicht-schirurgie 2001;5(1): 17-21.

[98] Lima GM, Soares MS, Penha SS, Romano MM. Comparison of the fracture torque of different Brazilian miniimplants. Brazilian Oral Research. 2011;25(2): 116-121.

[99] Barros SE, Janson G, Chiqueto K, Garib DG, Janson M. Effect of mini-implant diameter on fracture risk and selfdrilling efficacy. American Journal of Orthodontics and Dentofacial Orthopedics 2011;140(4): e181-192.

[100] Lee JS, Kim DH, Park YC, Kyung SH, Kim TK The efficient use of midpalatal miniscrew implants. Angle Orthodontist 2004; 74(5): 711-714.

[101] Park YC, Choi YJ, Choi NC, Lee JS. Esthetic segmental retraction of maxillary anterior teeth with a palatal appliance and orthodontic mini-implants. American Journal of Orthodontics and Dentofacial Orthopedics Orthop.2007;131(4): 537-544.

[102] Nienkemper M, Wilmes B, Lübberink G, Ludwig B, Drescher D. Extrusion of impacted teeth using mini-implant mechanics. Journal of Clinical Orthodontics 2012;46(3): 150-155.

[103] Takano-Yamamoto T, Kuroda S. Titanium screw anchorage for correction of canted occlusal plane in patients with facial asymmetry. American Journal of Orthodontics and Dentofacial Orthopedics 2007;132(2): 237-242.

[104] Aslan BI, Qasem M, Dinçer M. Maxillary Protraction of a Case with Mini-screw Bone Anchorage (Case Report). Journal of Orthodontic Research 2013;2(1): 77-81.

[105] Aslan BI, Kuçukkaraca E, Turkoz C, Dincer M. Treatment effects of the Forsus Fatigue Resistance Device used with miniscrew anchorage. Angle Orthodontist 2013;84(1): 76-87.

[106] Celenza F. Implant-enhanced tooth movement: indirect absolute anchorage. The International Journal of Periodontics and Restorative Dentistry 2003;23(6): 533-541.

[107] Isaacson RJ, Lindauer SJ. Closing anterior open bites: the extrusion arch. Seminars in Orthodontics 2001;7(1): 34-41.

[108] Roth A, Yildirim M, Diedrich P. Forced eruption with microscrew anchorage for pre-prosthetic leveling of the gingival margin: case report. Journal of Orofacial Orthopedics 2004;65(6): 513-519.

[109] Park HS, Kwon OW, Sung JH. Microscrew implant anchorage sliding mechanics. World Journal of Orthodontics 2005; 6(3): 265-274.

[110] Wehrbein H, Feifel H, Diedrich P. Palatal implant anchorage reinforcement of posterior teeth: a prospective study. American Journal of Orthodontics & Dentofacial Orthopedics 1999;116(6): 678-686.

[111] Byloff FK, Karcher H, Clar E, Stoff F. An implant to eliminate anchorage loss during molar distalization: a case report involving the Graz implant-supported pendulum. International Journal of Adult Orthodontics and Orthognathic Surgery 2000;15(2): 129-137.

[112] Keles A, Erverdi N, Sezen S. Bodily distalization of molars with absolute anchorage. Angle Orthodontist 2003;73(4): 471-482.

[113] Carano A, Velo S, Leone P, Siciliani G. Clinical applications of the miniscrew anchorage system. Journal of Clinical Orthodontics 2005; 39(1): 9-24.

[114] Karaman AI, Basçiftçi FA, Polat O. Unilateral distal molar movement with an implant-supported distal jet appliance. Angle Orthodontist 2002;72(2): 167-174.

[115] Gelgor IE, Buyukyilmaz T, Karaman AI, Dolanmaz D, Kalayci A. Intraosseous screw-supported upper molar distalization. Angle Orthodontist 2004;74(6): 838-850.

[116] Kircelli BH, Pektas ZO, Kircelli C. Maxillary molar distalization with a bone-anchored pendulum appliance. Angle Orthodontist 2006;76(4): 650-659.

[117] Lim SM, Hong RK. Distal Movement of Maxillary Molars Using a Lever-arm and Mini-implant System. Angle Orthodontist 2008;78(1): 167-175.

4

Dental Implant Placement in Inadequate Posterior Maxilla

Umit Karacayli, Emre Dikicier and Sibel Dikicier

1. Introduction

Hard tissue defects resulting from trauma, infection, or tooth loss often lead to an unfavorable anatomy of maxillary and mandibular alveolar processes. Dental implant placement in the edentulous posterior maxilla can present difficulties because of a horizontal or vertical alveolar ridge deficiency, unfavorable bone quality, or increased pneumatization of the maxillary sinus. The posterior maxilla has been known as the most difficult and problematic intraoral area for implant dentistry, requiring a maximum of attention for the achievement of successful surgery. Both anatomical structures and mastication dynamics contribute to the long term survival rates of endosseous dental implants in this region [1]. During the past 25 years, surgical procedures have been developed to increase the local bone volume, thus enabling the placement of implants [2]. The hard tissue augmentation techniques were separated into two anatomic sites, the maxillary sinus and alveolar ridge. Within the alveolar ridge augmentation procedures, different surgical approaches were developed and are currently used, including guided bone regeneration, onlay grafting, distraction osteogenesis, ridge splitting, free and vascularized autografts for discontinuity defects, and socket preservation. Among the variety of techniques have been described, the three that are the most widely used in maxilla are lateral approach, osteotome technique and ridge splitting [3].

2. Anatomy of the posterior maxilla

The maxillary sinus is a pyramid shaped cavity with an anterior wall corresponding to the facial surface of the maxilla. The size of the sinus is minimal until the eruption of permanent teeth. The average dimensions of the adult sinus are 2.5 to 3.5cm wide, 3.6 to 4.5 cm tall, and

3.8 to 4.5 cm deep. The size of the sinus will increase with age after extraction of the maxillary molar teeth. The extent of pneumatization varies from person to person and from side to side. The inner walls of the maxillary sinus is lined with the sinus membrane, also known as the Schneiderian membrane. This membrane consists of ciliated epithelium cells resting of the basement membrane. It is continuous with, and connects to, the nasal epithelium through the ostium in the middle meatus. The blood circulation to the maxillary sinus is primarily obtained from the posterior superior alveolar artery and the infraorbital artery, both being branches of the maxillary artery. Many anastomoses are occureed between these 2 arteries in the lateral antral wall. Among these arteries, the posterior superior alveolary artery and the infra-orbital artery also supply the buccal part of the maxillary sinus. However, because the blood supplies to the maxillary sinus are from terminal branches of peripheral vessels, to avoid bleeding complications, the branches of the maxillary artery should be taken into consideration. Nerve supply to the sinus is derived from the superior alveolar branch of the maxillary division of the trigeminal nerve [4].

The objective of sinus lift procedure is to compensate the bone loss by creating increased bone volume in the maxillary sinus and thus permitting the installation of implants in the posterior maxilla [4,5]. Membrane perforations and bleeding are procedure-related complications, seen in lateral wall sinus approach [6]. Therefore, the anatomy of the area should be carefully examined before surgical interventions.

3. Augmentation procedures

3.1. Vertical ridge augmentation

3.1.1. Sinus lifting procedure

Implant placement in the posterior maxilla is a challenging procedure when vertical deficiencies are occured. Maxillary sinus elevation technique is a main surgical procedure which permits to augment the sufficient bone volume in posterior maxilla in order to place implants.

To increase the amount of bone in the posterior maxilla, the sinus lift procedure, or subantral augmentation, originally presented in 1977 and subsequently published in 1980 [4]. After modifications of the surgical procedure, access was accomplished through the lateral wall of the maxilla. It is preferable techniques to adjust the low residual bone height in the posterior maxilla performed in two ways: A lateral window technique and an osteotome sinus floor elevation technique and placing bone-graft material in the maxillary sinus to increase the height and width of the available bone. Autogenic bone graft is often used in this method. The bone usually seems to be harvested from the iliac crest, although several anatomic areas have been used.

When the ridge bone height is more than 6 mm, the osteotome technique can be performed. In that case, implant placement is usually carried out simultaneously with elevation of the sinus floor.

3.1.1.1. Lateral approach

Lateral approach is also known as lateral antrostomy which is a predictable technique to increase vertically available bone volume of the edentulous posterior maxilla giving the possibility to place osseointegrated implants. The sinus floor is elevated and it can be augmented with either autologous or xenogeneic bone grafts following an opening bone window prepared on the facial buccal wall of the sinus.

The 2-step antrostomy is the treatment of choice when the residuel ridge bone height is less than 4 mm. As part of this approach, the implants are usually placed after a healing period of 6 to 18 months following sinus floor elevation [7]. The 1-step antrostomy is applied when the ridge bone height ranges from 4 to 6 mm. In this situation, implant placement is performed simultaneously with sinus floor elevation.

With respect to the grafting procedure, several grafting materials have successfully been used for elevating and stabilizing the sinus membrane: autogenous bone, allografts, xenografts and combination of these materials. Sinus floor elevation by lateral antrostomy has provided good implant survival rates, as reported in several studies. However, it is a demanding surgical procedure and is quite invasive. The 1-step antrostomy, in which implants are placed during the same surgical visit as elevation of sinus floor is performed, is similar to the 2-step technique with regard to advantages and disadvantages. The most important difference is that less time elapses before initiation of prosthetic therapy [7,8].

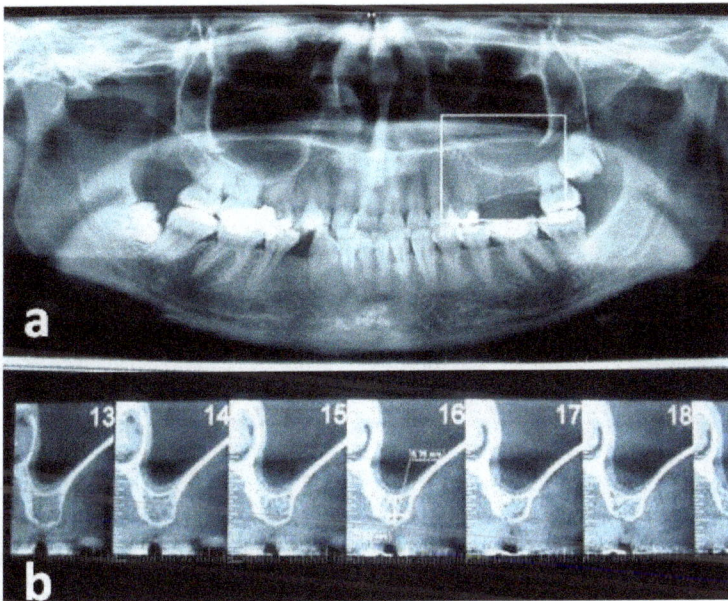

Figure 1. (a) Panoramic image before sinus augmentation procedure (b) Cone beam computerized image of the residual alveolar bone

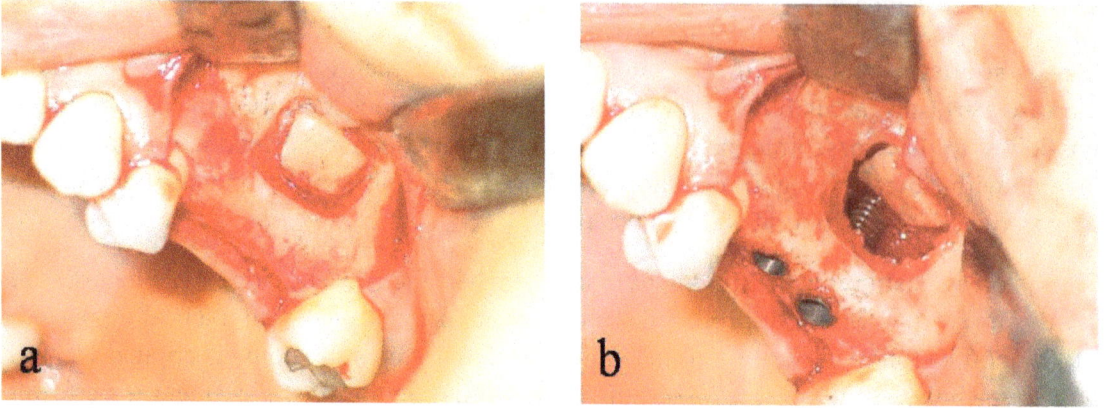

Figure 2. (a) Preparation of the bony window with a round bur (b) Medial rotation of the bone flap, elevation of the mucosa of the maxillary sinus and implant placement

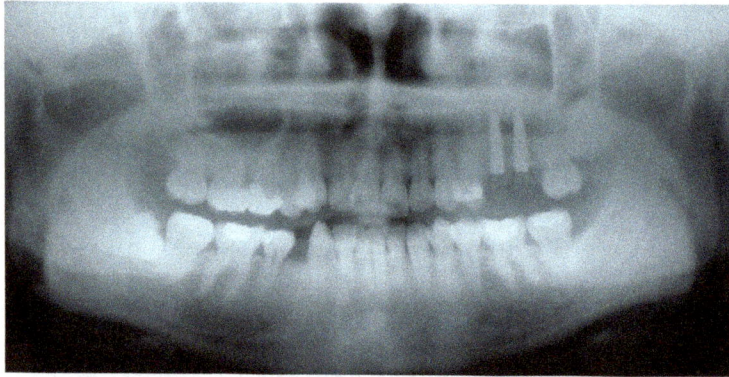

Figure 3. Postoperative radiographic view

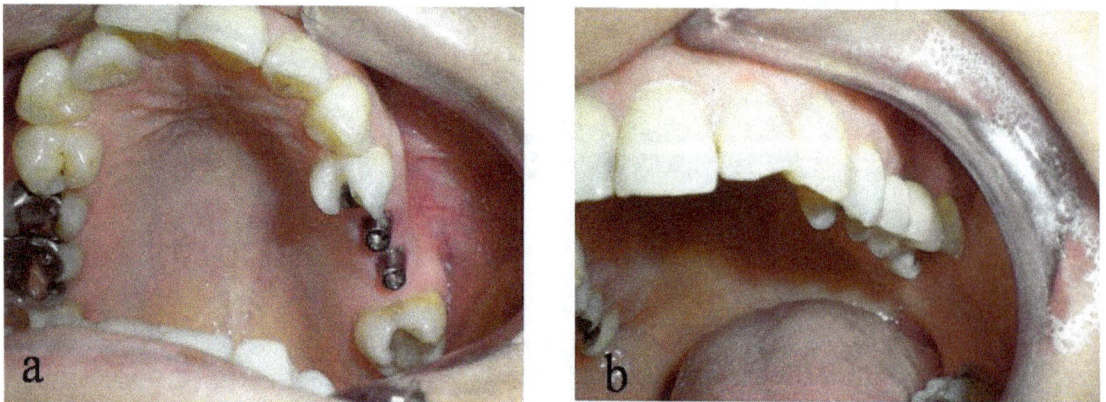

Figure 4. (a) Clinical view of the implants (b) Final prosthetic restoration

3.1.1.2. Osteotome sinus floor elevation technique

When the ridge bone height is more than 6 mm, the osteotome technique can be performed. In that case, implant placement is usually carried out simultaneously with elevation of the sinus floor. In the original approach, implants were placed after the controlled fracture of sinus floor and were submerged during the healing phase (Figure 5) [9].

Although the transcrestal approach is decided more conservative than the lateral approach, the main disadvantage is that the sinus lifting procedure must be performed blindly because of the impossibility to visualize the sinus floor [10]. In spite of this limitation, membrane perforation was reported to be less frequent in the osteotome-mediated procedure than in the lateral approach, for which such complication was occured in 7-35% of cases [11].

Osteotome-mediated sinus lift surgery may be performed with or without using many type of bone graft material as allograft, autogenous bone, or xenogeneic bone material [12]. No significant differences in terms of implant survival and surgical success rates were reported comparing the two methods [13]. Also, the use of platelet derivatives without any bone substitute is described in literature with the aim of allowing a better control of forces during sinus floor elevation and reducing the incidence of complications [13].

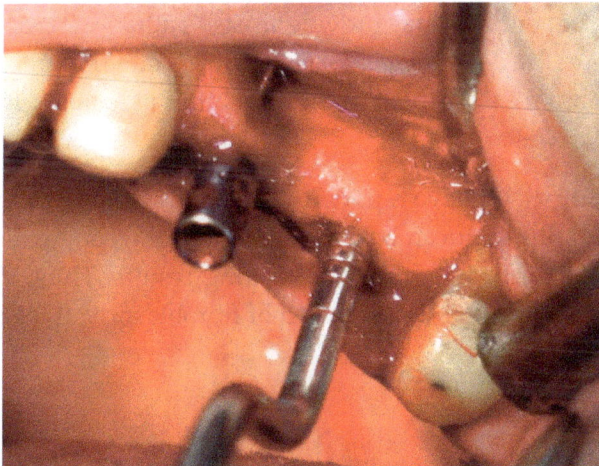

Figure 5. Osteotome sinus floor elevation technique

3.1.2. Titanium mesh

Natural hard and soft tissue contours allow both ideal implant placement and the emergence of a restoration. If there is large or small volume hard and soft tissue defects in these contours, these are prevent three-dimensional implant placement and aesthetic results [14]. Reconstructive efforts at aesthetic implant sites usually involve more than replacing missing hard and soft tissue. For reconstruction of these type of defects, the surgeon uses different techniques: (1) Distraction osteogenesis, which describes the surgical induction of a fracture and the subsequent gradual separation of the two bone ends to create spontaneous bone regeneration between the two fragments; (2) Osteoinduction, which employs appropriate growth factors and/or stem/osteoprogenitor cells to encourage new bone formation [15, 16]; (3) Osteoconduction, in which a grafting material serves as a scaffold for new bone formation; and (4) Guided bone regeneration (GBR), which provides spaces using barrier membranes that are to be subsequently filled with new bone [17, 18]. Guided bone regeneration was introduced as a therapeutic modality to achieve bone regeneration, via the use of barrier membranes and titanium mesh. Titanium mesh has been used for a variety of clinical applications in reconstructive implant surgery and reported positive results. Titanium mesh has excellent mechanical properties for the stabilization of bone grafts beneath the membrane [19]. Its rigidity provides extensive space maintenance and prevents contour collapse; its elasticity prevents mucosal compression; its stability prevents graft displacement; and its plasticity permits bending, contouring, and adaptation to any unique bony defect [20]. The common feature of commercially available titanium mesh membranes is its macroporosity (in the millimeter range). This is thought to play a critical role in maintaining blood supply and is believed to enhance regeneration by improving wound stability through tissue integration and allowing diffusion of extracellular nutrients across the membrane [21]. The most important advantage of this macroporosity is related to the attachment of soft tissues, which may stabilize and restrict the migration of epithelial cells. However, this makes the material difficult to remove at the second surgery. These macro- and multi-porous characteristics also create sharp spots when the material is cut or bent, and may provide an easy pathway for microbial contamination into the healing site. Thus, the development of less porous and micropore-sized titanium mesh membrane could alleviate some of the current difficulties associated with titanium mesh in dental applications [22].

Although many relevant articles have reported good clinical results without using resorbable membrane over titanium mesh, it can be considered that the combination of titanium mesh and resorbable membrane can demonstrate satisfying results. Thus, it was achieved space creation by using titanium mesh and prevention of fibroblastic cell migration into the defect site by using resorbable membrane.

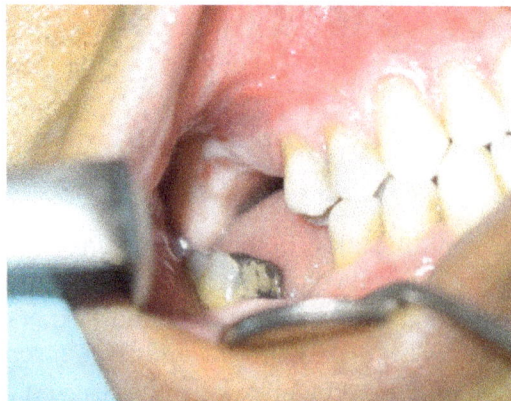

Figure 6. Pre-operative intraoral view

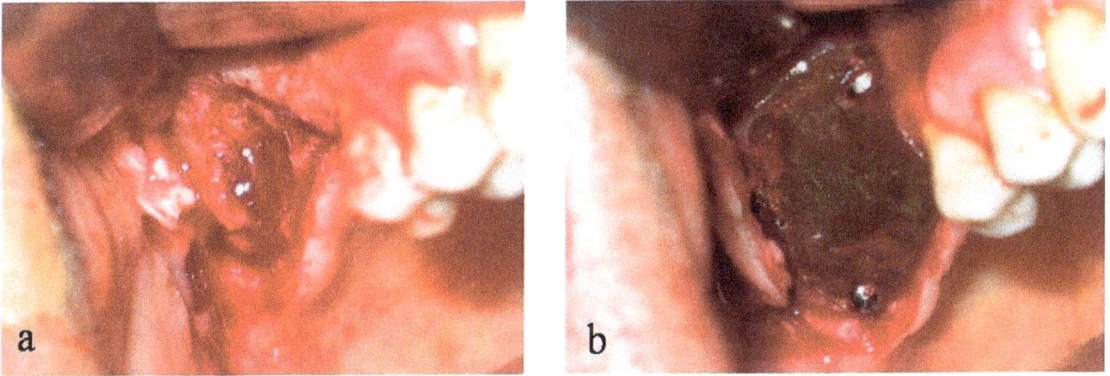

Figure 7. (a) Severe atrophy of right maxillar alveolar process (b) Titanium mesh

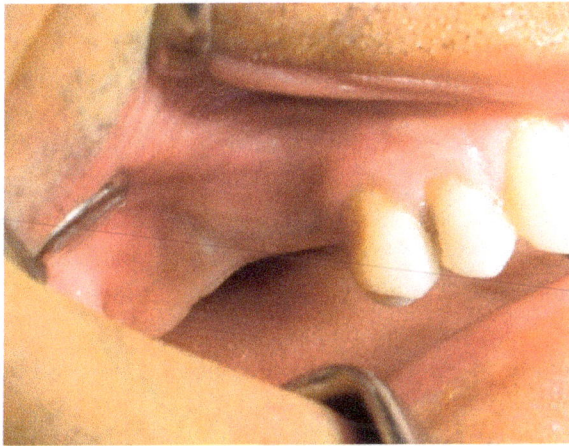

Figure 8. Post-operative 12 months intraoral view

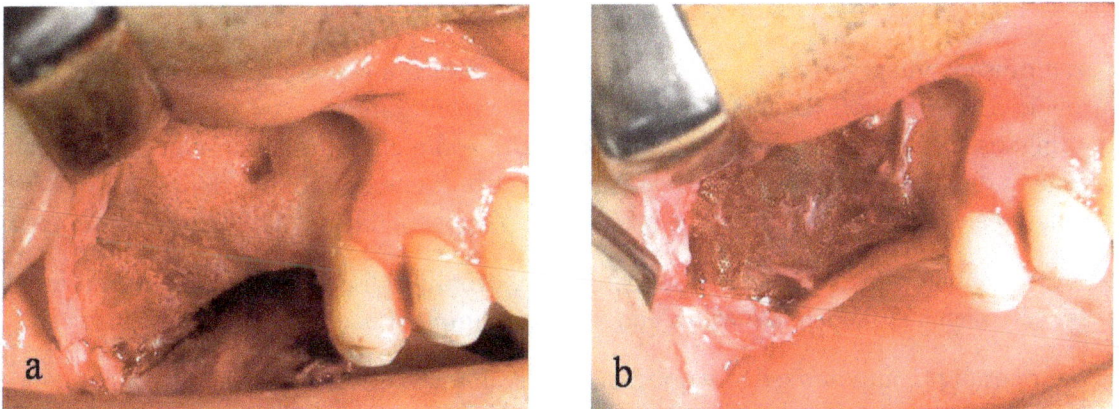

Figure 9. (a) Titanium mesh post-operative 12 months (b) Removal of titanum mesh.

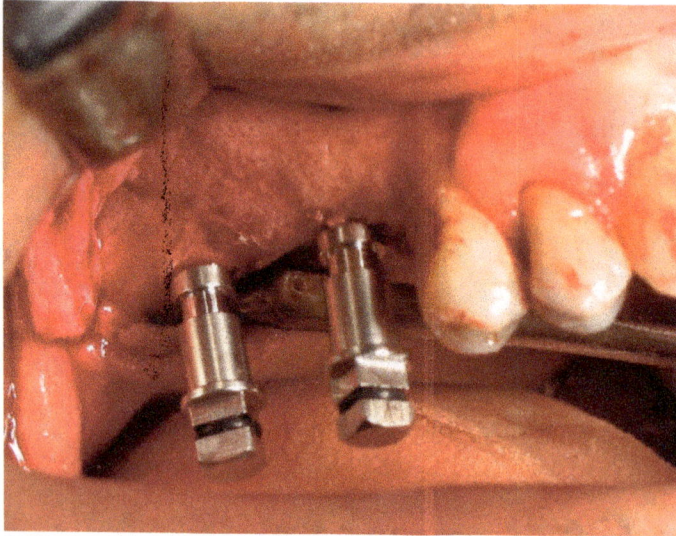

Figure 10. Implant placement

3.2. Lateral ridge augmentation

3.2.1. Ridge splitting

Alveolar bone splitting technique and immediate implant placement have been proposed for patients with narrow alveoalar ridge in the horizontal dimension. When the alveolar ridge is narrower than the optimally planned implant diameter, onlays of bone grafting material or guided bone regeneration are indicated [23]. This technique provides a selective cutting, minimal operative invasion and provides an acceptable inter-cortical gap for the placement of particulate bone grafting [24]. The obvious advantage of this technique is the absence of donor site morbidity associated to autologous bone harvesting. Crestal split augmentation involved a surgical osteotomy that was followed by alveolar crest split and augmentation after bucco-lingual bony plate expansion, prior to implantation [25].

Specific disadvantages have also been reported for each technique: resorption, limited amount of bone, damaging soft tissues, such as sinus floor membrane, nerves and vessels in bone grafting; tissue dehiscence, membrane displacement and membrane collapse in guided bone regeneration; and insufficiency of the distraction line, bone resorption, deficiency of bone formation and increased healing time for implant placement, in alveolar distraction [26-28].

50-year-old male patient referred to our clinic with atrophy of the alveolar rim in the posterior maxilla, which had inadequate width and height for implant placement (Figure 11).

A pre-operative computerized tomographic (CT) scan revealed 2.5-3 mm. of bone weightand-height of themolararareawas 5.64 mm. between the alveolar crest and maxillary sinus (Figures. 12a,b, 13a). We planned segmental split osteotomy, socket lifting and three dental implant placement at the same section without using any graft materials.

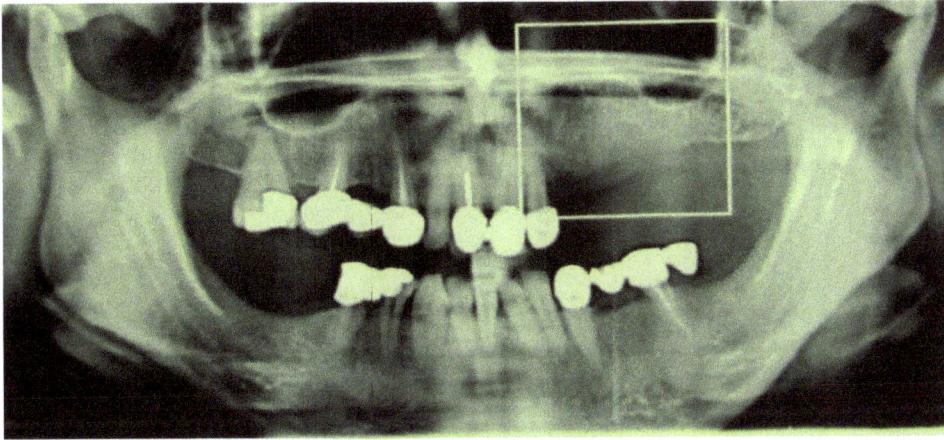

Figure 11. Pre-operative radiograph of the left posterior edentulous maxilla

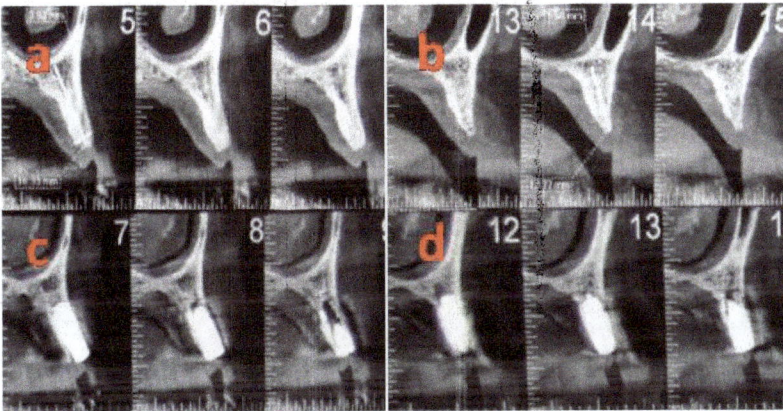

Figure 12. (a-b) Pre-operative CT scan (c-d) Post-operative CT scan

The surgical procedure was performed under local anesthesia. Full thickness muco-periostal flap was elevated with vertical and crestal incisions. Ridge splitting was applied with osteotome 8 mm/Obwegeser (Ace Surgical Supply Co., Brockton, MA, USA), after the crest being prepared with surgical diamond disc in straight high speed handpiece (Figure 14-15). One centimeter penetration of the osteotome blade in ridge crest would automatically expand the ridge. Since osteotome thickness increases from tip toward shaft further the osteotome penetrates, more the ridge will expand. Slight bucco-lingual movement of the osteotome increases the expansion. 3.5x12 mm implants were placed in the canine and first premolar region into the ridge splitted crest (Figure 16-17). Muco-periostal flap were sutured primerly by using 3.0 silk suture (Starmedix LLC, Miami, FL, USA).

The present study reports that the clinical results of narrow ridge splitting. Post-operative panoramic radiograph (Figure 8) and CT scan (Figure 13b) showed therewas not any complications around the implants and maxillary sinus. Five months after surgery, final fixed prosthetic restorations were accomplished.

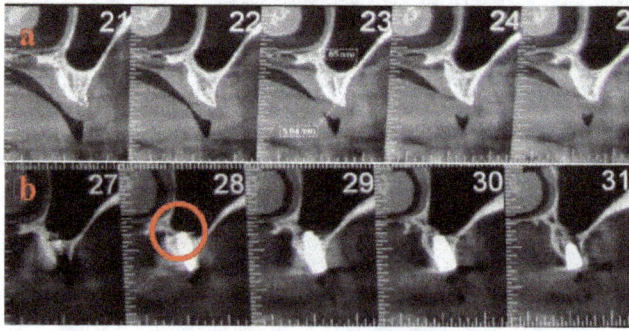

Figure 13. (a) Pre-operative CT scan (b) Post-operative CT scan

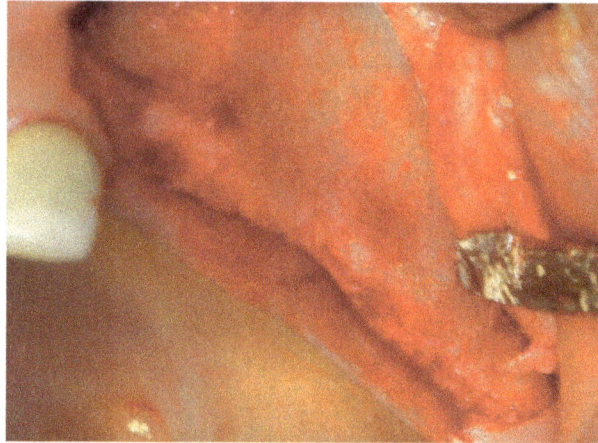

Figure 14. Pre-operative view of alveolar ridge

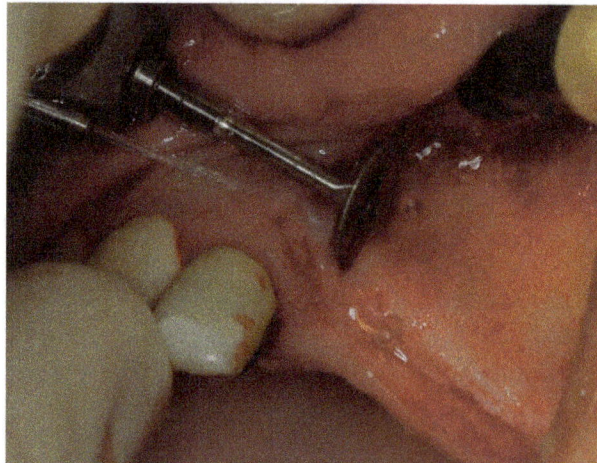

Figure 15. Ridge splitting procedure with diamond disc

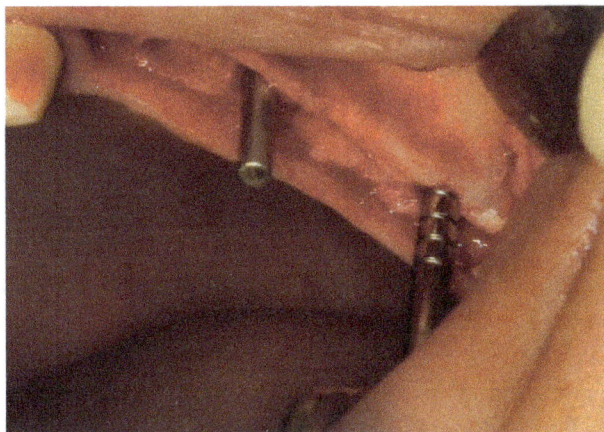

Figure 16. Implant placement

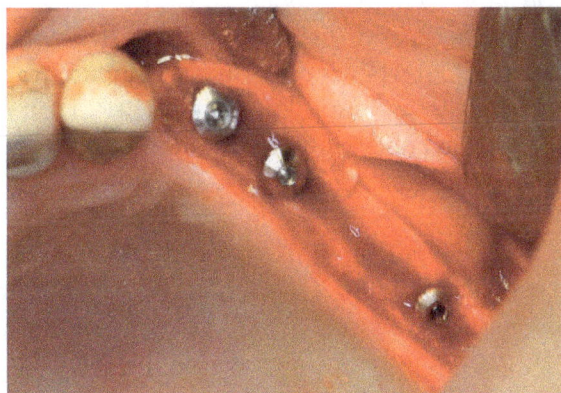

Figure 17. Post-operative view after implant placement

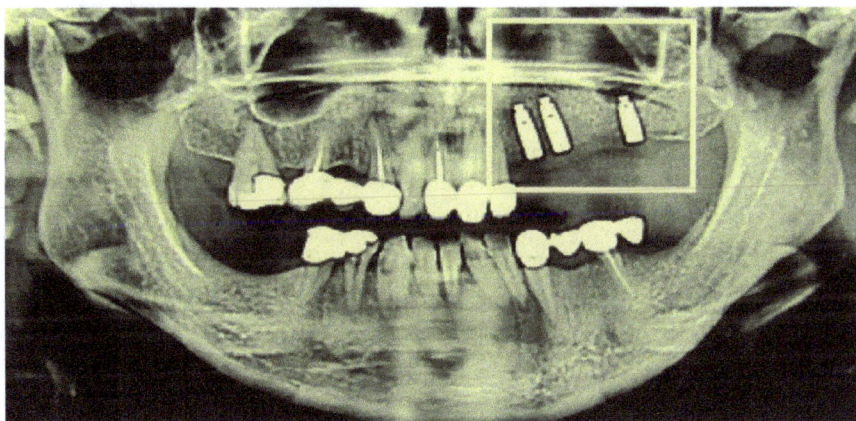

Figure 18. Post-operative panoramic radiograph

3.2.2. Autogenous block graft

Currently, various augmentation procedures have been introduced to rehabilitate of atrophic maxillary ridges in literature [29-32]. The grafting procedure using autogenous bone block is considered ideal by many researchers, as it shows osteogenic capability and deformation resistance [33]. A wide range of bone grafts and synthetic bone graft materials have been used in the last two decades for augmentation of inadequate alveolar ridge to facilitate the placement of dental implants of partially and completely edentulous patients. Various bone graft types, including autogenous, allogeneic (human), xenogeneic (porcine, equine, or bovine, and synthetic calcium-based materials (calcium phosphates [β-tricalcium phosphate/β-TCP, hydroxyapatite/HA], bioactive glasses), calcium sulfate, calcium hydroxide), and a combination of these with or without the use of membrane and screws have been employed for grafting procedure [34-37]. Although, allogeneic bone grafts do not have the drawbacks of autografts, the procedure is more delicate and less successful in clinical practice. They also display several other disadvantages: risk of disease transmission of the donour site, infection, difficulties in obtaining and processing, possible rapid resorption [38,39], and partial loss of mechanical strength after sterilization [40]. Xenogenic bone substitutes of porcine, bovine, or, more recently, equine origin are used because of their chemical and structural composition similarity when compared to human bone [32]. They represent an unlimited supply of available material and may reduce morbidity by eliminating the donor site [31]. Heat or other treatments are used to deproteinate bone particles and eliminate immunogenicity risks [40]. Synthetic calcium phosphate ceramics with their excellent biocompatibility are common alternatives to autogenous bone [41]. Autogenous bone grafts have been widely accepted as "gold standard" due to their compatibility and osteogenic potentials to form the new bone by processes of osteogenesis, osteoinduction, and osteoconduction. A particulate and block autogenous bone has been used to compensate of alveolar ridge deficiency [42]. Extraoral sites of autogenous block grafts are ilium, calvarium, tibia, rib, and others. The most widely used intraoral potential sites of autogenous block grafts include symphysis and retromolar-ramus areas. In the clinical practice, a maxillary tuberosity bone graft has been also used as a particulate graft for augmentation procedures in posterior maxilla prior to or simultaneously with implant insertion [43]. Some of advantages about the autogenous block graft procedure such as; intra- and extra-oral donor site morbidity, potential complications and risks associated with the harvesting procedures may have been reported [44].

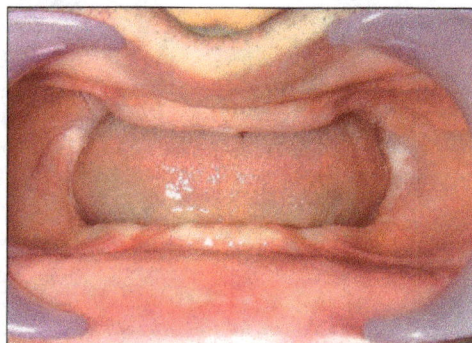

Figure 19. Pre-operative view

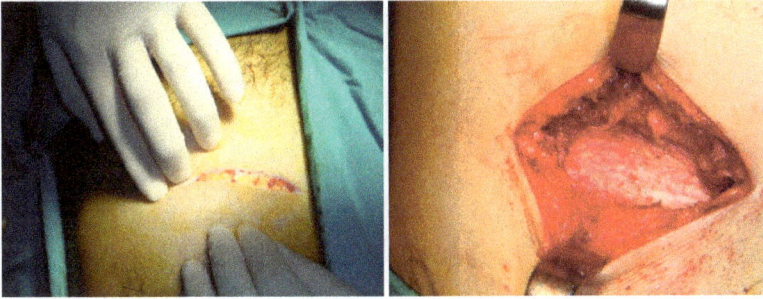

Figure 20. Operation site of the rib

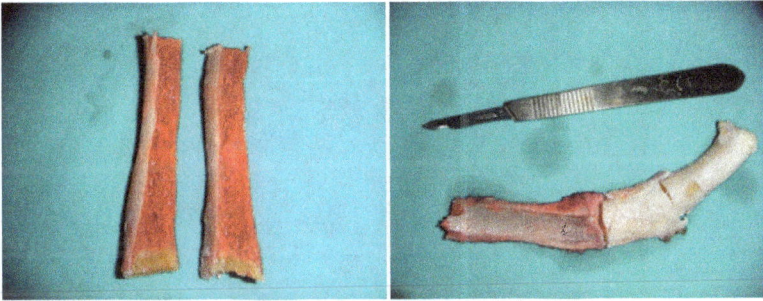

Figure 21. Autogenous rib block graft

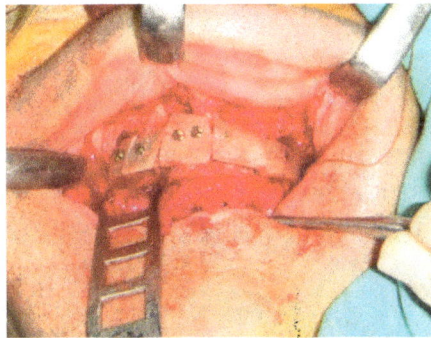

Figure 22. Lateral augmentation procedure of the maxilla with autogenous rib graft

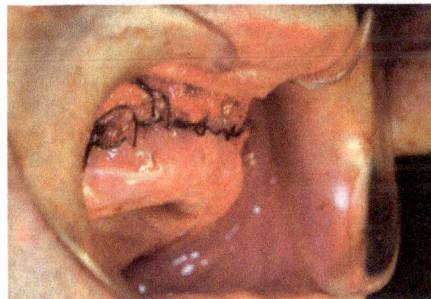

Figure 23. Post-operative intraoral view after rib grafting

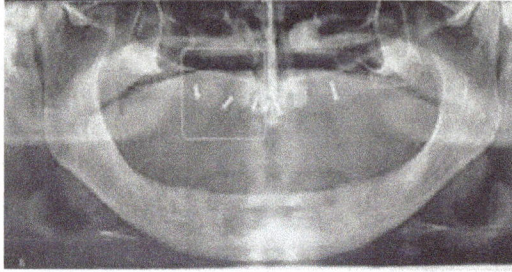

Figure 24. Post-operative panoramic radiograph of the graft

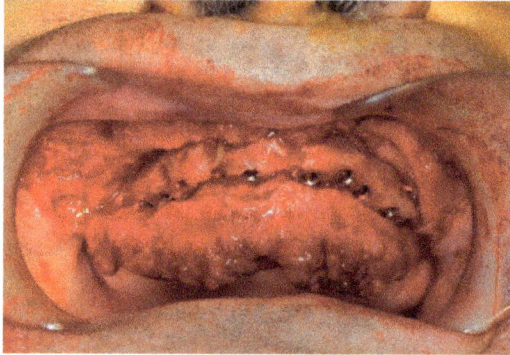

Figure 25. Implant placement four months after the augmentation procedure

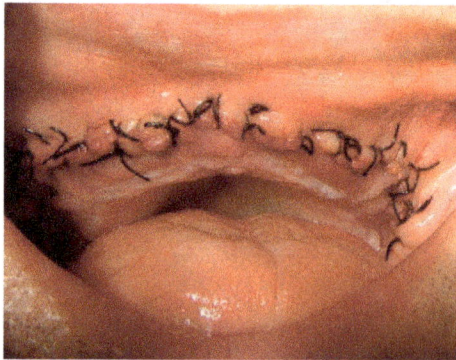

Figure 26. Post-operative intraoral view after implant surgery

4. Zygomatic implants

Maxillary posterior defects that occur after tumor resection or trauma are challenging to reconstruct and rehabilitate. The aim of rehabilitation is not only to provide a cosmetically acceptable appearance, but also to restore oral functions, such as deglutition, mastication, and phonation [45]. The impossibility of placing conventional implants in posterior maxilla due to maxillectomy, maxillary sinus pneumatization or the lack of bone volume is currently the main indication for the usage of zygomatic implants [46].

Various reconstructive approaches, involving differing surgical procedures, graft materials and endosseous implant systems, have been described for reconstruction of patients with severe resorption of alveolar bone, and also patients who have undergone maxillary resection for neoplastic disease. Restorative techniques have been emphasized such as; microvascular free flaps, local flaps, and obturator prosthesis [47,48]. However, significant obturator retention and stability problems occur when extensive defects remain following a maxillectomy. Zygomatic implants are an effective treatment alternative to limit free or vascularized bone graft procedures, employing the zygomatic bone as anchorage. When determining zygomatic implant rehabilitation, the patient must present not only resorbtion of posterior maxilla preventing the placement of additional fixations for supporting the prosthesis, but also sufficient bone volume in the anterior maxilla -with a 10 mm in height and a 4 mm in width- to allow the placement of 2-4 conventional fixations [49].

Zygomatic implants were firstly introduced by Branemark in 1998 to rehabilitate the masticatory and aesthetic functions in severe atrophied maxilla caused by trauma, congenital conditions, tumour resection or increased sinus pneumatization. Given the high success rate reported for zygomatic implant placement, this surgical technique can be considered as a valid alternative therapeutic approach to bone grafting and invasive surgery to restore function and improve the esthetic results for patients with atrophic edentulous maxilla [50,51]. The surgical manipulation may lead to potential risk because of the drill way is close to critical anatomical vital structures, such as the maxillary sinus, the nasal cavity, and the eyes [52]. However the limited intraoperative visibility, especially given the anatomical intricacies of the curved zygomatic bone, makes this kind of surgery a demanding procedure. Traditional complications of this surgery are secondary infection, sinusitis, pain, periimplantitis and bone resorption related to implant function [46,53]. The surgical approach consists of using the frontal part of the zygomatic bone as an anchorage for zygomatic implant, with support from the maxillary palatal or alveolar bone, without any bone augmentation. This offers a more simplified treatment approach, a decrease in biological impact and a more comfortable post-surgical period for the patient thanks to a quicker recovery time [49].

5. Angulated implants

Angulated implant treatment of the maxilla requires presurgical prosthetic treatment planning for high smile line esthetics to be acceptable [54]. This requires bone removal in the vast majority of dentate or edentulous patients who undergo full arch treatment.The use of angulated implants for short-span bridges or even long-span reconstructions to avoid bone grafts has been used for 10 years, although many of these were not immediately loaded [55]. However, with the advent of the angulated implant immediate function, this became consistently possible using a graftless protocol [56]. Angulated implant concept consists that to avoid the anatomical structures in the posterior regions by using implants just anterior to the maxillary sinus in the maxilla and anterior to mental foramen in the mandible by having them placed on a 30-45 degree angle. This concept solves the problem of insufficient bone and reduces the need for sinus and ridge augmentation.

Angulated implant treatment concept may not be considered or adopted as a conventional treatment modality by many clinicians. This treatment concept refers four implants to support a fixed prosthesis. However, long-term clinical results are inadequate on the effects of angulation on the development and distrubition of the loading stress within the implant [57].

Author details

Umit Karacayli[1*], Emre Dikicier[2] and Sibel Dikicier[3]

*Address all correspondence to: ukaracayli@gmail.com

1 Department of Oral and Maxillofacial Surgery, Gulhane Military Medical Academy, Ankara, Turkey

2 Department of Oral and Maxillofacial Surgery, Corlu Military Hospital, Tekirdag, Turkey

3 Department of Prosthodontics, Corlu Military Hospital, Tekirdag, Turkey

References

[1] Caudry, Landzberg M. Lateral window sinus elevation technique: Managing Challenges and complications. Journal of Canadian Dental Association 2013;79:d101. http://www.jcda.ca/article/d101

[2] Khojasteh A, Soheilifar S, Mohajerani H, Nowzari H. The effectiveness of barrier membranes on bone regeneration in localized bony defects. A systematic review. International Journal of Oral and Maxillofacial Implants 2013;28(4):1076-89.

[3] Rodoni LR, Glauser R, Feloutzis A, Hammerle CH. Implants in the posterior maxilla: a comparative clinical and radiologic study. International Journal of Oral and Maxillofacial Implants 2005;20(2):231-7.

[4] Bell GW, Joshi BB, Macleod RI. Maxillary sinus disease: diagnosis and treatment. Brazilian Dental Journal 2011;210(3):113-8.

[5] Troedhan A, Kurrek A, Wainwright M. Biological principles and physiology of bone regeneration under the schneiderian membrane after sinus lift surgery: A Radiological study in 14 patients treated with the transcrestal hydrodynamic ultrasonic cavitational sinus lift (Intralift). International Journal of Dentistry 2012; doi: 10.1155/2012/576238 [Epub ahead of print].

[6] Bensaha T. Evaluation of the capability of a new water lift system to reduce the risk of schneiderian membrane perforation during sinus elevation. International Journal of Oral and Maxillofacial Surgery 2011;40(8):815-20.

[7] Felice P, Pistilli R, Piattelli M, Soardi E, Barausse C, Esposito M. 1-stage versus 2-stage lateral sinus lift procedures: 1-year post-loading results of a multicentre randomised controlled trial. European Journal of Oral Implantology 2014;7(1):65-75.

[8] Pariente L, Dada K, Daas M. Mini-lateral windows for minimally invasive maxillary sinus augmentation: case series of a new technique. Implant Dentistry 2014;23(4): 371-7.

[9] Simon BI, Greenfield JL. Alternative to the gold standard for sinus augmentation: osteotome sinus elevation. Quintessence International 2011;42(10):863-71.

[10] Romero-Millan J, Martorell-Calatayud L, Penarrocha M, Garcia-Mira B. Indirect osteotome maxillary sinus floor elevation: an update. Journal of Oral Implantology 2012;38(6):799-804.

[11] Wen SC, Chan HL, Wang HL. Classification and management of antral septa for maxillary sinus augmentation. International Journal of Periodontics and Restorative Dentistry 2013;33(4):509-17.

[12] Calin C. Petre A. Drafta S. Osteotome-mediated sinus floor elevation: a systematic review and meta analysis. International Journal of Oral and Maxillofacial Implants 2014;29(3):558-76.

[13] Urban IA, Nagursky H, Church C, Lozada JL. Incidence, diagnosis, and treatment of sinus graft infection after sinus floor elevation: a clinical study. International Journal of Oral and Maxillofacial Implants 2012;27(2):449-57.

[14] Butura CC, Galindo DF. Implant placement in alveolar composite defects regenerated with rhBMP-2, anorganic bovine and titanium mesh: a report of eight reconstructed sites. International Journal of Oral and Maxillofacial Implants 2014;29(1):139-46.

[15] Sjöström T, McNamara LE, Meek RM, Dalby MJ, Su B. 2D and 3D nanopatterning of titanium for enhancing osteoinduction of stem cells at implant surfaces. Advanced Healthcare Materials 2013;2(9):1285-93.

[16] Egusa H, Sonoyama W, Nishimura M, Atsuta, Akiyama K. Stem cells in dentistry-Part II: Clinical applications. Journal of Prosthodontic Research 2012; 56(4):229-48.

[17] Rakhmatia YD, Avukawa Y, Furuhashi A, Koyano K. Current barrier membranes: titanium mesh and other membranes for guided bone regeneration in dental applications. Journal of Prosthodontic Research 2013;57(1):3-14.

[18] Miyamoto I, Funaki K, Yamauchi K, Kodama T, Takahashi T. Alveolar ridge reconstruction with titanium mesh and autogenous particulate bone graft: computed to-

mography-based evaluations of augmented bne quality and quantity. Clinical Implant Dentistry and Related Research 2012;14(2):304-11.

[19] Funato A, Ishikawa T, Kitajima H, Yamada M, Moroi H. A novel combined surgical approach to vertical alveolar ridge augmentation with titanium mesh, resorbable membrane, and rhPDGF-BB: a retrospective consecutive case series. International Journal of Periodontics and Restorative Dentistry 2013;33(4):437-45.

[20] Her S, Kang T, Fien MJ. Titanium mesh as an alternative to a membrane for ridge augmentation. Journal of Oral and Maxillofacial Surgery 2012;70(4):803-10.

[21] Moroi A, Ueki K, Okabe K, Marukawa K, Sotobori M, Mukozawa A, Miyazakia M. Comparison between unsintered hydroxyapatite/poly-L-lactic acid mesh and titanium mesh in bone regeneration of rabbit mandible. Implant Dentistry 2013;22(3): 255-62.

[22] Hirota M, Ikeda T, Tabuchi M, Iwai T, Tohnai I, Ogawa T. Effect of ultraviolet-mediated photofunctionalization for bone formation around medical titanium mesh. Journal of Oral and Maxillofacial Surgery 2014;72(9):1691-702.

[23] Cawood JI, Stoelinga PWJ, Blackburn TK. The evolution of pre implant surgery from pre prosthetic surgery. International Journal of Oral and Maxillofacial Surgery 2007;36(5):377–85.

[24] Rahpeyma A, Khajehahmadi S, Hosseini VR. Lateral ridge split and immediate implant placement in moderately resorbed alveolar ridges: How much is the added width? Dental Research Journal 2013;10(5):602-08.

[25] Kelly A, Flanagan D. Ridge expansion and immediate placement with piezosurgery and screw expanders in atrophic maxillary sites: two case reports. Journal of Oral Implantology 2013;39(1):85-90.

[26] Zakhary IE, El-Mekkawi HA, Elsalanty ME. Alveolar ridge augmentation for implant fixation: status review. Oral Surgery Oral Medicine Oral Pathology Oral Radiology and Endodontology 2012;114(5):179-89.

[27] Khairnar MS, Khairnar D, Bakshi K. Modified ridge splitting and bone expansion osteotomy for placement of dental implant in esthetic zone. Contemporary Clinical Dentistry 2014;5(1):110-4.

[28] Funaki K, Takahashi T, Yamuchi K. Horizontal alveolar ridge augmentation using distraction osteogenesis: comparison with a bone-splitting method in a dog model. Oral Surgery Oral Medicine Oral Pathology Oral Radiology and Endodontology 2009;107(3):350-8.

[29] Di Stefano DA, Artese L, Iezzi G, Piatelli A, Pagnutti S, Piccirilli M, Perrotti V. Alveolar ridge regeneration with equine spongy bone: a clinical, histological, and immunohistochemical case series. Clinical Implant Dentistry and Related Research 2009;11(2): 90-100.

[30] Davidas JP. Looking for a new international standard for characterization, classification and identification of surfaces in implantable materials: the long march for the evaluation of dental implant surfaces has just began. Periodontology, Oral Surgery, Esthetic & Implant Dentistry Open Journal 2014;2(1):1-5. http://www.poseido.info/publication/volume-2-2014/poseido-2014211-5-davidas.pdf

[31] Toeroek R, Ehrenfest DMD. The concept of Screw-Guided Bone Regeneration (S-GBR). Part 3: Fast Screw-Guided Bone Regeneration (FS-GBR) in the severely resorbed preimplant posterior mandible using allograft and Leukocyte-and Platelet-Rich Fibrin (L-PRF): a 4-year follow-up. Periodontology, Oral Surgery, Esthetic & Implant Dentistry Open Journal 2013;1(2):85-92. http://www.poseido.info/publication/volume-1-2013/poseido-20131285-92-toeroek.pdf

[32] Traini T, Piatelli A, Caputi S, Degidi M, Mangano C, Scarano A, Perrotti V, Iezzi G. Regeneration of human bone using different bone substitute biomaterials. Clinical Implant Dentistry and Related Research 2013 doi: 10.1111/cid.12089 [Epub ahead of print]

[33] Margonar R, dos Santos PL, Queiroz TP, Marcantonio E. Rehabilitation of atrophic maxilla using the combination of autogenous and allogeneic bone grafts followed by protocol-type prosthesis. Journal of Craniofacial Surgery 2010;21(6):1894-6.

[34] Tadic D, Epple M. A thorough physicochemical characterization of 14 calciun phosphate-based bone substitution materials in comparison to natural bone. Biomaterials 2004;25(6):987-94.

[35] Pietak AM, Reid JW, Stott MJ, Sayer M. Silicon substitution in the calcium phosphate bioceramics. Biomaterials 2007;28(28):4023-32.

[36] Lee MJ, Sohn SK, Kim KT. Effect of hydroxyapatite on bone integration in a rabbit tibial defect model. Clinics in Orthopedic Surgery 2010;2(1):90-7.

[37] Berberi A, Samarani A, Nader N, Noujeim Z, Dagher M, Kanj W, Mearawi R, Salemeh Z, Badran B. Physicochemical characteristics of bone substitutes used in oral surgery in comparison to autogenous bone. Biomedical Research International 2014; doi: 10.1155/2014/320790 [Epub ahead of print]. http://www.hindawi.com/journals/bmri/2014/320790/

[38] Gomes KU, Martins WD, Ribas Mde O. Horizontal and vertical maxillary osteotomy stability, in cleft lip and palate patients, using allogeneic bone graft. Dental Press Journal of Orthodontics 2013;18(5):84-90.

[39] da Silva Filho OG, Ozawa TO, Bachega C, Bachega MA. Reconstruction of alveolar cleft with allogenous bone graft: Clinical considerations. Dental Press Journal of Orthodontics 2013;18(6):138-47.

[40] Glovacki J. A review of osteoinductive testing methods and sterilization processes for demineralized bone. Cell and Tissue Banking 2005;6(1):3-12.

[41] Hing KA, Wilson LF, Buckland T. Comparative performance of three ceramic bone substitutes. Spine Journal 2007;7(4):475-90.

[42] McAllister BS, Haghighat K. Bone Augmentation techniques. Journal of Periodontology 2007;78:377-96.

[43] Tolstunov L. Maxillary tuberosity block bone graft: innovative technique and case report. Journal of Oral and Maxillofacial Surgery 2009;67(8):1723-9.

[44] Sullivan JP. Implant placement in the aesthetic zone following an autogenous bone graft from an intraoral site: a case study. Primary Dental Journal 2013;2(4):49-55.

[45] Sudhakar J, Ali SA, Karthikeyan S. Zygomatic implants – A Review. Journal of Indian Academy of Dental Specialists 2011;2(2):24-8.

[46] Aparicio C, Manresa C, Francisco K, Ouazzani W, Claros P, Potau JM. The long-term use of zygomatic implants: a 10-year clinical and radiographic report. Clinical Implant Dentistry Related Research 2014;16(3):447-59.

[47] Zwahlen RA, Gratz KW, Oechslin CK, Studer SP. Survival rate of zygomatic implants in atrophic or partially resected maxillae prior to functional loading: a retrospective clinical report. International Journal of Oral and Maxillofacial Implants 2006;21(3):413-20.

[48] Pi Urgell J, Revilla Gutierrez V, Gay Escoda CG. Rehabilitation of atrophic maxilla: a review of 101 zygomatic implants. Medicina Oral Patologia Oral y Cirugia Bucal 2008;13(6):363-70.

[49] Sorni M, Guarinos J, Peñarrocha M. Implants in anatomical buttresses of the upper jaw. Medicina Oral Patologia Oral y Cirugia Bucal 2005;10(2):163-8.

[50] Stievenart M, Malevez C. Rehabilitation of totally atrophied maxilla by means of four zygomatic implants and fixed prosthesis: a 6-40 months follow-up. International Journal of Oral and Maxillofacial Surgery 2010;39(4):358–63.

[51] Aparicio C, Ouazzani W, Hatano N. The use of zygomatic implants for prosthetic rehabilitation of the severely resorbed maxilla. Periodontology 2000 2008;47:162-71.

[52] Becktor JP, Isaksson S, Abrahamsson P, Sennerby L. Evaluation of 31 zygomatic implants and 74 regular dental implants used in 16 patients for prosthetic reconstruction of the atrophic maxilla with cross-arch fixed bridges. Clinical Implant Dentistry Related Research 2005;7(3):159–65.

[53] Branemark PI, Gröndahl K, Ohrnell LO, Nilsson P, Petruson B, Svensson B, Engstrand P, Nannmark U. Zygoma fixture in the management of advanced atrophy of the maxilla: technique and long-term results. Scandinavian Journal of Plastic and Reconstructive Surgery and Hand Surgery 2004;38(2):70-85.

[54] Jivraj S, Chee W. Treatment planning of implants in the aesthetic zone. Brazilian Dental Journal 2006;201(2):77-89.

[55] Jensen OT, Adams MW, Cottam JR, Parel SM, Phillips WR. The All-on-4 Shelf: Maxilla. Journal of Oral and Maxillofacial Surgery 2010;68(10):2520-7.

[56] Khatami AH, Smith CR. All-on-four immediate function concept and clinical report of treatment of an edentulous mandible with a fixed complete denture and milled titanium framework. Journal of Prosthodontics 2008;17(1):47-51.

[57] Agliard E, Panigatti S, Clerico M, Vila C, Malo P. Immediate rehabilitation of the edentulous jaws witfull fixed prostheses supported by four implants: interim results of a single cohort prospective study. Clinical Oral Implants Research 2010;21(5): 459-65.

5

Bone Substitute Materials in Implant Dentistry

Sybele Saska, Larissa Souza Mendes,
Ana Maria Minarelli Gaspar and
Ticiana Sidorenko de Oliveira Capote

1. Introduction

Although bone autografts have been routinely used as "gold standard" for reconstruction/ replacement bone defects, because they have osteogenic, osteoinductive, osteoconductive properties, they have a high number of viable cells and are rich in growth factors. However, the use of autograft is limited by several factors, being one of them the insufficient amount of donor tissue. Therefore, bone substitute materials have been extensively studied in order to develop an ideal material for substitution of bone grafts, due to some disadvantages presented by autografts, allografts and xenografts, such as poor bone quality, an inadequate amount of bone and possible immunogenicity for allografts and xenografts, which limit the use of these grafts in specific surgical protocols. These disadvantages have led tissue engineering and biotechnology to develop new materials and promising methods for tissue repair, especially for bone tissue. Thus, bone substitutes, synthetic and/or biotechnologically processed have become potential materials for clinical applications in different areas of health.

An ideal bone substitute (BS) material should provide a variety of shapes and sizes with suitable mechanical properties to be used in sites where there are impact loading; moreover, these materials should be biocompatible, osteoconductive, preferably being resorbable and replaced by new bone formation. In general, resorbable BS materials are preferred, since these materials are expected to preserve the increased bone volume during the reconstruction and simultaneously are gradually replaced by newly formed bone.

Synthetic materials, denominated as alloplastics, may act as scaffolds for bone cells providing tissue growth inside the respective material.

A scaffold must be highly porous with interconnected pores and have adequate mechanical properties. The surface of a scaffold should be similar to extracellular matrix (ECM). These properties enable the scaffold to act as a matrix for tissue regeneration to maintain and improve tissue/organs functions; therefore, it is considered the key element for the success in tissue engineering. Numerous physicochemical features of scaffolds, such as surface chemistry, surface roughness, topography, mechanical properties and interfacial free energy (hydrophobic/hydrophilic balance) are important for cell attachment, proliferation and differentiation. These factors are also critically important to the overall biocompatibility and bioactivity of a particular material [1-3].

Resorption of a biomaterial is related to several factors, such as, particle size, porosity, chemical structure (composition and crystallinity), and pH of body fluids [4, 5]. Particles with nanometric sizes are reabsorbed faster than micrometric particles, because osteoclasts or macrophages act faster on a biomaterial surface. Biomaterial crystallinity also changes the resorption rate, since highly crystalline structures are more resistant to resorption than an amorphous or semi-crystalline structure. Moreover, the chemical composition is also important. Impurities such as calcium carbonate promote faster resorption [6]. The failure or the success of a material for bone fill or replacement may be related to the resorption rate of the material, as well as the regenerative capacity of bone tissue. This process can occur in three forms: 1. insufficient permanence of the material to promote bone apposition and to allow the osteoconductivity; 2. premature destabilization of newly formed bone due to the complete degradation of the material; 3. an exaggerated inflammatory response due to the degradation of the material [7]. Thus, bone substitute materials must have suitable resorption rate in accordance with the rate of tissue formation.

Despite recent advances in the development of new BS for bone tissue engineering, there is still a search for a material or a composite with mechanical properties and physicochemical characteristics similar to autograft and a structure closer to the natural ECM.

2. Ceramic-based bone substitutes

Ceramics are compounds between metallic and nonmetallic elements. Ceramic materials have a several of attractive advantages comparing to other materials. These include high melting points, great hardness, low densities and chemical and environmental stability. However, ceramics are severely affected by lack of toughness; they are extremely brittle, and are highly susceptible to fracture. They are most frequently oxides, nitrides, and carbides, for example, some of the common ceramic materials include aluminum oxide (or alumina, Al_2O_3) and silicon dioxide (or silica, SiO_2), in addition, some traditional ceramics are referred as those composed of clay minerals (i.e., porcelain), as well as cement and glass [8].

The ability of ceramic materials to bond to the bone tissue is a unique property of bioactive ceramics. This property has been led their wide clinical application in both areas as orthopedics and dentistry. The use of ceramics for hard tissues reconstitution has been performed for centuries, but in clinical practice the use of these materials only began in the late eighteenth

century with the use of porcelain for making dental prostheses. On the other hand, in orthopedics the use of ceramic materials happened in the late nineteenth century with the use of
plaster of Paris (calcium sulfate hemihydrate, $CaSO_4$ $\frac{1}{2}H_2O$) for bone defects filling [9].

The term "bioceramic" refers to biocompatible ceramic materials applied to biomedical and
clinical use due to certain characteristics such as biocompatibility, excellent tribological
properties and high chemical stability, which is superior to metals in different applications,
moreover excellent osteoconductive [10].

Among bioceramics, calcium phosphates are ceramics with Ca/P molar ratio ranging from 0.5
to 2.0 and are found in different types [11], in which the best known form is hydroxyapatite
(HA), a natural mineral component representing 30 to 70% of the mass of bones and teeth [12].
The chemical structure of biological HA is very complex, because it not presents a totally pure
composition (non-stoichiometric), being frequently calcium-deficient hydroxyapatite enriched
with carbonate ions forming the carbonate-apatite [13]. Some calcium phosphates of biological
relevance are: amorphous calcium phosphate (ACP), dicalcium phosphate dihydrate (DCPD),
dicalcium phosphate (DCP), octacalcium phosphate (OCP), tricalcium phosphate (TCP),
calcium pyrophosphate (CPP) and hydroxyapatite (HA).

Pure HA, calcium hydroxyapatite specifically, is a stoichiometric composition of
$(Ca)_{10}(PO_4)_6(OH)_2$ (Ca/P = 1.67). It is main inorganic component of bone tissue and teeth. For
many years, different types of synthesis and applications of these calcium phosphates have
been researched for regeneration/reconstruction of bone structures. Synthetic HA has been
used for this purpose, because they are bioactive material and can have a Ca/P molar ratio less
than 1.67; thus, they are more effective clinically due to its similarities with the composition
of bone tissue and their osteoconductive properties [13, 14].

Bioceramics have different rates of *in vitro* solubility, which reflects in the *in vivo* degradation,
i.e., as greater the Ca/P molar ratio lower is the solubility of bioceramics [15]. However, the
rate of dissolution is not only influenced by Ca/P molar ratio, but also may be influenced by
other factors such as local pH, chemical composition, crystallinity, particle size and porosity
of material [5].

Bioceramics when in contact with body fluids and tissues, in this interface material-tissue,
suffer reactions at the molecular scale of type dissolution preferably by the release of Ca^{2+} and
PO_4^{3-} ions; however, in this interface there is an increase of local pH promoted by Ca^{2+} ion
release. This increase in pH stimulates alkaline phosphatase activity in pre-existing osteoblastic cells and in newly-differentiated active osteoblasts to synthesize more alkaline phosphatase,
type I collagen, non-collagen proteins and others. Therefore, pH at the material-tissue interface
is gradually reestablished, while occurs the nucleation of crystals of calcium phosphate to the
collagen fibers until forming a chemically phase more stable. This event is related to PO_4^{3-} ion
release from ATP molecules, pyrophosphate and others, which contain PO_4^{3-} ion from adjacent
tissues. Moreover the action of biological buffers containing HCO^{3-} ion, which favor the
precipitation of carbonate-apatite as well as the decrease of chemical mediators locally,
produced by leukocytes [13]. Table 1 shows the occurrence of calcium phosphates in biological
systems.

Apatite phase	Formula	Ca/P
Monocalcium phosphate monohydrate - MCPH	$Ca(H_2PO_4)_2 \cdot H_2O$	0.5
Monocalcium phosphate anhydrous - MCP	$Ca(H_2PO_4)_2$	0.5
Dicalcium phosphate dihydrate (Brushite) - DCPD	$CaHPO_4 \cdot 2H_2O$	1.0
Dicalcium phosphate anhydrous (Monetite) - DCP	$CaHPO_4$	1.0
Octacalcium phosphate - OCP	$Ca_8H_2(PO_4)6 \cdot 5H_2O$	1.33
Amorphous calcium phosphate - ACP	$Ca_x(PO_4)_y \cdot nH_2O$	1.2 - 2.2
α or β-Tricalcium phosphate - TCP	$Ca_3(PO_4)_2$	1.48 - 1.50
Calcium-deficient hydroxyapatite - CDHA	$Ca_9(HPO_4)(PO_4)5(OH)$	1.5
Hydroxyapatite - HA	$Ca_{10}(PO_4)6(OH)_2$	1.67

Table 1. Main calcium phosphate phases. Apatite phase, chemical formula and Ca/P molar ratio.

Bioactive ceramics have been used as bone substitute materials for maxillary sinus lift, alveolar ridge augmentation, inlay bone grafting and as coatings for titanium and their respective alloys. However, bioceramics present a limitation in clinical application due to their low mechanical properties, for instance, low elastic modulus, when compared to other metallic and polymeric biomaterials. Therefore, these ceramic materials cannot be used in sites where there is a high mechanical loading, but can be used for bone fill materials and coatings of metallic surfaces or materials of high mechanical properties [16, 17]. These coatings may accelerate initial stabilization of implants and stimulating bone appositions on the implant surface, promoting a rapid fixation of these devices [18].

The bioceramics may be employed in dense and porous forms. Despite the increase in porosity decrease the mechanical strength of ceramics, the existence of isolated pores with suitable dimensions can favor the ingrowth of tissue through of these pores, promoting a strong entanglement between the material and newly formed tissue [19], moreover this porosity may promote circulation of biological fluids, increases the specific surface area, and thus accelerating the biodegradability.

Bioceramics can be single crystals (sapphire), polycrystalline [alumina, hydroxyapatite (HA), tricalcium phosphate (TCP)] or semi-crystalline structure as glass-ceramics (Ceravital® or A/W glass-ceramic) and composites, which have an amorphous phase and one or more crystalline phases. In addition, bioactive glasses (Bioglass®, PerioGlas®, BioGran®) which are a group of glass-ceramic consist in a structure of amorphous solids.

The initial medical applications of CS were documented in 1961 [20]. This material, plaster of Paris, was used in many bone defects of trauma. In the dental field, one of the first reports of the use of CS was in 1961 by Lebourg and Biou [21]. These authors implanted CS in alveoli after extraction of third molars, even in other bone defects in the mandible and maxilla. After three to four weeks it has been observed that the material had been completely resorbed, and bone healing was accelerated in the treated areas in comparison with the control. The authors concluded that CS was a favorable material for the treatment of bone defects and they justify it by the ability of the material to supply essential inorganic ions for the repair process.

Clinical studies showed positive results regarding the use of CS as material for bone fill and barrier to the preservation of alveolar ridge, post-dental extraction, providing a barrier which stabilizes the clot, assisting in the healing and bone regeneration of the local to receive the implant. The use of CS hemihydrates (CS) (powder, particulate or cement form) and CS associated with demineralized freeze-dried bone (DFDB) in bone defects, post-extraction dental and periodontal defects, promotes the increase of the quality and quantity of newly formed bone preserving the dimensions of alveolar ridge [22-24]. Moreover, CS or CS associated with DFDB when used to maxillary sinus lift, this bone substitute, favors a good primary stability of dental implants and with relative bone density [25-27]. In addition to these advantages, CS is a BS rapidly resorbable and promotes angiogenesis [27-29]; however, in some clinical situations this rapid absorption *in vivo*, may be a disadvantage, due to its degradation which often occurs before the new bone formation.

Other the bioactive ceramics most commonly investigated as bone substitute materials are HA, β-TCP and bioactive glasses. Synthetic HA, β-TCP and biphasic calcium phosphates (HA:β-TCP) are routinely employed as BS in block or granule forms. Furthermore, cements based on HA and/or β-TCP are excellent bone fill materials, due to their easy manipulation and favor the bone contour, moreover, are clinically used by their similarity to the bone inorganic composition and by osteoconductive property. On the other hand, bioactive glasses are most commonly used in granule forms.

For several years, synthetic HA was used as the main method in the reconstruction of bone defects involving the craniofacial region, oral surgery, orthopedic and implant dentistry [14, 30-32]. HA presents some disadvantages related to its resorption, because it is hardly absorbed, which hampers the remodeling and the new bone formation, and results in poor local stability or permanent stress concentration. Currently, biphasic calcium phosphates, mixtures containing HA/TCP (α-TCP or β-TCP) are preferably used in clinical practice with varied proportions between HA and TCP [33-38] due to their considerably difference in the resorption rate, which HA reabsorbs very slowly compared with TCP. The difference in the resorption rate influences in the osteoconductive property of these materials, TCPs are more osteoconductive than HA, due to their greater biodegradability rate in relation to HA [13, 39, 40]. Clinical and experimental studies have shown that mixture HA/TCP promotes intense activity of bone formation with high osteoconductivity [34, 41-43], whose mixture has demonstrated to be an excellent material for sinus lift [34, 37, 38]. However, even the resorption rate of TCP being faster than HA, clinical studies that used just TCP reported presence of TCP particles after long-term postoperative of maxillary sinus lift and mandible defects [44-49]. Results show that β-TCP is a good material for grafting [44-51], on this account also promotes stability of implants increasing the survival rate [48].

Furthermore, these bioceramics when associated with biopolymers as hyaluronic acid [49] and collagen [52, 53] or other osteoinductive biomolecules (growth factors: bone morphogenetic protein-2 (BMP-2); fibroblast growth factor-2 (FGF-2)) [54-59] have displayed promising results for bone regeneration. These associations have promoted a better quality and quantity of newly formed bone [49, 52, 53, 56, 57, 59], consequently they can improve the primary stability of implants.

Other subgroups of bioceramics quite used as BS material are bioactive glasses and glass-ceramics. Silica glasses are generally classified as a subgroup of ceramics. The glass-ceramics are materials formed by a glass matrix reinforced by ceramic crystals obtained from controlled crystallization processes [60]. This crystallization process can take place by heat treatment, resulting in a material containing various crystal phases and controlled grain sizes [10]. The glass-ceramic materials have relatively high mechanical strengths, low coefficients of thermal expansion and good biological compatibility. Possibly the most attractive attribute of this class of materials is the ease with which they may be fabricated, in which conventional glass-forming techniques may be used [8]. On the other hand, bioactive glasses present limitations in certain mechanical properties such as low strength and toughness.

In the late 1960s and early 1970s, the several researches for developing implant materials with a better biocompatibility resulted in the new concept of bioceramic materials, which could mimic natural bone tissue. During this period, Hench and coworkers [61] developed a new biocompatible material, silica-based melt-derived glass, for bonding fractured bones, a bioactive glass denominate 45S5 Bioglass®. This denomination was given because the material mimicked normal bone and to stimulate the new bone formation between the fractures [62]. Bioglass® is a commercially available family of bioactive glasses, based on SiO_2, Na_2O, CaO and P_2O_5 in specific proportions, and was one of the first materials completely synthetic with excellent osteoconductive properties, which seamlessly binds to bone [61, 63]. The bioactive glasses, since their discovered, have been widely used in dentistry for bone defects repair/reconstruction, because these glasses exhibit bone bonding, a phenomenon also observed with other bioactive ceramics [64]. Bioglass offers advantages such as control of resorption rate, excellent osteoconductivity, bioactivity, and capacity for delivering cells. This process is a result of the surface reactive silica, calcium, and phosphate groups that are characteristic of these materials. Silica is believed to play a critical role in bioactivity [64].

In the 1970s, Brömer and coworkers [65] developed a glass-ceramic, Ceravital® through reduction of alkali oxides in the composition and the phase precipitation of the glass matrix by heat treatment of Bioglass®. Ceravital® has been used for small bone defects/structure reconstruction as dentistry [66] as other medical applications, *e.g.* tympanoplasties [67].

The use of bioactive glasses as alloplastic bone graft materials for alveolar ridge augmentation [68-71] and maxillary sinus lift [72-74] procedures has received increasing attention in implant dentistry. Besides Bioglass® other commercial types of bioactive glass have been used for bone repair such as PerioGlas® [70, 75, 76] and BioGran® [71-73]. Studies have reported presence of bioactive glass long-term postoperative (1-2 years) [72, 73].

Moreover, several studies have shown that bioactive glasses and glass ceramics stimulates the secretion of angiogenic growth factors on fibroblasts and endothelial cell proliferation [77, 78].

Although they are quite biocompatible and exhibit bone bonding, bioactive glasses are not osteoinductive and are not capable of forming bone in ectopic sites (although they can be used to deliver osteopromotive growth factors) [64].

Another glass-ceramic with potential for application in implant dentistry is apatite/wollastonite (A/W), which was developed by Kokubo et al., in 1982 [79]. This material presents a great capacity for bone bonding and moderate mechanical strength [80], with excellent results in orthopedic applications [81-83]. The resorption rate of this glass-ceramic can be increased when associated with β-TCP [84]. According to Carrodeguas et al. (2008) [85] the report that the new ceramics containing wollastonite did not exhibit toxicity in cell culture with human fibroblasts. Moreover, they are biocompatible, resorbable and bioactive releasing ions of silica and calcium in the physiological environment, which are capable of stimulating cells to produce bone matrix [86, 87].

Biosilicate®, glass-ceramic developed by Zanotto and coworkers in 2004 [88], which is highly crystalline (~100%), has an elastic modulus value close to cortical bone, and displays high level of bioactivity [89-91]. It is biocompatible and provides efficient new bone formation in sockets preserving alveolar bone ridge height and allowing osseointegration of implants [92].

Table 2 summarizes some bioceramics used in clinical practice.

Material	Application	Results	Ref.
Calcium Sulphate	Sinus lift	Promote new bone formation with new vessels	[27-29, 93]
		High resorption in 1 month	
HA	Bone graft	Promote new bone formation	[30, 31, 94, 95]
	Sinus lift	Produce avoid space for blood clot	
		Increase bone volume in 8 weeks	
		Promote direct mineralized bone-to-implant contact in the augmented area	
β-TCP	Guide bone regeneration	No induce inflammation	[37, 38, 42-49]
	Sinus Lift	Osteoconductive	
	Bone graft	Highly degraded by macrophages and osteoclast	
Biphasic calcium phosphate (HA:β-TCP)	Bone graft	Increase bone volume in 8 weeks	[33-38, 40, 41]
	Sinus lift	Osteoconductive	
		Promote stability of implants	
		Promote new bone formation	
Bioglass®	Bone graft	Increase bone volume	[68, 69, 93]
	Sinus lift	High bioactivity	
		Promote new bone formation	
BONITmatrix®	Bone graft	Stimulate IGF-1 gene expression	[96]
		Enhance Coll-1 expression	
Biocoral®	Bone graft	Promote formation of fibrovascular tissue	[93, 97]
	Sinus lift	New formed bone 39% highly mineralized	
Fisiograft®	Sinus lift	Increase bone volume 33%	[93]
		High absorption	
OSSANOVA	Bone graft	Stimulate IGF-1 expression	[96]

Table 2. Some bioceramics used in clinical practice.

3. Composite and polymer-based bone substitutes

Composite materials are described as those that have at least two components or two phases with distinct physical and chemical properties that are separated by an interface. The purpose of developing composites is to associate different materials to produce a single device with superior properties compared with the isolated components [10]. Separately the constituents of the composite maintains their features, however when mixed they constitute a compound with their own properties inherent to the new composition. Two examples of natural fiber composites are: 1. wood, which is basically formed of cellulose fibers and lignin (amorphous resin which binds the cellulose fibers); 2. bone tissue, which is formed by an inorganic phase, essentially carbonate-apatite, placed in an organic matrix, whose composition is about 95% type I collagen. Therefore, the composites are formed by the matrix, which is the continuous phase ("fiber network") and involves the other phase, the dispersed one. Among the several types of composites, polymer composites exhibit some advantages such as: low weight, corrosion resistance, high temperature resistance and good mechanical properties when compared to conventional engineering materials [98].

However, the current goal of tissue engineering is the development of polymer composites, metal-free, with mechanical properties similar to living tissue, especially bone tissue, for partial or total replacement or reconstruction of the organ or tissue being repaired.

Polymers can be classified as natural or synthetic and degradable or non-degradable. These compounds provide versatility in their structure and can modulate the mechanical properties of other compounds like ceramics. Degradable polymers may be advantageous in certain clinical situations.

Composites produced from a combination of natural polymers (collagen, cellulose, polyhydroxybutyrate), or synthetic [poly (lactic-*co*-glycolic acid) (PLGA), poly(lactic acid) (PLA), poly(ε-caprolactone) (PCL)] associated with bioceramics have been highlighted in academic community [99-106] because they are biocompatible, excellent osteoconductors, bioactives, have satisfactory mechanical properties, and are absorbable, therefore they are potential materials for application in regenerative medicine therapies.

Natural polymers or biopolymers have attractive properties for the construction of 3D scaffolds, such as biocompatibility and biodegradability. Bioactivity of these polymers, if you need to improve, can also be controlled by the addition of chemicals, proteins, peptides, and cells. The most commonly studied natural polymers for the purpose of bone engineering are collagen/gelatin, chitosan, silk, alginate, hyaluronic acid, and peptides [107].

Currently, the most BS, available commercially, for clinical application in implant dentistry based on polymers are barrier membranes for guided bone regeneration (GBR) or collagen sponge/BMPs (INFUSE®) for bone reconstruction.

At the beginning of the use of the GBR the treatment was preferably with non-resorbable membranes based on expanded polytetrafluoroethylene (e-PTFE) [108, 109], because of its inert characteristic and their biological effective and predictable results as a mechanical barrier.

However, resorbable membranes have been widely used to the development of new bioma-terials, due to the predictable and similar results compared to the non-resorbable membranes [110-112], moreover resorbable membranes can be used on peri-implant defects, *i. e.,* an advantage in relation to non-resorbable membranes. Among the membranes the most used as resorbable membranes are: collagen, PLA and PLGA [110-113].

The type I collagen is an example of biopolymers quite used to the development of BS. It is a matrix that provides a favorable environment for induction of osteoblasts differentiation *in vitro* and osteogenesis *in vivo* [114]. Type III collagen constitutes the reticular fibers of the tissues and is also widely used in the manufacture of membranes for GBR. The non-mineral-ized collagen membranes are usually weak (low tensile strength) making their clinical manipulation difficult. The great advantage of them is the excellent cell affinity stimulating the chemotaxis of fibroblasts and acting as support migration of these cells (osteoconduction). Other advantages are: good adaptation to bone surfaces, especially to dental roots and hemostatic effect [113]. When embedded in the bone matrix they are gradually metabolized by the action of collagenase, or can be partially embedded in the bone matrix.

The resorption of collagen occurs parallel to bone formation as well as by the formation of new periodontal tissue such as cementum and periodontal ligament. The resorption time ranges from 06 to 08 weeks depending on the strength of the material, however it can last from 04 to 06 months [115]. In this case, the new bone is protected against the growth of connective tissue within the defect area. Despite prevent cellular infiltration, this membrane is permeable to nutrients, and the degradation occurs through enzymatic reactions without irritating the surrounding tissues. These membranes have adequate mechanical resistance [116]; moreover, they can facilitate the maintenance of the space to be regenerated, similar to the non-resorbable membranes.

The collagen membranes developed in recent years have shown optimal physicochemical characteristics for clinical application [117-121]. According to the literature, the determination of the density of crosslinking reaction (cross-linking) directly influences the physical properties of collagen matrices, *i. e.,* the increased crosslinking of collagen fibrils provides increased tensile strength and enzymatic degradation, and higher thermal stability [118, 119, 121, 122].

The membrane Bio-Gide® has been the most membrane widely used for GBR in the last years [113, 123-126], which is composed of type I and III collagen from porcine. This membrane has a bilayer structure with a compact layer and other porous. The porous layer (inner face) promotes a three-dimensional matrix for bone integration. The natural collagen structure of the Bio-Gide ® is ideal for tissue adhesion, while the newly formed bone is protected against the growth of connective tissue into the defect region; while preventing cellular infiltration this membrane is permeable to nutrients, and the degradation occurs through enzymatic reactions without irritating the surrounding tissues.

Studies with collagen membrane for GBR have reported satisfactory results *in vivo,* for example, the rate of bone regeneration has a similar efficacy to the e-PTFE membranes. This occurred due to the advent of collagen membranes with good mechanical strength. In the past, it was difficult to obtain such satisfactory and predictable results due to the difficulty of producing collagen membranes with these characteristics [123, 127].

4. New perspectives for bone substitutes

4.1. Bone tissue engineering

In recent years, a new generation of bone substitutes have been developed in an attempt to obtain materials closer to the autograft standard by using biomaterials capable of inducing specific cellular responses at the molecular level, by integrating the bioactivity and biodegradability of these materials [107]. These BS are being based on the concept of bone tissue engineering. Tissue engineering/regenerative medicine has emerged as an interdisciplinary field that includes cell-based therapies and use of porous-bioactive materials for development of functional substitutes for the repair or replacement of damaged tissues or organs [128]. Tissue engineering has achieved great progress in the development of three-dimensional materials (scaffolds) for repair or replacement of damaged tissues or organs, including alloplastic materials such as bioceramics, bioactive glasses and polymers [60, 61, 63, 129, 130] in association to the signaling pathway, molecular and/or biophysical stimulation. Thus, tissue engineering is based on three elements that must be in synergism: matrix (scaffolds), cells and signals (mechanical and/or molecules: proteins, peptides and cytokines) [131, 132]; the absence or dysfunction of one element will halt or delay tissue regeneration. Furthermore, the tissue formation inside the scaffolds is directly influenced by porosity rate and pore size. In the case of bone formation, scaffolds should preferably have pores greater than 300 μM for promoting a good vascularization and a new bone formation, preventing hypoxia and induction of endochondral formation before the osteogenesis [133].

Porous scaffolds have been developed by variety of conventional methods from alloplastic materials, such as particle/salt leaching, chemical/gas foaming, fiber bonding, solvent casting, melting molding, phase separation and freeze drying [134, 135]. However, these methods present some limitations due to their lack of the controlled formation of pores and do not produce interconnected structures to favoring cell growth inside the structure. For overcome these disadvantages, additive manufacturing (AM), also otherwise known as three-dimensional (3D) printing, is a promising option for the production of scaffolds particularly for bone substitutes.

This technique consists in constructing 3D scaffolds by a tool for direct digital fabrication that selectively prints a respective material (layer-by-layer) into/onto a bed, whose shape is given by CAD specifications [136]. A distinctive feature of this layer-by-layer printing process, is the printing of structures with high geometric complexity and well-defined architecture as well as patient-specific implant designs, which are not possible to be constructed by any other manufacturing method (Figure 1).

Some of the commercially available AM techniques are 3DP (ExOne, PA), fused deposition modeling (FDM, Stratasys, MN), selective laser sintering (SLS, 3D Systems, CA), stereolithog-

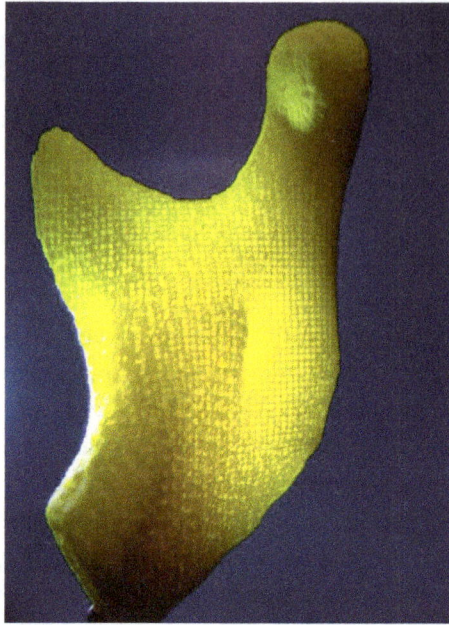

Figure 1. Printed mandibular condyle by Fused Deposition Modeling (FDM) process. *Image provided by Centro de Tecno-logia de Informação (CTI) – Renato Archer (Campinas, Brazil).*

raphy (3D Systems, CA), 3D plotting (Fraunhofer Institute for Materials Research and BeamTechnology, Germany), as well as various methods [135]. These AM techniques can be classified as – (a) extrusion (deformation + solidification), (b) polymerization, (c) laser-assisted sintering, and (d) direct writing-based processes [135, 136].

Recently, some researches have performed using 3D printed scaffolds for bone regeneration. Among them we can highlight the use of this 3D printed BS based on bioceramics for vertical bone augmentation as onlay graft. The results shown by these studies are promising and efficient as bone graft compared to autografts [137-139]. Li et al (2011) [140] reported a case report of a 3D printed mandibular condyle implant made of nano-hydroxyapatite/polyamide. The clinical results suggest that this type of 3D printed implant can be a viable alternative to the autografts for maxillofacial defects. 3D printed scaffolds base on PLGA have also demonstrated good results for bone regeneration [141]. So far, as signaling pathway, growth factor and drug delivery, have been reported the use recombinant human BMP-2 (rhBMP-2) [142] and alendronate [143]. PCL/PLGA/gelatin scaffolds containing rhBMP-2 did not induce the osteogenic differentiation of mesenchymal stem cells *in vitro*, however, in the preclinical experiements, PCL/PLGA/collagen/rhBMP-2 showed the best bone healing quality at both weeks (4 and 8 after implantation) without inflammatory response. On the other hand, a large number of macrophages indicated severe inflammation caused by burst release of rhBMP-2 [142]. In addition, a study about 3D-printed bioceramic scaffolds containing alendronate shows that *in vivo* local alendronate delivery from PCL-coated 3DP TCP scaffolds could further induce increased early bone formation [143].

4.2. Growth factors

Osteoprogenitor cells, osteoblasts and osteoclasts are under growth factors activity. The role of growth factors is not only to stimulate cell proliferation through cell cycle regulation by initiating mitosis but also to maintain cell survival and to stimulate the migration, differentiation and apoptosis as well. Osteoblasts proliferate mediated by growth factors released by themselves and by the bone during the resorption process. Among the most important are the TGF-β and the factors released by the bone matrix, such as growth factor similar to insulin (IGF-1 and 2), the fibroblast growth factor (FGF-2) and growth factor derived from platelets (PDGF) [144, 145] which are potent mitogens [146, 147].

Moreover, other factors are secreted during the repair process, such as BMPs and angiogenic factors (vascular endothelial growth factor - VEGF) [147]. TGF-β presents activity in embryonic development, cell differentiation, hormone secretion and immune function, and acts synergistically with TGF-α in the induction of phenotypic transformation [146]. The TGF-β superfamily includes TGF-β1, TGF-β2, TGF-β3 and other important factors, such as BMPs 1-8, which promote several stages of intramembranous and endochondral ossification during bone repair [148].

Among these several growth factors, BMP-2 has received attention from the scientific community due its use in combination with different scaffolds to promote bone repair, especially in tissue engineering. The literature, in the constant search for developing a biomaterial with excellent osteoinductive properties, such as autogenous bone for reconstructive surgery, has recently shown that some polymers and bioceramics can be great carriers for BMPs, especially the collagen [54, 57, 59, 143, 149-152].

The concept of osteoinduction was first described by Urist in 1965 [153] when he observed new bone formation inside the demineralized bone matrices. Since then, these proteins, BMPs, have been reported as factors responsible for bone neoformation [149, 154]. BMPs attract mesenchymal cells to the site of bone formation by chemotaxis, and induces the conversion of these cells to a pre-osteoblastic lineage. BMP-2, 6 and 9 are described as important for the initiation of the differentiation of mesenchymal cells into pre-osteoblasts, while BMP-4 and 7 promote the differentiation of pre-osteoblasts into osteoblasts [155].

Clinical studies with rhBMP-2 using collagen as a carrier for surgical protocol of vertebral column showed similar or better results compared to autografts [150, 156-158]. However, the cost-effectiveness ratio of BMPs is questionable because of the large required amount (12 mg, 1.5 mg.mL^{-1} therapeutic dose of INFUSE®) to obtain an effective bone repair in comparison to conventional surgical techniques [159].

In recent years, the use of synthetic peptides has been highlighted due to the ease of recognition and binding to specific sites of the extracellular matrix proteins increasing the material-cell interaction and for do not promote an immunogenic reaction. In this context, the specific amino acid sequence Arg-Gly-Asp (RGD) of the extracellular matrix proteins, such as fibronectin and osteopontin is recognized by the transmembrane receptors (integrins) [160, 161], and promotes better adhesion, and consequently a greater proliferation of osteoblastic cells. This RGD sequence has been widely used for functionalization of biomaterials in order to stimulate the initial process of cell adhesion [162-164].

5. Cytototoxic, genotoxic and mutagenic tests of biomaterials

Biomaterials may have low, medium or high potential risk to human safety, depending on the type and extent of the patient contact. Safety assessments of medical biomaterials are guided by the toxicological guidelines recommended by the International Organization of Standardization (ISO 10993-1/EN 30993-1). One of the recommended and appropriate steps for the biological assessment of potential medical biomaterials consists of an *in vitro* evaluation of cytotoxicity and genotoxicity [165].

It is important to consider the possible impact of the composition on processes linked to cell proliferation and survival. It is essential to ensure that the proportional amounts of each component do not impoverish the cytocompatibility of the final composite, due to the release of toxic or irritating components. Therefore, *in vitro* cytotoxicity tests represent critical requirements previous to the clinical application of such materials (ISO 10993-12; [166])The choice of one or more cytotoxic tests depends on the nature of the sample to be evaluated, the potential site of use and the nature of the use (ISO 10993-5).

Cytotoxicity can be evaluated regarding the cell viability. XTT is a soluble variation of the widely employed MTT test, which accounts for mitochondrial activity in the tested material [166, 167]. Dimethyl sulfoxide solubilization of cellular-generated 3-(4,5-dimethylthiazol-2-yl)-2,5-diphenyltetrazolium bromide (MTT) - formazan presents several inherent disadvantages of this assay, including the safety hazard of personnel exposure to large quantities of dimethyl sulfoxide, the deleterious effects of this solvent on laboratory equipment, and the inefficient metabolism of MTT by some human cell lines [167, 168]. Recognition of these limitations prompted development of possible alternative microculture tetrazolium assays utilizing a different tetrazolium reagent, 2,3-bis(2-methoxy-4-nitro-5-sulfophenyl)-5-[(phenyl-amino)carbonyl]-2H-tetrazolium hydroxide (XTT), which is metabolically reduced in viable cells to a water-soluble formazan product. This reagent allows direct absorbance readings, therefore eliminating a solubilization step and shortening the microculture growth assay procedure [167]. Therefore, in XTT test mitochondrial dehydrogenase activity is measured by the ability of such enzymes to reduce the reagent XTT to soluble formazan salts, with differing color.

To evaluate cell survival, Neutral Red uptake cytotoxicity test detects membrane intact viable cells by incorporation of the dye in their lysosomes [166, 169]. It is one of the most used cytotoxicity tests with many biomedical and environmental applications and most primary cells and cell lines from diverse origin may be used [169]. The procedure is cheaper and more sensitive than other cytotoxicity tests (tetrazolium salts, enzyme leakage or protein content) [169].

Bone substitute and implant materials have been evaluated regarding cytotoxicity by different assays [166, 170-173].

It is inherent in the provision of safe medical devices that the risk of serious and irreversible effects, such as cancer or second-generation abnormalities, can be minimized to the greatest extent feasible. The assessment of mutagenic, carcinogenic and reproductive hazards is an essential component of the control of these risks (ISO 10993-3). An international standard (ISO 10993) lays down specific requirements for biocompatibility, including the tests based on the nature of the contact and the duration of implantation of the biomaterial. The standard stipulates that all materials that will be in contact with mucous, bone, or dentinal tissue if the contact exceeds 30 days, as well as all implantable devices if the contact exceeds 24h, must undergo genotoxicity testing [174].

A useful approach for assessing genotoxic activity is the single cell gel electrophoresis (SCGE) or Comet assay. Singh et al. (1988) [175] introduced a microgel technique involving electrophoresis under alkaline conditions for detecting DNA damage in single cells which led to a sensitive version of the assay that could assess both double- and single-strand DNA breaks as well as the alkali labile sites expressed as frank strand breaks in the DNA. In this technique, cells are embedded in agarose gel on microscope slides, lysed by detergents and high salt, and then electrophoresed for a short period under alkaline conditions [175]. The assay is called a comet assay because the damaged cells look like a comet under a microscope. Cells with increased DNA damage display increased migration of DNA from the nucleus toward anode [176], so it appears like a comet tail that moves away from the unbroken DNA ("comet head") (Figure 2). Cells with increased DNA damage display increased migration of DNA from the nucleus toward anode [175]. Staining with different fluorescent dyes like ethidium bromide, propidium iodide, SYBR green quantifies the migrating DNA [176]. The most flexible approach for collecting comet data involves the application of image analysis techniques to individual cells, and several software programs are commercially available [176].

Some advantages of the SCGE assay is its sensitivity for detecting low levels of DNA damage, the requirement for small numbers of cells per sample, its flexibility and the short time needed to complete a study [176].

The SCGE assay has the capability to assess an increasing genotoxicity of a biomaterial model, whatever the cause and mechanism of the genotoxicity [174].

The *in vitro* micronucleus assay is well established in the field of toxicology for screening the effects of physical and chemical agents that may damage the DNA of eukaryotic cells [177]. The micronucleus assays have emerged as one of the preferred methods for assessing chromosome damage because they enable both chromosome loss and chromosome breakage to be measured reliably [178]. Because of the uncertainty of the fate of micronuclei following more than one nuclear division it is important to identify cells that have completed one nuclear division only [178]. In the cytokinesis-block micronucleus (CBMN) assay the cytokinesis is blocked using cytochalasin-B (Cyt-B). Cyt-B is an inhibitor of actin polymerization required for the formation of the microfilament ring that constricts the cytoplasm between the daughter nuclei during cytokinesis [178].

Micronuclei (MNi) are acentric chromosome fragments or whole chromosomes that are left behind during mitotic cellular division and appear in the cytoplasm of interphase cells as small additional nuclei [179]. MNi are morphologically identical to nuclei but smaller (Figure 3). The diameter of MNi usually varies between 1/16th and 1/3rd of the mean diameter of the main nuclei [180]. The number of micronuclei in 1000 binucleated cells should be scored and the frequency of MN per 1000 binucleated cells calculated [178].

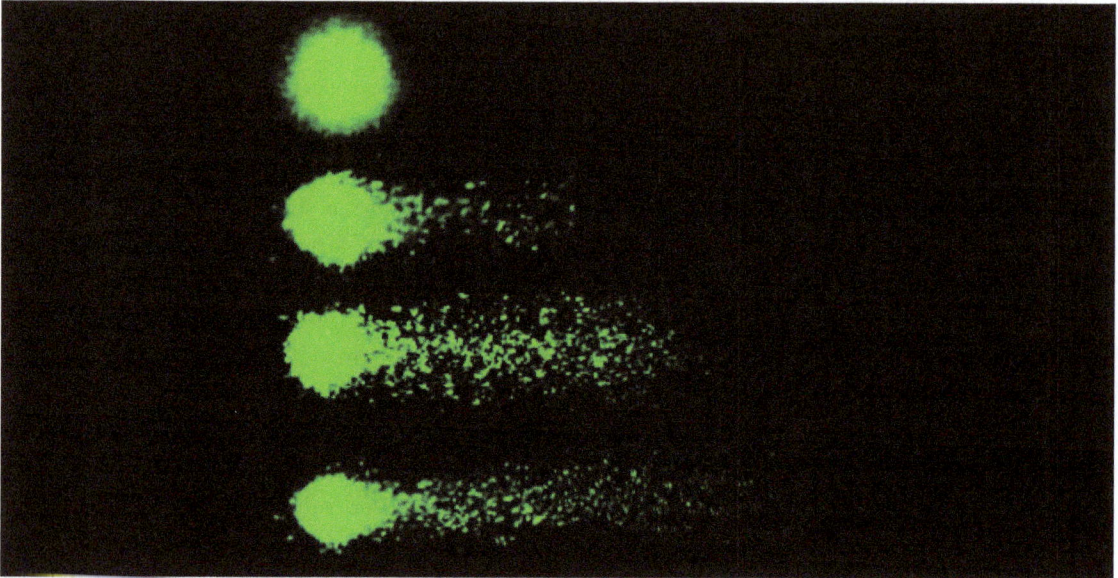

Figure 2. CHO-K1 cells exposed to different treatments. We can observe cells with different quantity of DNA damage obtained from Comet Assay. CHO-K1 cells stained by SYBR green. The cell located more superiorly presents minimal damage (about 5%) and the other cells show higher DNA damage. The longer is the tail of the "comet", the greater is the migration of damaged DNA.

Due to CBMN assay reliability and good reproducibility, it has become one of the standard cytogenetic tests for genetic toxicology tests in human and mammalian cells [180].

The measurement of nucleoplasmic bridges (NPBs), nuclear buds (NBUDs) and MNi of binucleated cells led the development of the concept of the cytokinesis-block micronucleus cytome (CBMN Cyt) assay [180]. The frequency of binucleated cells with MNi, NPBs or NBUDs provides a measure of genome damage and/or chromosomal instability. An NPB is a contin-uous DNA-containing structure linking the nuclei in a binucleated cell which originates from dicentric chromosomes (resulting from misrepaired DNA breaks or telomere end fusions) in which the centromeres are pulled to opposite poles during anaphase [180]. NBUDs represent the mechanism by which a nucleus eliminates amplified DNA and DNA repair complexes. They are similar to MNi in appearance with the exception that they are connected with the nucleus by a bridge [180]. Figure 3 shows NPB and NBUD in binucleated cells.

Since no single test has proved to be capable of detecting mammalian mutagens and carcino-gens with an acceptable level of precision and reproducibility, a battery of tests is needed (ISO 10993-3).

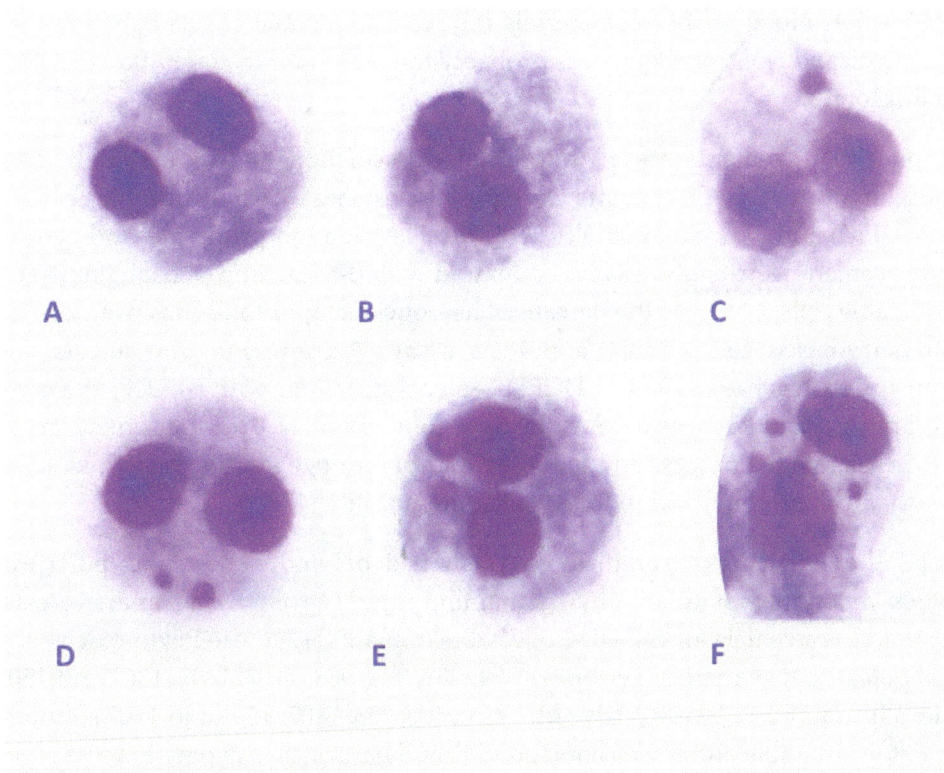

Figure 3. CHO-K1 cells after CBMN assay. We can observe binucleated cells (A, B); a binucleated cell with one micronucleus (C); a binucleated cell with two micronuclei (D); a binucleated cell with NBUDs (E); a binucleated cell with micronuclei and a NPB between the main nuclei.

5.1. Some biomaterial studies — Cytotoxic, genotoxic, mutagenic assays

Because of the low biodegradation rates of hydroxyatatite (HA), beta-tricalcium phosphate was added to HA, generating a biphasic calcium phosphate (BCP) composite, which may play an important role during assisted bone regeneration [166]. The authors [166] evaluated the cytocompatibility of dense HA, porous HA, dense BCP and porous BCP by three different cell viability parameters (XTT, Crystal Violet Dye Elution, Neutral Red assay) on human mesenchymal cells. No significant differences on mitochondrial activity (XTT) or cell density (Crystal Violet Dye Elution) were observed among groups. Dense materials induced lower levels of total viable cells by Neutral Red assay. It was concluded that porous BCP has shown better results than dense materials and these ceramics are suited for further studies [166].

Authors [165] evaluated cytotoxic, genotoxic and mutagenic effects of fluor- hydroxyapatite (FHA) and fluorapatite (FA) eluates on Chinese hamster V79 cells and compared them with the effects of hydroxyapatite (HA) eluate. The results showed that the highest test concentrations of the biomaterials (100% and 75% eluates) induced very weak inhibition of colony growth (about 10%). On the other hand, the reduction of cell number per colony induced by these concentrations was in the range from 43% to 31%. The comet assay showed that biomaterials induced DNA breaks, which increased with increasing test concentrations in the order

HA < FHA < FA. None of the biomaterials induced mutagenic effects compared with the positive control; and DNA breakage was probably the reason for the inhibition of cell division in V79 cell colonies.

Calcium phosphate cements are an important class of bone repair materials. Dicalcium phosphate dihydrate (DCPD) cements were prepared using monocalcium phosphate mono-hydrate (MCPM) and hydroxyapatite (HA) [170]. Degradation properties and cytocompati-bility of this cement were analyzed and compared with β-tricalcium phosphate (β-TCP). The percent of viable cells as well as the percent of necrotic and apoptotic ones were evaluated by flow cytometry-based cell viability/apoptosis assay. According to the results, although conversion to HA has been noted in DCPD cements prepared with β-TCP, the conversion occurred rapidly when HA was used as the base component. HA during cement preparation seemed to accelerate the process and led to a rapid pH drop, extensive mass loss, a complete loss of mechanical integrity, and reduced cytocompatibility [170].

Authors [173] evaluated poloxamines, i.e., X-shaped poly(ethylene oxide)-poly(propylene oxide) block copolymers with an ethylenediamine core (Tetronic®), as an active osteogenic component and as a vehicle for rhBMP-2 injectable implants [173]. After cytotoxicity screening of various poloxamine varieties, Tetronic® 304, 901, 904, 908, 1107, 1301, 1307 and 150R1 and poloxamer Pluronic® F127 were analyzed. Tetronic® 908, 1107, 1301 and 1307 solutions were the most cytocompatible and it was concluded that the intrinsic osteogenic activity of polox-amines offers novel perspectives for bone regeneration using minimally invasive procedures (i.e., injectable scaffolds) and overcoming the safety and the cost/effectiveness concerns associated with large scale clinical use of recombinant growth factors [173].

Recombinant human bone morphogenetic protein 2 (rhBMP-2) has been widely employed for the induction of bone growth in animal models and in clinical trials [177]. Authors [177] prepared their own rhBMP-2 and the micronucleus assay was used to evaluate the genotoxic effect of it. It was concluded that author's preparations of recombinant human BMP-2 prepared in E. coli do not promote DNA damage in the concentration range tested.

A fully crystallized bioactive glass–ceramic material (Biosilicate®) for bone repair was developed and the biocompatibility was evaluated by means of histopathological (after subcutaneous test), cytotoxic (MTT) and genotoxic analysis (Comet assay). Neonatal murine calvarial osteoblastic (OSTEO-1) and murine fibroblasts (L929) were employed in this study. The results indicated that Biosilicate® scaffolds was biocompatible and noncytotoxic and did not induce DNA strand breaks at any evaluated period [172].

Polymethyl methacrylate (PMMA) is an acrylic resin which is widely used as a biomaterial due to its excellent biocompatibility and haemocompatibility [181]. *In vitro* micronucleus (MN) induction by PMMA bone cement was analyzed in cultured human lymphocyte [181]. The results showed a highly significant increase in MN frequency in human lymphocytes treated with PMMA and consequently a genotoxic effect of this substance or of the aphorised residual ingredients, which continue to be released in small amounts from the polymer. According to the authors, after the polymerization process, small quantities of ingredients usually present in self-curing methacrylate bone cements are released and their rate of diffusion depends on storage conditions.

Titanium has been one of the most clinically applicable metals in bone tissue to serve as fracture fixation devices and also as endosseous implants for the rehabilitation of various parts of human body, especially in the oral maxillofacial region [182]. Piozzi et al. (2009) [182] evaluated whether liver, kidney, and lung of rats were particularly sensitive organs for DNA damaging (Comet assay) and cytotoxicity (histopathological changes) following implantation of internal fixture materials composed by titanium alloy in rats. No histopathological changes in cells of lung, kidney or liver were observed in the negative control group and in the experimental groups. The liver, lung and kidney cells did not show any genotoxic effects along the time course experiment. In the same way, no cytotoxic effects were present since neither tissue alterations nor signals of metals deposition were evidenced in these organs, even after 180 days of titanium exposure [182].

Metallic implants can release not only biocompatible ions but also some particles from mechanical wear or degradation. After corrosion or mechanical wear, these metal biomaterials release toxic elements such as ions or particles to the environment. Biodegradable metals seem to be the suitable material for orthopedic applications. Screws and plates made of magnesium alloys may work as stable biodegradable implants, which avoids the instance of a second operation. However, despite their use in novel technology, there is no available information about the possible toxic effects of magnesium particles (MP) from wear debris on human health [171]. Authors [171] used Mg powder to simulate the presence of MP wear debris within a cell culture and cytotoxic and genotoxic effects (comet assay and micronucleus induction) were analyzed. Neutral red (NR) incorporation and acridine orange/ethidium bromide (AO/EB) staining techniques were used to analyze the cytotoxic effects at 25–1000 µg/mL concentration range. Changes in lysosome activity were observed after 24 h only at 1000 µg/mL. Accordingly, AO/EB staining showed a significant decrease in the number of living cells at 500 µg/mL. A significant dose-dependent increase in MN frequencies was observed at 25–100 µg/mL range (nontoxic range). DNA damage induction was observed by comet assay only at 500 µg/mL. Therefore, authors verified a dose-dependent cytotoxic and genotoxic effects of MP on UMR106 cells with different threshold values of MP concentration.

6. Summary

This chapter approaches the most current bone substitute materials used in implant dentistry, as in research as in clinical application, for alveolar ridge augmentation, maxillary sinus lift and guided bone regeneration, such as: alloplastic materials (bioceramics, bioactive glasses, glass-ceramics, polymers and composites) and bioactive molecules (peptides and growth factors). In addition, concepts of tissue engineering used for the development of the new materials and techniques for implant dentistry were approached. Moreover, this chapter approached some cytotoxic, genotoxic and mutagenic assays used to evaluate the safety of biomaterials. Some studies that evaluated cytotoxicity, genotoxicity and/or mutagenicity of biomaterials were presented.

Thus, the use of bone substitutes continues to increase along with the availability of new technologies. Many alternatives for the replacement of autografts, allografts and xenografts are emerging. Rigorous preclinical and clinical studies are necessary to confirm the cost-effectiveness of these approaches over traditional bone grafts methods with benefits of technological advancement exceeding risks to the patient and costs of implantation.

Author details

Sybele Saska[1*], Larissa Souza Mendes[1], Ana Maria Minarelli Gaspar[2] and Ticiana Sidorenko de Oliveira Capote[2]

*Address all correspondence to: sybele_saska@yahoo.com.br

1 Institute of Chemistry, São Paulo State University-UNESP, Araraquara – SP, Brazil

2 Dental School at Araraquara, São Paulo State University-UNESP, Department of Morphology, Araraquara – SP, Brazil

References

[1] Li P. Biomimetic nano-apatite coating capable of promoting bone ingrowth. Journal of Biomedical Materials Research A. 2003;66:79-85.

[2] Vance RJ, Miller DC, Thapa A, Haberstroh KM, Webster TJ. Decreased fibroblast cell density on chemically degraded poly-lactic-co-glycolic acid, polyurethane, and poly-caprolactone. Biomaterials. 2004;25:2095-2103.

[3] Liu H, Webster TJ. Nanomedicine for implants: a review of studies and necessary experimental tools. Biomaterials. 2007;28:354-369.

[4] Kovaleva ES, Kuznetsov AV, Soin AV, Veresov AG, Putlyaev VI, Tret'Yakov YD. Study of materials bioactivity with the use of model media. Doklady Chemistry. 2005;405:213-216.

[5] Misch CE. Contemporary Implant Dentistry 2nd ed. St Louis: Mosby; 2006.

[6] Saska S, Barud HS, Gaspar AMM, Marchetto R, Ribeiro SJL, Messaddeq Y. Bacterial cellulose-hydroxyapatite nanocomposites for bone regeneration. International Journal of Biomaterials. 2011; doi:10.1155/2011/175362.

[7] Hing KA, Wilson LF, Buckland T. Comparative performance of three ceramic bone graft substitutes. The Spine Journal. 2007;7:475-490.

[8] Callister Jr. WD, Rethwisch DG. Materials Science and Engineering: An Introduction. 8th ed. New York: John Wiley & Sons, Inc.; 2009.

[9] Thomas MV, Puleo DA. Calcium sulfate: properties and clinical applications. Journal of Biomedical Materials Research Part B: Applied Biomaterials. 2008; 88(2):597–610.

[10] Oréfice RL, Pereira MM, Mansur HS. Biomaterais: Fundamentos & Aplicações. 1ª ed ed. Rio de Janeiro: Cultura Médica; 2006.

[11] Driessens FCM, Boltong MG, Bermudez G, Planell JA. Formulation and setting times of some calcium orthophosphate cements: A pilot study. Journal of Materials Science: Materials in Medicine. 1993;4(5):503-508.

[12] Junqueira LC, Carneiro J. Tecido ósseo. In: ed, editor. Histologia Básica. Rio de Janeiro: Guanabara Koogan; 2004.

[13] Mann S. Biomineralization: Principles and concepts in bioinorganic materials chemistry. United Kingdom: Oxford - University Press; 2005.

[14] Reikeras O, Gunderson RB. Long-term results of HA coated threaded versus HA coated hemispheric press fit cups: 287 hips followed for 11 to 16 years. Archives of Orthopaedic and Trauma Surgery. 2006;126:503-508.

[15] Le Guehennec L, Layrolle P, Daculsi G. A review of bioceramics and fibrin sealant. European Cells and Materials. 2004;8:1-10.

[16] Liu H, Webster TJ. Nanomedicine for implants: A review of studies and necessary experimental tools. Biomaterials. 2007;28(2):354-369.

[17] Chevalier J, Gremillard L. Ceramics for medical applications: A picture for the next 20 years. Journal of the European Ceramic Society. 2009;29:1245-1255.

[18] Knabe C, Berger G, Gildenhaar R, Klar F, Zreiqat H. The modulation of osteogenesis in vitro by calcium titanium phosphate coatings. Biomaterials. 2004;25:4911-4919.

[19] Kawachi EY, Bertran CA, Dos Reis RR, Alves OL. Bioceramics: Tendencies and perspectives of an interdisciplinary area. Quimica Nova. 2000;23:518-522.

[20] Peltier LF. The use of plaster of Paris to fill defects in bone. Clinical Orthopaedics Journal. 1961;21:1-31.

[21] Labourg L, Biou C. The embedding of plaster of paris in surgical cavities of the jaws. Semaine des hôpitaux. Therapeutique. 1961;37:1195-1197.

[22] Sottosanti JS. Aesthetic extractions with calcium sulfate and the principles of guided tissue regeneration. Practical Periodontics and Aesthetic Dentistry. 1993;5:61-69.

[23] Anson D. Calcium sulfate: a 4-year observation of its use as a resorbable barrier in guided tissue regeneration of periodontal defects. Compendium of Continuing Education in Dentistry. 1996;17:895-899.

[24] Vance GS, Greenwell H, Miller RL, Hill M, Johnston H, Scheetz JP. Comparison of an allograft in an experimental putty carrier and a bovine-derived xenograft used in ridge preservation: a clinical and histologic study in humans. The International Journal of Oral and Maxillofacial Implants. 2004;19:491-497.

[25] De Leonardis D, Pecora GE. Prospective study on the augmentation of the maxillary sinus with calcium sulfate: histological results. Journal of Periodontology. 2000;71:940-947.

[26] Andreana S, Cornelini R, Edsberg LE, Natiella JR. Maxillary sinus elevation for implant placement using calcium sulfate with and without DFDBA: six cases. Implant Dentistry. 2004;13:270-277.

[27] Iezzi G, Fiera E, Scarano A, Pecora G, Piattelli A. Histologic evaluation of a provisional implant retrieved from man 7 months after placement in a sinus augmented with calcium sulphate: a case report. Journal of Oral Implantology. 2007;33:89-95.

[28] Scarano A, Orsini G, Pecora G, Iezzi G, Perrotti V, Piattelli A. Peri-implant bone regeneration with calcium sulfate: a light and transmission electron microscopy case report. Implant Dentistry. 2007;16:195-203.

[29] Urban RM, Turner TM, Hall DJ, Inoue N, Gitelis S. Increased bone formation using calcium sulfate-calcium phosphate composite graft. Clinical Orthopaedics and Related Research. 2007;459:110-117.

[30] Sepulveda P, Bressiani AH, Bressiani JC, Meseguer L, Konig B, Jr. *In vivo* evaluation of hydroxyapatite foams. Journal of Biomedical Materials Research. 2002;62:587-592.

[31] Cho YR, Gosain AK. Biomaterials in craniofacial reconstruction. Clinics in Plastic Surgery. 2004; 31(3):377-385.

[32] Kveton JF, Coelho DH. Hydroxyapatite cement in temporal bone surgery: a 10 year experience. Laryngoscope. 2004;114:33-37.

[33] Nery EB, LeGeros RZ, Lynch KL, Lee K. Tissue response to biphasic calcium phosphate ceramic with different ratios of HA/beta TCP in periodontal osseous defects. Journal of Periodontology. 1992;63:729-735.

[34] Kolerman R, Goshen G, Joseph N, Kozlovsky A, Shetty S, Tal H. Histomorphometric analysis of maxillary sinus augmentation using an alloplast bone substitute. Journal of Oral and Maxillofacial Surgery. 2012;70:1835-1843.

[35] Lomelino Rde O, Castro S, II, Linhares AB, Alves GG, Santos SR, Gameiro VS, Rossi AM, Granjeiro JM. The association of human primary bone cells with biphasic calcium phosphate (betaTCP/HA 70:30) granules increases bone repair. Journal of Materials Science: Material in Medicine. 2012;23:781-788.

[36] Mangano C, Perrotti V, Shibli JA, Mangano F, Ricci L, Piattelli A, Iezzi G. Maxillary sinus grafting with biphasic calcium phosphate ceramics: clinical and histologic eval-

uation in man. The International Journal of Oral and Maxillofacial Implants. 2013;28:51-56.

[37] Mangano C, Sinjari B, Shibli JA, Mangano F, Hamisch S, Piattelli A, Perrotti V, Iezzi G. A human clinical, histological, histomorphometrical and radiographical study on biphasic HA-Beta-TCP 30/70 in maxillary sinus augmentation. Clinical Implant Dentistry and Related Research. 2013; doi: 10.1111/cid.12145.

[38] Ohayon L. Maxillary sinus floor augmentation using biphasic calcium phosphate: a histologic and histomorphometric study. The International Journal of Oral & Maxillofacial Implants. 2014;29:1143-1148.

[39] LeGeros RZ. Calcuim phophastes in oral biology and medicine. Basel: Karger; 1991.

[40] Rojbani H, Nyan M, Ohya K, Kasugai S. Evaluation of the osteoconductivity of alpha-tricalcium phosphate, beta-tricalcium phosphate, and hydroxyapatite combined with or without simvastatin in rat calvarial defect. Journal of Biomedical Materials Research A. 2011;98:488-498.

[41] Farina NM, Guzon FM, Pena ML, Cantalapiedra AG. *In vivo* behavior of two different biphasic ceramic implanted in mandibular bone of dogs. Journal of Materials Science: Materials in Medicine. 2008;19:1565-1573.

[42] Zyman Z, Glushko V, Dedukh N, Malyshkina S, Ashukina N. Porous calcium phosphate ceramic granules and their behavior in differently loaded areas of skeleton. Journal of Materials Science: Materials in Medicine. 2008;19:2197-2205.

[43] Sanda M, Shiota M, Fujii M, Kon K, Fujimori T, Kasugai S. Capability of new bone formation with a mixture of hydroxyapatite and beta-tricalcium phosphate granules. Clinical Oral Implants Research. 2014;doi: 10.1111/clr.12473.

[44] Zerbo IR, Bronckers AL, de Lange GL, van Beek GJ, Burger EH. Histology of human alveolar bone regeneration with a porous tricalcium phosphate. A report of two cases. Clinical Oral Implants Research. 2001;12:379-384.

[45] Zerbo IR, Zijderveld SA, de Boer A, Bronckers AL, de Lange G, ten Bruggenkate CM, Burger EH. Histomorphometry of human sinus floor augmentation using a porous beta-tricalcium phosphate: a prospective study. Clinical Oral Implants Research. 2004;15:724-732.

[46] Knabe C, Koch C, Rack A, Stiller M. Effect of beta-tricalcium phosphate particles with varying porosity on osteogenesis after sinus floor augmentation in humans. Biomaterials. 2008;29:2249-2258.

[47] Chappard D, Guillaume B, Mallet R, Pascaretti-Grizon F, Baslé MF, Libouban H. Sinus lift augmentation and β-TCP: A microCT and histologic analysis on human bone biopsies. Micron. 2010;41:321-326.

[48] Uckan S, Deniz K, Dayangac E, Araz K, Ozdemir BH. Early implant survival in posterior maxilla with or without beta-tricalcium phosphate sinus floor graft. Journal of Oral and Maxillofacial Surgery. 2010;68:1642-1645.

[49] Stiller M, Kluk E, Bohner M, Lopez-Heredia MA, Muller-Mai C, Knabe C. Performance of beta-tricalcium phosphate granules and putty, bone grafting materials after bilateral sinus floor augmentation in humans. Biomaterials. 2014;35:3154-3163

[50] Nemeth Z, Suba Z, Hrabak K, Barabas J, Szabo G. Autogenous bone versus beta-tricalcium phosphate graft alone for bilateral sinus elevations (2-3D CT, histologic and histomorphometric evaluations). Orvosi Hetilap. 2002;143:1533-1538.

[51] Trisi P, Rao W, Rebaudi A, Fiore P. Histologic effect of pure-phase beta-tricalcium phosphate on bone regeneration in human artificial jawbone defects. International Journal of Periodontics & Restorative Dentistry. 2003;23:69-77.

[52] Gotterbarm T, Breusch SJ, Jung M, Streich N, Wiltfang J, Berardi Vilei S, Richter W, Nitsche T. Complete subchondral bone defect regeneration with a tricalcium phosphate collagen implant and osteoinductive growth factors: a randomized controlled study in Gottingen minipigs. Journal of Biomedical Materials Research B Applied Biomaterial. 2014;102:933-942.

[53] Kato E, Lemler J, Sakurai K, Yamada M. Biodegradation property of beta-tricalcium phosphate-collagen composite in accordance with bone formation: a comparative study with Bio-Oss Collagen(R) in a rat critical-size defect model. Clinical Implant Dentistry and Related Research. 2014;16:202-211.

[54] Sohier J, Daculsi G, Sourice S, de Groot K, Layrolle P. Porous beta tricalcium phosphate scaffolds used as a BMP-2 delivery system for bone tissue engineering. Journal of Biomedical Materials Research A. 2010;92:1105-1114.

[55] Fukunaga K, Minoda Y, Iwakiri K, Iwaki H, Nakamura H, Takaoka K. Early biological fixation of porous implant coated with paste-retaining recombinant bone morphogenetic protein 2. Journal of Arthroplasty. 2012;27:143-149.

[56] Lee JH, Ryu MY, Baek HR, Lee KM, Seo JH, Lee HK, Ryu HS. Effects of porous beta-tricalcium phosphate-based ceramics used as an E. coli-derived rhBMP-2 carrier for bone regeneration. Journal of Materials Science: Materials in Medicine. 2013;24:2117-2127.

[57] Hanseler P, Ehrbar M, Kruse A, Fischer E, Schibli R, Ghayor C, Weber FE. Delivery of BMP-2 by two clinically available apatite materials: In vitro and in vivo comparison. Journal of Biomedical Materials Research A. 2014; doi: 10.1002/jbm.a.35211.

[58] Tanaka T, Kumagae Y, Chazono M, Komaki H, Kitasato S, Kakuta A, Marumo K. An Injectable Complex of beta-tricalcium Phosphate Granules, Hyaluronate, and rhFGF-2 on Repair of Long-bone Fractures with Large Fragments. The Open Biomedical Engineering Journal. 2014;8:52-59.

[59] Wang Z, Wang K, Lu X, Li M, Liu H, Xie C, Meng F, Jiang O, Li C, Zhi W. BMP-2 encapsulated polysaccharide nanoparticle modified biphasic calcium phosphate scaffolds for bone tissue regeneration. Journal of Biomedical Materials Research A. 2014; doi: 10.1002/jbm.a.35282.

[60] Dubok VA. Bioceramics - Yesterday, today, tomorrow. Powder Metallurgy and Metal Ceramics. 2000;39:381-394.

[61] Hench LL. The story of Bioglass®. Journal of Materials Science: Materials in Medicine. 2006;17:967-978.

[62] Cao W, Hench LL. Bioactive materials. Ceramics International. 1996;22:493-507.

[63] Krishnan V, Lakshmi T. Bioglass: A novel biocompatible innovation. Journal of Advanced Pharmaceutical Technology & Research. 2013;4:78-83.

[64] Thomas MV, Puleo DA, Al-Sabbagh M. Bioactive glass three decades on. Journal of Long-Term Effects of Medical Implants. 2005;15(6): 585-597.

[65] Brömer H, Pfeil E, Kos M. Ceravital® glass–ceramics for clinical use. "German Patent". No 2,326,100. (1973).

[66] Bunte M, Strunz V. Ceramic augmentation of the lower jaw. Journal of Maxillofacial Surgery. 1977;5:303-309.

[67] Reck R, Helms J. The bioactive glass ceramic Ceravital in ear surgery. Five years' experience. American Journal of Otolaryngology. 1985;6:280-283.

[68] Stanley HR, Hall MB, Colaizzi F, Clark AE. Residual alveolar ridge maintenance with a new endosseous implant material. Journal of Prosthetic Dentistry. 1987;58:607-613.

[69] Wilson J, Clark AE, Hall M, Hench LL. Tissue response to Bioglass endosseous ridge maintenance implants. Journal of Oral Implantology. 1993;19:295-302.

[70] Suzuki KR, Misch CE, Arana G, Rams TE, Suzuki JB. Long-term histopathologic evaluation of bioactive glass and human-derived graft materials in Macaca fascicularis mandibular ridge reconstruction. Implant Dentistry. 2011;20:318-322.

[71] Margonar R, Queiroz TP, Luvizuto ER, Marcantonio E, Lia RC, Holzhausen M, Marcantonio-Júnior E. Bioactive glass for alveolar ridge augmentation. Journal of Craniofacial Surgery. 2012;23:e220-222.

[72] Tadjoedin ES, de Lange GL, Holzmann PJ, Kulper L, Burger EH. Histological observations on biopsies harvested following sinus floor elevation using a bioactive glass material of narrow size range. Clinical Oral Implants Research. 2000;11:334-344.

[73] Tadjoedin ES, de Lange GL, Lyaruu DM, Kuiper L, Burger EH. High concentrations of bioactive glass material (BioGran) vs. autogenous bone for sinus floor elevation. Clin Oral Implants Res. 2002;13:428-36.

[74] Jodia K, Sadhwani BS, Parmar BS, Anchlia S, Sadhwani SB. Sinus elevation with an alloplastic material and simultaneous implant placement: a 1-stage procedure in severely atrophic maxillae. Journal of Oral and Maxillofacial Surgery. 2014;13:271-280.

[75] Karatzas S, Zavras A, Greenspan D, Amar S. Histologic observations of periodontal wound healing after treatment with PerioGlas in nonhuman primates. International Journal of Periodontics & Restorative Dentistry. 1999;19:489-499.

[76] Cancian DC, Hochuli-Vieira E, Marcantonio RA, Garcia Junior IR. Utilization of autogenous bone, bioactive glasses, and calcium phosphate cement in surgical mandibular bone defects in Cebus apella monkeys. The International Journal of Oral & Maxillofacial Implants. 2004;19:73-79.

[77] Day RM. Bioactive glass stimulates the secretion of angiogenic growth factors and angiogenesis in vitro. Tissue Engineering. 2005;11:768-777.

[78] Keshaw H, Forbes A, Day RM. Release of angiogenic growth factors from cells encapsulated in alginate beads with bioactive glass. Biomaterials. 2005;26:4171-4179.

[79] Kokubo T, Shigematsu M, Nagashima Y, Tashiro M, Yamamuro T, S H. Apatite and wollastonite-containing glass-ceramics for prosthetic application. Bulletin of the Institute for Chemical Research. 1982; 60:260-268.

[80] De Aza PN, De Aza AH, Pena P, De Aza S. Bioactive glasses and glass-ceramics. Boletin de la Sociedad Española de Cerámica y Vidrio. 2007;46:45-55.

[81] Fujita H, Iida H, Ido K, Matsuda Y, Oka M, Nakamura T. Porous apatite-wollastonite glass-ceramic as an intramedullary plug. Journal of Bone and Joint Surgery. 2000;82:614-618.

[82] Barone DTJ, Raquez JM, Dubois P. Bone-guided regeneration: from inert biomaterials to bioactive polymer (nano) composites. Polymers for Advanced Technologies. 2011;22(5): 463–475.

[83] So K, Kanatani KT, Kuroda Y, Nakamura T, Matsuda S, Akiyama H. Good short-term outcome of primary total hip arthroplasty with cementless bioactive glass ceramic bottom-coated implants: 109 hips followed for 3-9 years. Acta Orthopaedica. 2012;83:599-603.

[84] Teramoto H, Kawai A, Sugihara S, Yoshida A, Inoue H. Resorption of apatite-wollastonite containing glass-ceramic and beta-tricalcium phosphate in vivo. Acta Medica Okayama. 2005;59:201-207.

[85] Carrodeguas RG, De Aza AH, Jimenez J, De Aza PN, Pena P, López-Bravo A, De Aza S. Preparation and in vitro characterization of wollastonite doped tricalcium phosphate bioceramics. Key Engineering Materials. 2008;361-363:237-240.

[86] Carrodeguas RG, De Aza AH, De Aza PN, Baudin C, Jimenez J, Lopez-Bravo A, Pena P, De Aza S. Assessment of natural and synthetic wollastonite as source for bioceramics preparation. Journal of Biomedical Materials Research A. 2007;83:484-495.

[87] Minarelli Gaspar AM, Saska S, Carrodeguas RG, De Aza AH, Pena P, De Aza PN, De Aza S. Biological response to wollastonite doped alpha-tricalcium phosphate implants in hard and soft tissues in rats. Key Engineering Materials. 2009;396-398:7-10.

[88] Dutra Zanotto E, Ravagnani C, Peitl Filho O, Panzeri H, Guimaraes Lara EH, Peitl O, et al. Preparation of particulate and resorbable biosilicates useful for treating oral ailments e.g. dentine hypersensitivity, comprises thermal treatment of vitreous plates or frits to crystalline silicates and milling. US Patent No. 2006251737-A1.

[89] Moura J, Teixeira LN, Ravagnani C, Peitl O, Zanotto ED, Beloti MM, Panzeri H, Rosa AL, de Oliveira PT. *In vitro* osteogenesis on a highly bioactive glass-ceramic (Biosilicate®). Journal of Biomedical Materials Research - Part A. 2007;82:545-557.

[90] Siqueira RL, Zanotto ED. Biosilicate®: historical of a highly bioactive brazilian glass-ceramic. Quimica Nova. 2011;34:1231-1241.

[91] Pinto KN, Tim CR, Crovace MC, Matsumoto MA, Parizotto NA, Zanotto ED, Parizotto NA. Effects of Biosilicate® scaffolds and low-level laser therapy on the process of bone healing. Photomedicine and Laser Surgery. 2013;31:252-260.

[92] Roriz VM, Rosa AL, Peitl O, Zanotto ED, Panzeri H, de Oliveira PT. Efficacy of a bioactive glass-ceramic (Biosilicate) in the maintenance of alveolar ridges and in osseointegration of titanium implants. Clinical Oral Implants Research. 2010;21:148-155.

[93] Sacarano A, Degidi M, Iezzi G, Pecora G, Piattelli M, Orsini G, Caputi S, Perrotti V, Mangano c, Piattelli A. Maxillary sinus augmentation with different biomaterials: a comparative histologic and histomorphometric study in man. Implant Dentistry. 2006;15(2):197-207.

[94] Allegrini Jr S, Yoshimoto M, Salles MB, Kfnig Jr B. The effects of bovine BMP associated to HA in maxillary sinus lifting in rabbits. Annals of Anatomy. 2003;185:343-349.

[95] Quinones C, Hürzeler M, Schüpbach P, Kirsch A, Blum P, Caffesse RG, Strub JR. Maxillary sinus augmentation using different grafting materials and osseointegrated dental implants in monkeys. Part II. Evaluation of porous hydroxyapatite as a grafting material. Clinical Oral Implants Research. 1997; 8:487–496.

[96] Gredes T, Heinemanna F, Dominiak M, Mack H, Gedrangee T, Spassova A, Klinkec T, Kunert-Keil C. Bone substitution materials on the basis of BONITmatrix® up-regulate mRNA expression of IGF1 and Col1a1. Annals of Anatomy. 2012;194:179-184.

[97] Wikesjo, UME, Lim WH, Razi SS, Sigurdsson TJ, Lee MB, Tatakis DN, Hardwick WR. Periodontal repair in dogs: a bioabsorbable calcium carbonate coral implant enhan-

ces space provision for alveolar bone regeneration in conjunction with guided tissue regeneration. Journal of Periodontology. 2003; 74:957-964.

[98]   Contant S, Lona LL, Calado VMA. Predição do comportamento térmico de tubos compósitos através de redes neurais. Polímeros: Ciência e Tecnologia. 2004;14:295-300.

[99]   Honda Y, Kamakura S, Sasaki K, Suzuki O. Formation of bone-like apatite enhanced by hydrolysis of octacalcium phosphate crystals deposited in collagen matrix. Journal of Biomedical Materials Research B Applied Biomaterial. 2007;80:281-289.

[100] Hutchens SA, Benson RS, Evans BR, Rawn CJ, O'Neill H. A resorbable calcium-deficient hydroxyapatite hydrogel composite for osseous regeneration. Cellulose. 2009;16:887-898.

[101] Song JH, Kim HE, Kim HW. Collagen-apatite nanocomposite membranes for guided bone regeneration. Journal of Biomedical Materials Research - Part B Applied Biomaterials. 2007;83:248-257.

[102] Wiegand C, Elsner P, Hipler UC, Klemm D. Protease and ROS activities influenced by a composite of bacterial cellulose and collagen type I in vitro. Cellulose. 2006;13:689-696.

[103] Zhang LJ, Feng XS, Liu HG, Qian DJ, Zhang L, Yu XL, Cui FZ. Hydroxyapatite/collagen composite materials formation in simulated body fluid environment. Materials Letters. 2004;58:719-722.

[104] Chen GQ, Wu Q. The application of polyhydroxyalkanoates as tissue engineering materials. Biomaterials. 2005;26(33):6565-6578.

[105] Yu H, Matthew HW, Wooley PH, Yang SY. Effect of porosity and pore size on microstructures and mechanical properties of poly-epsilon-caprolactone- hydroxyapatite composites. Journal of Biomedical Materials Research B Applied Biomaterial. 2008;86B:541-547.

[106] Cardoso GBC, Ramos ACD, Higa OZ, Zavaglia CAC, Arruda ACF. Scaffolds of poly(caprolactone) with whiskers of hydroxyapatite. Journal of Materials Science. 2010;45:4990-4993.

[107] Polo-Corrales L, Latorre-Esteves M, Ramirez-Vick JE. Scaffold design for bone regeneration. Journal of Nanoscience and Nanotechnology. 2014;14:15-56.

[108] Bosch C, Melsen B, Vargervik K. Guided bone regeneration in calvarial bone defects using polytetrafluoroethylene membranes. The Cleft Palate-Craniofacial Journal. 1995;32:311-317.

[109] Kay SA, Wisner-Lynch L, Marxer M, Lynch SE. Guided bone regeneration: integration of a resorbable membrane and a bone graft material. Practical Periodontics and Aesthetic Dentistry 1997;9:185-194.

[110] Strietzel FP, Khongkhunthian P, Khattiya R, Patchanee P, Reichart PA. Healing pattern of bone defects covered by different membrane types - a histologic study in the porcine mandible. Journal of Biomedical Materials Research, Part B: Applied Biomaterials. 2006;78B:35-46.

[111] Chen ST, Darby IB, Adams GG, Reynolds EC. A prospective clinical study of bone augmentation techniques at immediate implants. Clinical Oral Implants Research. 2005;16:176-184.

[112] Van der Zee E, Oosterveld P, Van Waas MAJ. Effect of GBR and fixture installation on gingiva and bone levels at adjacent teeth. Clinical Oral Implants Research. 2004;15:62-65.

[113] Duskova M, Leamerova E, Sosna B, Gojis O. Guided tissue regeneration, barrier membranes and reconstruction of the cleft maxillary alveolus. Journal of Craniofacial Surgery. 2006;17(6):1153-1160.

[114] Mizuno M, Shindo M, Kobayashi D, Tsuruga E, Amemiya A, Kuboki Y. Osteogenesis by bone marrow stromal cells maintained on type I collagen matrix gels in vivo. Bone. 1997;20(2):101-107.

[115] Hürzeler MB, Kohal RJ, Naghshbandi J, Mota LF, Conradt J, Hutmacher D, Caffesse RG. Evaluation of a new bioresorbable barrier to facilitate guided bone regeneration around exposed implant threads. An experimental study in the monkey. International Journal of Oral and Maxillofacial Surgery. 1998;27:315-320.

[116] Coïc M, Placet V, Jacquet E, Meyer C. Mechanical properties of collagen membranes used in guided bone regeneration: A comparative study of three models. Propriétés Mécaniques des Membranes de Collagne. 2010;111:286-290.

[117] Forti FL, Bet MR, Goissis G, Plepis AMG. 1,4-Dioxane enhances properties and biocompatibility of polyanionic collagen for tissue engineering applications. Journal of Materials Science: Materials in Medicine. 2011;22(8):1-12.

[118] Rodrigues FT, Martins VCA, Plepis AMG. Porcine skin as a source of biodegradable matrices: Alkaline treatment and glutaraldehyde crosslinking. Polimeros. 2010;20:92-97.

[119] Charulatha V, Rajaram A. Influence of different crosslinking treatments on the physical properties of collagen membranes. Biomaterials. 2003;24:759-767.

[120] Goissis G, Piccirili L, Goes JC, Plepis AMDG, Das-Gupta DK. Anionic collagen: Polymer composites with improved dielectric and rheological properties. Artificial Organs. 1998;22:203-209.

[121] Yunoki S, Nagai N, Suzuki T, Munekata M. Novel biomaterial from reinforced salmon collagen gel prepared by fibril formation and cross-linking. Journal of Bioscience and Bioengineering. 2004;98:40-47.

[122] Park SN, Park JC, Kim HO, Song MJ, Suh H. Characterization of porous collagen/ hyaluronic acid scaffold modified by 1-ethyl-3-(3-dimethylaminopropyl)carbodiimide cross-linking. Biomaterials. 2002;23:1205-1212.

[123] Juodzbalys G, Raustia AM, Kubilius R. A 5-year follow-up study on one-stage implants inserted concomitantly with localized alveolar ridge augmentation. Journal of Oral Rehabilitation. 2007;34:781-789.

[124] Urban IA, Nagursky H, Lozada JL, Nagy K. Horizontal ridge augmentation with a collagen membrane and a combination of particulated autogenous bone and anorganic bovine bone-derived mineral: a prospective case series in 25 patients. The International Journal of Periodontics & Restorative Dentistry. 2013;33:299-307.

[125] Ella B, Laurentjoye M, Sedarat C, Coutant JC, Masson E, Rouas A. Mandibular ridge expansion using a horizontal bone-splitting technique and synthetic bone substitute: an alternative to bone block grafting? The International journal of oral & maxillofacial implants. 2014;29:135-140.

[126] Pang C, Ding Y, Zhou H, Qin R, Hou R, Zhang G, et al. Alveolar ridge preservation with deproteinized bovine bone graft and collagen membrane and delayed implants. Journal of Craniofacial Surgery. 2014; 25:1698-1702

[127] Caporali EH, Rahal SC, Morceli J, Taga R, Granjeiro JM, Cestari TM, Mamprim MJ, Correa MA. Assessment of bovine biomaterials containing bone morphogenetic proteins bound to absorbable hydroxyapatite in rabbit segmental bone defects. The Journal Acta Cirurgica Brasileira. 2006;21: 366-373.

[128] Langer R, Vacanti JP. Tissue engineering. Science. 1993;260:920-926.

[129] Klein M, Glatzer C. Individual CAD/CAM fabricated glass-bioceramic implants in reconstructive surgery of the bony orbital floor. Plastic and Reconstructive Surgery. 2006;117:565-570.

[130] Li L, Bao CY, Ou GM, Chen WC, Zhang XJ, Yang DJ, et al. Guiding bone regeneration with a novel biodegradable polymeric membrane and bioceramic bone grafts around dental implants. Key Engineering Materials. 2007;330-332:1417-1420.

[131] Marx RE. Applications of Tissue Engineering: Principles to Clinical Practice. In: Lynch SE, Marx RE, Nevins M, Wisner-Lynch LA, editors. Tissue Engineering - Applications in Oral and Maxillofacial Surgery and Periodontics. second ed. Chicago: Quintessence Publishing Co; 2008. p. 47-63.

[132] Estes BT, Gimble JM, Guilak F. Mechanical signals as regulators of stem cell fate. Current Topics in Developmental Biology. 2004;60:91-126.

[133] Karageorgiou V, Kaplan D. Porosity of 3D biomaterial scaffolds and osteogenesis. Biomaterials. 2005;26:5474-5491.

[134] Park S, Kim G, Jeon YC, Koh Y, Kim W. 3D polycaprolactone scaffolds with controlled pore structure using a rapid prototyping system. Journal of Materials Science: Materials in Medicine. 2009;20:229-234.

[135] Bose S, Vahabzadeh S, Bandyopadhyay A. Bone tissue engineering using 3D printing. Materials Today. 2013;16:496-504.

[136] Utela B, Storti D, Anderson R, Ganter M. A review of process development steps for new material systems in three dimensional printing (3DP). Journal of Manufacturing Processes. 2008;10:96-104.

[137] Torres J, Tamimi F, Alkhraisat MH, Prados-Frutos JC, Rastikerdar E, Gbureck U, et al. Vertical bone augmentation with 3D-synthetic monetite blocks in the rabbit calvaria. Journal of Clinical Periodontology. 2011;38:1147-1153.

[138] Tamimi F, Torres J, Al-Abedalla K, Lopez-Cabarcos E, Alkhraisat MH, Bassett DC, et al. Osseointegration of dental implants in 3D-printed synthetic onlay grafts customized according to bone metabolic activity in recipient site. Biomaterials. 2014;35:5436-5445.

[139] Habibovic P, Gbureck U, Doillon CJ, Bassett DC, van Blitterswijk CA, Barralet JE. Osteoconduction and osteoinduction of low-temperature 3D printed bioceramic implants. Biomaterials. 2008;29:944-953.

[140] Li J, Hsu Y, Luo E, Khadka A, Hu J. Computer-aided design and manufacturing and rapid prototyped nanoscale hydroxyapatite/polyamide (n-HA/PA) construction for condylar defect caused by mandibular angle ostectomy. Aesthetic Plastic Surgery. 2011;35:636-640.

[141] Ge Z, Tian X, Heng BC, Fan V, Yeo JF, Cao T. Histological evaluation of osteogenesis of 3D-printed poly-lactic-co-glycolic acid (PLGA) scaffolds in a rabbit model. Biomedical materials. 2009;4:021001.

[142] Shim JH, Kim SE, Park JY, Kundu J, Kim SW, Kang SS, et al. Three-dimensional printing of rhBMP-2-loaded scaffolds with long-term delivery for enhanced bone regeneration in a rabbit diaphyseal defect. Tissue Engineering - Part A. 2014;20:1980-1992.

[143] Tarafder S, Bose S. Polycaprolactone-coated 3D printed tricalcium phosphate scaffolds for bone tissue engineering: In vitro alendronate release behavior and local delivery effect on in vivo osteogenesis. ACS Applied Materials and Interfaces. 2014;6:9955-9965.

[144] Amadei SU, Silveira VAS, Pereira AC, Carvalho YR, da Rocha RF. Influência da deficiência estrogênica no processo de remodelação e reparação óssea. Journal Brasileiro de Patologia e Medicina Laboratorial. 2006;42:5 -12.

[145] Tsiridis E, Upadhyay N, Giannoudis P. Molecular aspects of fracture healing: which are the important molecules? Injury. 2007;38(1):S11-25.

[146] Assoian RK, Komoriya A, Meyers CA, Miller DM, Sporn MB. Transforming growth factor-beta in human platelets. Identification of a major storage site, purification, and characterization. The Journal of Biological Chemistry. 1983;258:7155-7160.

[147] Bielby R, Jones E, McGonagle D. The role of mesenchymal stem cells in maintenance and repair of bone. Injury. 2007;38(1):S26-32.

[148] Cho TJ, Gerstenfeld LC, Einhorn TA. Differential temporal expression of members of the transforming growth factor beta superfamily during murine fracture healing. Journal of Bone and Mineral Research. 2002;17:513-20.

[149] Eppley BL, Pietrzak WS, Blanton MW. Allograft and alloplastic bone substitutes: a review of science and technology for the craniomaxillofacial surgeon. Journal of Craniofacial Surgery. 2005; 16(6):981-989.

[150] Singh K, Smucker JD, Gill S, Boden SD. Use of recombinant human bone morphogenetic protein-2 as an adjunct in posterolateral lumbar spine fusion: a prospective CT-scan analysis at one and two years. Journal of Spinal Disorders & Techniques. 2006;19: 416-423.

[151] Jung UW, Choi SY, Pang EK, Kim CS, Choi SH, Cho KS. The effect of varying the particle size of beta tricalcium phosphate carrier of recombinant human bone morphogenetic protein-4 on bone formation in rat calvarial defects. Journal of Periodontology. 2006;77:765-772.

[152] Pang EK, Im SU, Kim CS, Choi SH, Chai JK, Kim CK, Han SB, Cho KS. Effect of recombinant human bone morphogenetic protein-4 dose on bone formation in a rat calvarial defect model. Journal of Periodontology. 2004;75:1364-1370.

[153] Urist MR. Bone: Formation by autoinduction. Science. 1965;150:893-899.

[154] Veillette CJ, McKee MD. Growth factors - BMPs, DBMs, and buffy coat products: are there any proven differences amongst them? Injury. 2007;38:S38-48.

[155] Chen H, Jiang W, Phillips FM, Haydon RC, Peng Y, Zhou L, Luu HH, An N, Breyer B, Vanichakarn P, Szatkowski JP, Park JY, He TC. Osteogenic activity of the fourteen types of human bone morphogenetic proteins (BMPs). The Journal of Bone and Joint Surgery. 2003;85:1544-1552.

[156] Boden SD, Zdeblick TA, Sandhu HS, Heim SE. The use of rhBMP-2 in interbody fusion cages. Definitive evidence of osteoinduction in humans: a preliminary report. Spine. 2000;25:376-381.

[157] Boden SD, Kang J, Sandhu H, Heller JG. Use of recombinant human bone morphogenetic protein-2 to achieve posterolateral lumbar spine fusion in humans: a prospective, randomized clinical pilot trial. Spine. 2002;27:2662-2673.

[158] Glassman SD, Carreon LY, Djurasovic M, Campbell MJ, Puno RM, Johnson JR, Dimar JR. RhBMP-2 versus iliac crest bone graft for lumbar spine fusion: a randomized, controlled trial in patients over sixty years of age. Spine. 2008;36:2843-2849.

[159] Epstein NE. Pros, cons, and costs of INFUSE in spinal surgery. Surgical Neurology International. 2011;2:10. doi: 10.4103/2152-7806.76147

[160] Olivier V, Faucheux N, Hardouin P. Biomaterial challenges and approaches to stem cell use in bone reconstructive surgery. Drug Discovery Today. 2004;9:803-811.

[161] Kim TI, Jang JH, Kim HW, Knowles JC, Ku Y. Biomimetic approach to dental implants. Current Pharmaceutical Design. 2008;14:2201-2211.

[162] Fink H, Ahrenstedt L, Bodin A, Brumer H, Gatenholm P, Krettek A, Risberg B. Bacterial cellulose modified with xyloglucan bearing the adhesion peptide RGD promotes endothelial cell adhesion and metabolism--a promising modification for vascular grafts. Journal of Tissue Engineering and Regenerative Medicine. 2011;5:454-463.

[163] Jung HJ, Ahn KD, Han DK, Ahn DJ. Surface characteristics and fibroblast adhesion behavior off RGD-immobilized biodegradable PLLA films. Macromolecular Research. 2005;13:446-452.

[164] Hu Y, Winn SR, Krajbich I, Hollinger JO. Porous polymer scaffolds surface-modified with arginine-glycine-aspartic acid enhance bone cell attachment and differentiation *in vitro*. Journal of Biomedical Materials Research A. 2003;64:583-590.

[165] Jantova S, Theiszova M, Letasiova S, Birosova L, Palou TM. *In vitro* effects of fluorhydroxyapatite, fluorapatite and hydroxyapatite on colony formation, DNA damage and mutagenicity. Mutation Research. 2008;652:139-144.

[166] Mitri F, Alves G, Fernandes G, Konig B, Rossi AJ, Granjeiro J. Cytocompatibility of porous biphasic calcium phosphate granules with human mesenchymal cells by a multiparametric assay. Artificial Organs. 2012;36:535-542.

[167] Scudiero DA, Shoemaker RH, Paull KD, Monks A, Tierney S, Nofziger TH, et al. Evaluation of a soluble tetrazolium/formazan assay for cell growth and drug sensitivity in culture using human and other tumor cell lines. Cancer Research. 1988;48:4827-4833.

[168] Alley MC, Scudiero DA, Monks A, Hursey ML, Czerwinski MJ, Fine DL, et al. Feasibility of drug screening with panels of human tumor cell lines using a microculture tetrazolium assay. Cancer Research. 1988;48:589-601.

[169] Repetto G, del Peso A, Zurita JL. Neutral red uptake assay for the estimation of cell viability/cytotoxicity. Nature Protocols. 2008;3:1125-1131.

[170] Alge DL, Goebel WS, Chu TM. In vitro degradation and cytocompatibility of dicalcium phosphate dihydrate cements prepared using the monocalcium phosphate monohydrate/hydroxyapatite system reveals rapid conversion to HA as a key

mechanism. Journal of biomedical materials research Part B, Applied biomaterials. 2012;100:595-602.

[171] Di Virgilio AL, Reigosa M, de Mele MF. Biocompatibility of magnesium particles evaluated by in vitro cytotoxicity and genotoxicity assays. Journal of Biomedical Materials Research Part B, Applied biomaterials. 2011;99:111-119.

[172] Kido HW, Oliveira P, Parizotto NA, Crovace MC, Zanotto ED, Peitl-Filho O, et al. Histopathological, cytotoxicity and genotoxicity evaluation of Biosilicate(R) glass-ceramic scaffolds. Journal of Biomedical Materials Research A. 2013;101:667-673.

[173] Rey-Rico A, Silva M, Couceiro J, Concheiro A, Alvarez-Lorenzo C. Osteogenic efficiency of in situ gelling poloxamine systems with and without bone morphogenetic protein-2. European Cells and Materials Journal. 2011;21:317-340.

[174] Chauvel-Lebret DJ, Auroy P, Tricot-Doleux S, Bonnaure-Mallet M. Evaluation of the capacity of the SCGE assay to assess the genotoxicity of biomaterials. Biomaterials. 2001;22:1795-1801.

[175] Singh NP, McCoy MT, Tice RR, Schneider EL. A simple technique for quantitation of low levels of DNA damage in individual cells. Experimental Cell Research. 1988;175:184-191.

[176] Tice RR, Agurell E, Anderson D, Burlinson B, Hartmann A, Kobayashi H, et al. Single cell gel/comet assay: guidelines for in vitro and in vivo genetic toxicology testing. Environmental and Molecular Mutagenesis. 2000;35:206-221.

[177] Rumpf HM, Dopp E, Rettenmeier AW, Chatzinikolaidou M, Jennissen HP. Absence of genotoxic effects after exposure of mammalian cells to the recombinant human bone morphogenetic protein 2 (BMP-2) prepared from E. coli. Materialwiss Werkst. 2003;34:1101-1105.

[178] Fenech M. The in vitro micronucleus technique. Mutation Research. 2000;455:81-95.

[179] Surralles J, Xamena N, Creus A, Catalan J, Norppa H, Marcos R. Induction of micronuclei by five pyrethroid insecticides in whole-blood and isolated human lymphocyte cultures. Mutation Research. 1995;341:169-184.

[180] Fenech M. Cytokinesis-block micronucleus cytome assay. Nature Protocols. 2007;2:1084-1104.

[181] Bigatti MP, Lamberti L, Rizzi FP, Cannas M, Allasia G. In vitro micronucleus induction by polymethyl methacrylate bone cement in cultured human lymphocytes. Mutation Research. 1994;321:133-137.

[182] Piozzi R, Ribeiro DA, Padovan LEM, Filho HN, Matsumoto MA. Genotoxicity and cytotoxicity in multiple organs induced by titanium miniplates in Wistar rats. Journal of Biomedical Material Research A. 2009;88A:342-347.

6

Minimally Invasive Implant Treatment Alternatives for the Edentulous Patient — Fast & Fixed and Implant Overdentures

Elena Preoteasa, Laurentiu Iulian Florica,
Florian Obadan, Marina Imre and
Cristina Teodora Preoteasa

1. Introduction

Edentulism, defined as the loss of all natural teeth, is a severe chronic irreversible medical condition that associates extensive oral changes and has a negative impact on general health, psychological comfort, social functioning and on the overall quality of life. Despite the efforts made, edentulism still has a high prevalence, about 7 to 69% in the adult population worldwide, projections displaying a high rate of occurrence in the next decades, especially in the elderly population [1,2].

The most common treatment option for complete edentulism is still the conventional complete denture, an alternative which rather often does not fulfill patients' needs and is regarded as having multiple shortcomings, mainly in relation to its instability. The use of implant prostheses, fixed or removable, provides a better treatment outcome, with a significant improvement of oral function and quality of life [3].

Implant prosthesis in edentulous patients, despite their increasing use, still register low prevalence, which is most probably linked to oral, systemic and social factors. Frequently, the edentulous patients are elderly and face barriers to treatment access (e.g., limited financial means, transportation difficulties, communication problems linked to loss of hearing or visual acuity) [4,5]. They show less willingness to accept complex treatment options, with major surgical interventions, such as bone grafting, or sometimes even implant placement. Often elderly have systemic comorbidities that are sometimes risk factors for developing complications. Considering the previous, simpler treatments with high predictability and easy main-tenance procedures are preferred.

Despite these factors that limit usage of implant prosthetic rehabilitations in edentulous patients, due to their better treatment outcome compared to conventional dentures or root overdentures, in the future most likely they will be standard treatment options widely used. Supporting the previous, McGill consensus states that two-implant overdenture is the minimum standard of care for mandibular edentulism, taking into account performance, patient satisfaction, cost and clinical time [6]. Implant use for prosthetic rehabilitation will probably increase over time in relation to the advancement of research and technology in the dental field, combined with decrease of the implant treatment costs and increase of the acceptance for this treatment option by the general public.

Out of the variety of implant prosthetic options that can be used, the minimally invasive implant treatment alternatives may be more appropriate for the aged edentulous patients, considering their oral and systemic status, needs, expectations and barriers [7-9]. Usage of fewer and less invasive surgical procedures (e.g., avoiding bone grafting; using flapless technique for implant placement; using a reduced number of implants) is beneficial due to a shorter healing period and a decreased patient discomfort, represented by either pain or stress [10]. Additionally, the possibility of immediate implant loading with the regain of function-ality, the decreased clinical time needed for their execution and the relatively moderate treatment burden are all positive aspects that should be considered [11-13].

Subsequently, two minimally invasive implant treatment options for the edentulous patient, one fixed, namely Sky Fast & Fixed (concept derived from All-on-4), and one removable, namely implant overdentures, will be presented. These are perceived as being minimally invasive compared to other implant treatment options, with regards to the limited surgical interventions (they usually don't require bone grafting; a reduced number of implants are placed; when appropriate, flapless technique is used) and reduced clinical time, favoring rapid healing and functionality regaining through immediate implant loading. Both fixed and removable treatment option were chosen considering patient's needs and expectations. Therefore, fixed prosthetic restorations are more appropriate for younger patients, who usually don't easily accept removable prosthesis, and have better dexterity that is needed in order to properly maintain the oral hygiene. The implant overdentures are more appropriate for older edentulous patients, especially for the ones dissatisfied with the conventional dentures, ensuring a satisfying performance and esthetic rehabilitation, requiring simpler procedures for oral hygiene maintenance [14].

2. SKY Fast & Fixed — Fixed-prosthetic implant restoration

General presentation. Sky Fast & Fixed defines an option of immediate fixed-prosthetic implant restoration for complete edentulism, with specific protocol and materials, developed by Bredent Medical (Senden, Germany). Basically, this treatment concept is derived from All-on-4 and All-on-6 concepts, previously developed by Professor Paulo Malo, together with

Nobel Biocare (Göteborg, Sweden) [15-17]. Sky Fast & Fixed differs mainly through the particularities of the system components, such as implant and abutment design.

The main characteristics of Sky Fast & Fixed treatment concept are presented below:

- It is designed for complete edentulism, as current or imminent condition.

- It can be applied in one or both jaws.

- This treatment concept uses 6 implants in the maxilla and 4 implants in the mandible. The distal implants are placed tilted, and the other implants are placed axial. Placement of the distal implants tilted is due to several aspects. It associates a decrease of clinical time and number of appointments, through avoiding extensive bone grafting, frequently needed in the posterior area of the jaws in order to have sufficient bone for implant placement and to avoid maxillary sinus or the inferior alveolar nerve injury. An increase of the prosthesis' implant bearing area occurs-as prosthesis' dental arch length, that reduces the need of using cantilever extremities, and as the occlusal tooth-surface areas that ensures good load distribution to the dental arch. Tilted position of the distal implants associates an increase of the osseointegration surface and using longer implants favors a good primary stability [18,19].

- A rigid fixed provisional prosthesis, without cantilever extensions, is used through immediate implant loading. Therefore, for the dentate patients, edentulism treated by removable prosthesis can be avoided-teeth extraction, implant placement and provisional prosthesis are done during one appointment. The prosthesis is usually designed as a shortened dental arch, comprising the anterior teeth and the premolars.

- A rigid fixed prosthesis that splints the implants, provides cross arch stabilization, designed with or without cantilever extensions, is used for definitive restoration [20]. Usually it is designed as a shortened dental arch, comprising the anterior teeth, the premolars and the first molars.

- Treatment implementation requires a well-trained team, with knowledge of the treatment concept that must include a dentist with clinical experience in prosthodontics and implantology, and a dental technician.

- Sky Fast & Fixed implies the use of some specific materials, components and instruments of Bredent Medical, some of them developed especially for this concept, such as the implants and the abutments. The distal implants that are meant to be placed tilted are designed with length of 14 or 16 mm and diameters over 4 mm. The axial implants should have a length of at least 10 mm and a diameter over 3.5mm. For implant divergence, compensation abutments are designed with angulations of 0°, 17.5° and 35°, and an outer cone of 17.5° Also, the abutments have an unique platform of 4mm and are designed for variable gingiva heights, from 0.9 mm to 3.6 mm.

- Ensures a simpler and fast oral rehabilitation, with limited surgical procedures performed during one single appointment and with reduced costs, compared to conventional fixed-prosthetic implant restorations.

Time sequence of the main phases of Sky Fast & Fixed can be observed in figure 1.

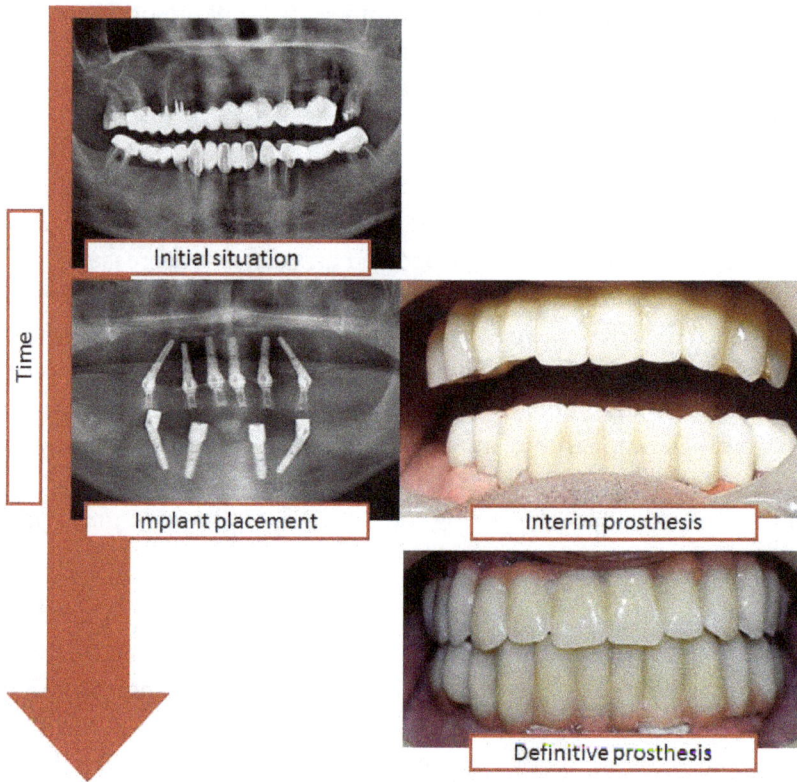

Figure 1. Sky Fast & Fixed – time sequence of the main treatment phases

Clinical phases. Sky Fast & Fixed is implemented following the regular steps of fixed-prosthetic implant restorations, with some specific aspects related to this concept and to patient features. Some of the aspects that should be accounted in treatment planning are synthetized in table 1, followed by a more detailed presentation.

Patient evaluation should comprise information regarding the oral and systemic health, considering anatomical and functional aspects, in order to accurately collect diagnostic data, essential for treatment planning and execution.

Oral examination must consider, among others, the initial dental condition (as dentulous or edentulous), maxillomandibular relationship, the vertical interarch space (restorative space), bone features (quality, quantity, anatomical limitations) and plaque control. Dentate patients, compared to the edentulous ones, present an increased treatment time, linked to the procedures performed previous to implant placement (teeth extraction, bone leveling, removal of infected tissue), that may have specific complications. Even so, it may be a more favorable clinical situation considering implants associate a reduction of bone resorption, it is possible to register the maxillomandibular relationship and identify some of the patient's natural esthetic particularities. In edentulous patients, severity of bone resorption and its consequen-

Diagnostic procedures	• oral and systemic health assessment • facial esthetic evaluation • analyze of radiographs and computed tomography • wax-up • informed consent
Preoperative interventions and instructions	• instruction and motivation on maintaining a proper oral hygiene (antibacterial mouthwash, such as Chlorhexidine 0.12%, is recommended) • record of maxillomandibular relations and occlusion • impression used for fabricating the provisional prosthesis • surgical template (guide) • medication - antibiotics (amoxicillin with clavulanic acid, administered for 5-7 days, starting 1 hour prior to surgical intervention) and sometimes sedatives
Anesthesia	• local anesthesia is usually required
Preprosthetic surgery	• teeth extraction, bone leveling, removal of infected tissue • alveolectomy, when ridge crest is displayed during smiling • bone grafting procedures
Implant placement	• implant number, position and design (diameter, length) • usually, first the mesial implants are placed and last the distal implants • exposure of implant site - flap or flapless technique
Additional surgical procedures	• bone grafting (socket grafting; with autograft and synthetic alternatives; with or without membrane) • suture
Interim prosthesis	• abutments selection (angulation) • impression and record of maxillomandibular relationship • design - dental arch length (number of teeth) • materials – as acrylic or Visio.lign
Postoperative instructions	• radiological exam • instructions for oral hygiene, diet (soft diet, for at least 10 weeks) and medication (antibiotics, analgesic drugs) • informing about the need to make an appointment if bleeding, pain, implant mobility, detachment or damage of the prosthesis occur • establishing the next appointment
Definitive prosthesis	• design – dental arch length (number of teeth, usage of cantilever extremities); occlusion scheme; fixation type, as occlusal screw-retained • materials
Maintenance	• regular check-ups • addressing complications

Table 1. Main coordinates of the clinical interventions of Sky Fast & Fixed

ces (e.g., deficient lip support), particularities of maxillomandibular relationship are important to be correctly acknowledged in order to obtain an aesthetic and functional outcome. Additionally to alveolar ridge particularities (bone width, vertical ridge orientation and aspect of the surface-uniform or with irregularities), the characteristics of the mucosa, such as resilience and amount of keratinized mucosa, may be decision-factors for using either a flap or a flapless technique for implant placement. In dentate patients, registration of maxillomandibular relations for the implant prosthesis can be eased by initial records or preservation of posterior occluding teeth. Bone assessment is essential for establishing if this treatment option is viable, and if it is, it's very important for treatment planning, as for deciding upon implant number, position and design (diameter and length). In this respect, a quantitative and qualitative bone evaluation is required, which includes aspects like ridge width, ridge height, anatomical limitations and bone density, additional to panoramic radiographies, computed tomography being highly recommended. Considering that oral hygiene is an important prognosis factor for all implant prosthesis, patient's behavior in this respect should be assessed and deficiencies of it addressed by mechanisms as awareness, motivation and training.

Facial appearance with this type of prosthetic restoration must be assessed and predicted, in order to provide an adequate esthetic result. The analysis should start with the evaluation of initial situation (natural teeth or prosthetic rehabilitation), acknowledging also patient's perception and preferences. Difficulties in this regard are mainly found in edentulous patients that have severe facial changes related to tooth loss and bone resorption, especially in the maxilla due to the centripetal bone resorption. Assessment of facial and lip support can be done comparing the facial appearance with and without the dentures or using a wax try-in without the buccal flange [21]. In patients with severe ridge resorption, if between the ideal artificial teeth location and the ridge there is an increased sagittal discrepancy, in order to obtain a satisfactory esthetic outcome, a removable denture with a buccal flange may be more appropriate. For a natural appearance, vertical bone loss is addressed also through the use of pink acrylic or ceramic.

Implementing this treatment concept should be done in patients with good overall health, considering the inherent risks of the surgical intervention, but also the considerable physical and psychological stress related to the increased number of clinical procedures done in only one day. Therefore, acknowledgement of patient general health status is needed and constant monitoring of the blood pressure and pulse rate in the dental office is recommended.

The surgical phase mainly comprises preprosthetic procedures and implants placement.

Preprosthetic surgery aims to obtain optimal conditions for implant placement and for the prosthetic reconstruction (Figure 2). Teeth extraction and related interventions, alveolectomy, bone grafting, excision of hyperplasic lesions and bone leveling may be included.

Implant placement may be done using a flap or flapless technique. Flap technique is usually selected, due to the better assessment of available bone and thickness of the crestal area, but flapless surgery has also numerous advantages related to preservations of circulation and bone tissue volume at implant site, decrease of surgical time and accelerated healing [22]. In edentulous patients that do not require preprosthetic surgery and a flapless technique is used, the interim prosthesis can be done prior to the surgical phase, and minor adjustment are needed, contributing to a considerable decrease of the clinical time.

Implant placement should be done according to the treatment plan; for a more accurate position a surgical template can be used. Usually, the axial implants are placed first (Figure

3), and then the tilted ones (Figure 4). For verifying implant angulation, parallelizing pins can be used.

Immediate implant loading requires a good primary stability for achieving a successful osseointegration. This is related to multiple factors, such as bone density, implant diameter and length and insertion torque of 45 N cm or more. Using the long titled implants favors a good primary stability due to the fact that they follow a dense bone structure-the anterior wall of the sinus [23].

After the selected abutments are placed, the sutures follow. Therefore, there is no need for another surgical phase, as there is in the case of using healing abutments.

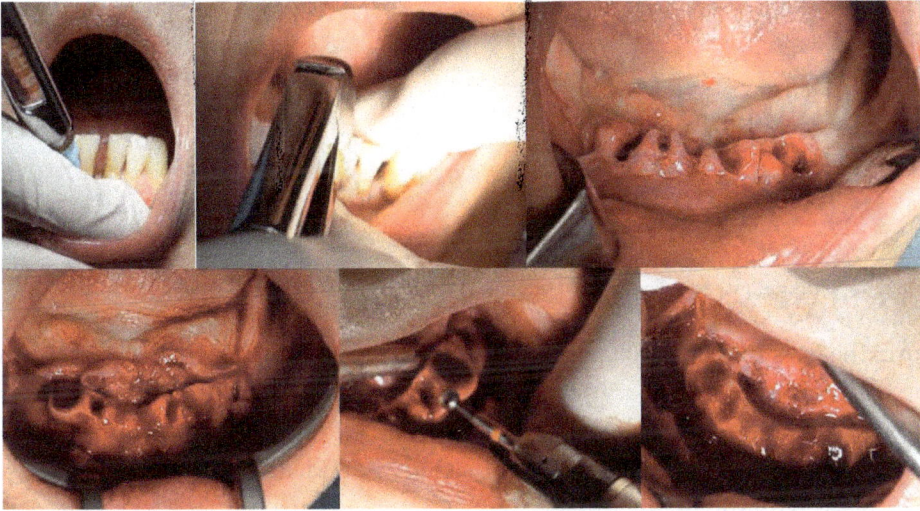

Figure 2. Preprosthetic surgery that included teeth extraction and bone leveling

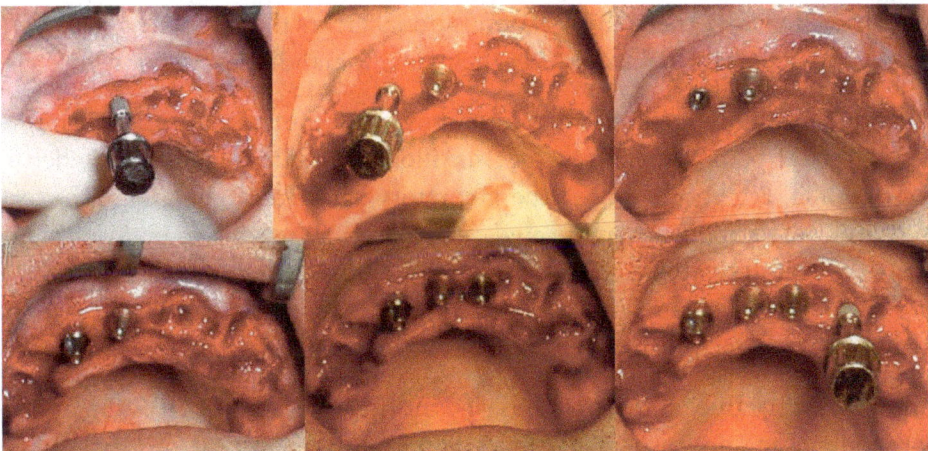

Figure 3. Axial implant are placed first

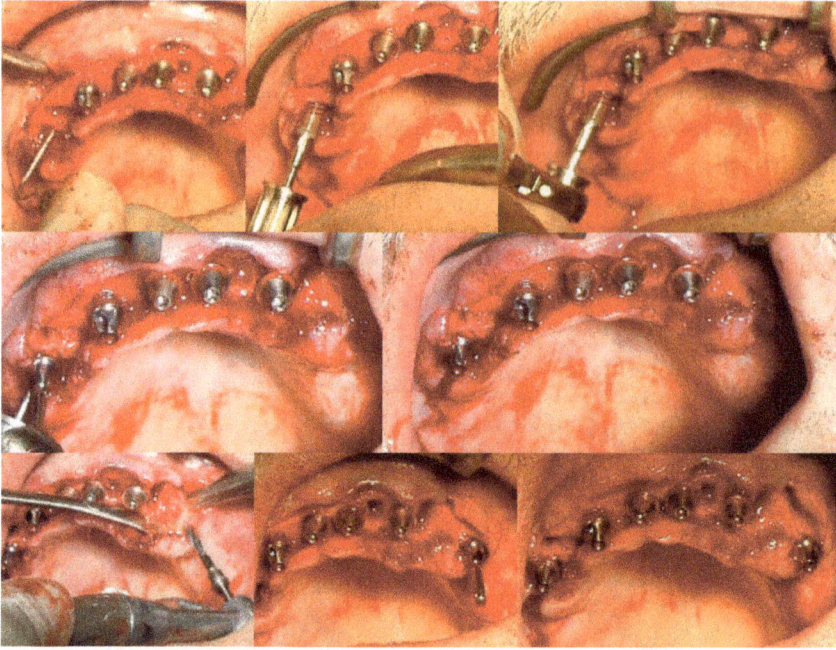

Figure 4. Tilted implants are placed second

Interim prosthesis is fixed, usually made from rigid acrylic material and splints the implants, protecting them from adverse loading and reducing the stress in the bone around the implant [20,24]. It is manufactured and placed in the same day with implant insertion. Therefore, it is mandatory to include a dental technician in the team that, ideally, has the dental laboratory in the same location with the dental office.

Manufacturing the interim prosthesis basically follows the same steps as other fixed-prosthetic implant restoration. After placement of abutments and suture, an impression is taken with a closed or open tray (Figure 5). The impression copings are attached to the implant abutment without splinting, that associates the risk of positional errors that are reflected as deficiencies on all forthcoming laboratory phases. After that, maxillomandibular relationship is recorded.

The dental technician manufactures the interim prosthesis, the procedure being simpler, faster and better adapted to patient's features (e.g., maxillomandibular relationship) when a wax-up is previously made. For shortening of the laboratory phase and obtaining a better esthetic outcome, composite or acrylic prefabricated veneers can be used. The prefabricated veneers are used for a wax set-up, followed by manufacturing a positioning template for them, through the use of a silicone impression. Finishing of the interim prosthesis is achieved by transferring the set-up, adding rigid acrylic material, and fixation of only one implant coping (Figure 6).

After manufacturing of the interim prosthesis by the dental technician, fixation of the remaining implant copings and adjustments are made in the dental office. All implant copings except one are fixed insitu, directly intraorally by the dentist, in order to address coping errors and to ensure passive fit and tension-free placement. Only after that occlusal adjustments are made.

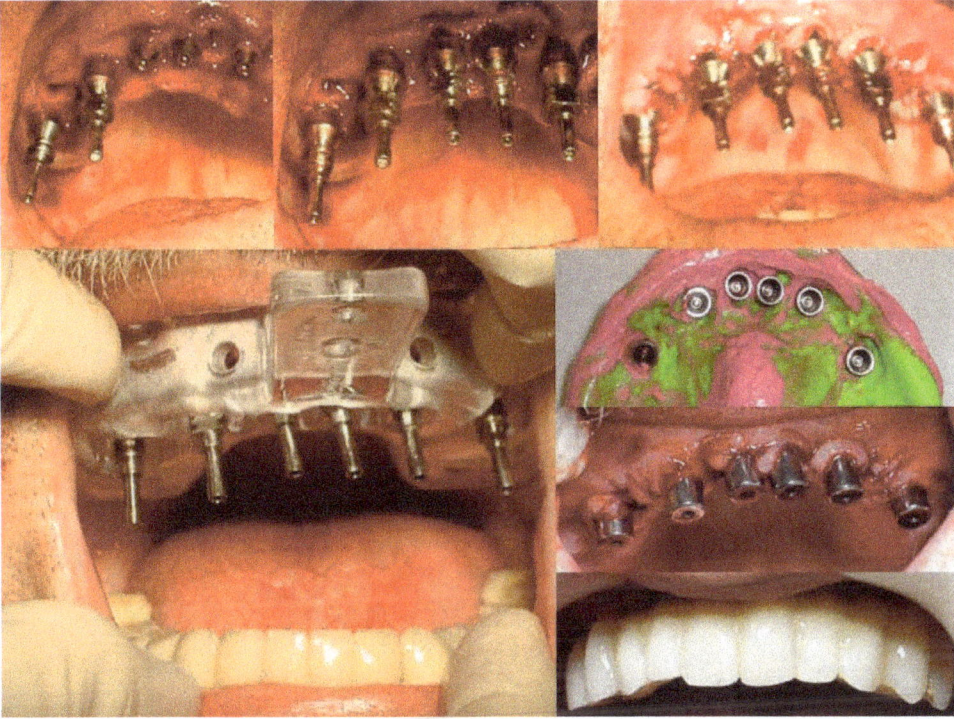

Figure 5. Interim prosthesis – clinical phases

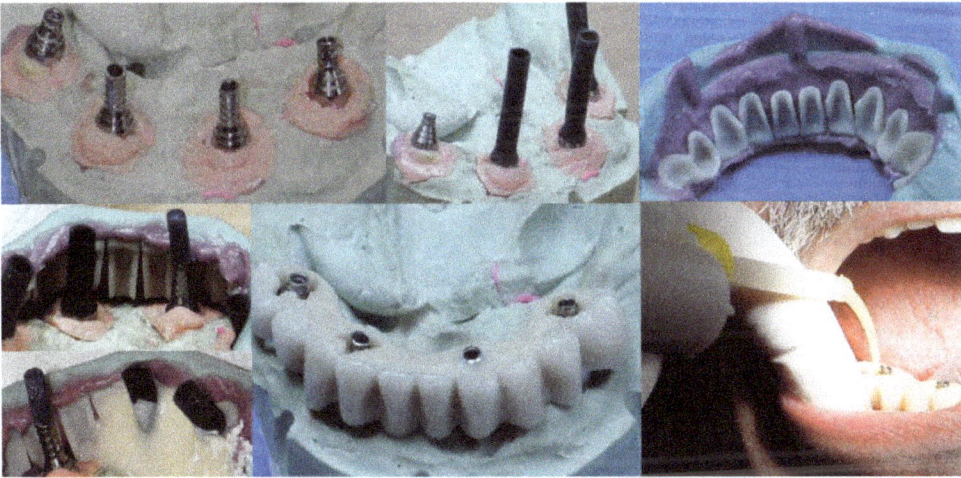

Figure 6. Interim prosthesis – laboratory phases

Therefore, during the osseointegration phase, a comfortable fixed interim restoration is used, that ensures esthetic and functional rehabilitation, which can be used for a moderate period of time. Also, during this interim phase, the patient has the time to analyze and form his own opinion about the esthetic outcome, and declare his own requirements about the changes desired for the definitive prosthesis.

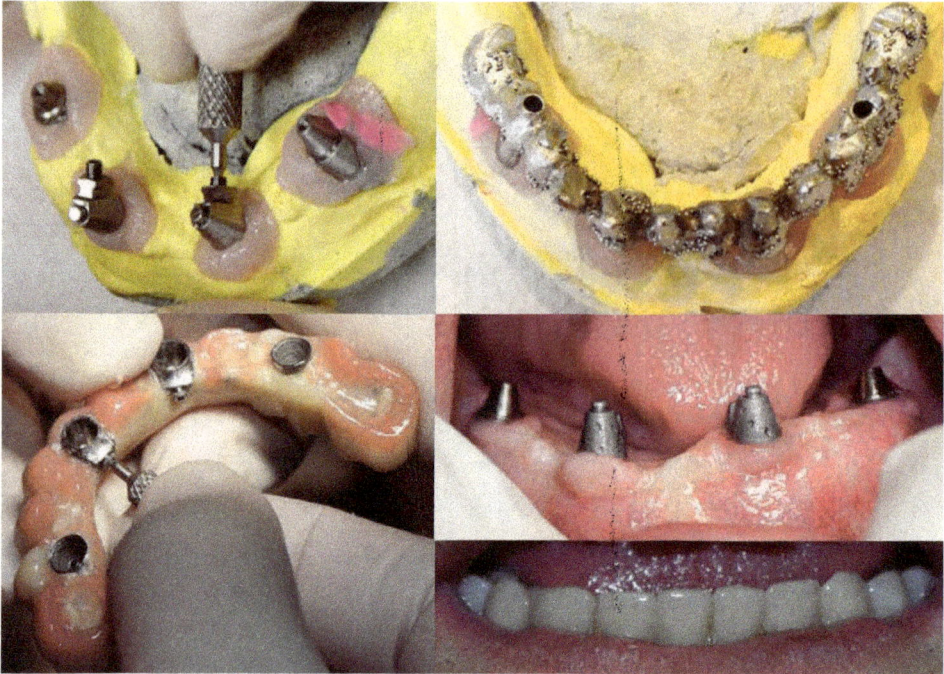

Figure 7. Definitive prosthesis execution

Postoperative instructions target mainly postoperative medications, the adequate plaque control and using a soft diet during the first weeks. In the next appointment, scheduled in the following days after surgery, occlusal adjustments should be done, considering their impact on the prognosis..

The definitive prosthesis is a splinted implant fixed restoration, by a rigid metal-based ceramic or acrylic prosthesis. It is manufactured after at least 4 months after surgery in the maxilla, respectively after at least 3 months in the mandible.

Clinical phase of definitive prosthesis manufacture are similar to those used for fixed-prosthetic implant restorations (Figure 7). If desired, implant abutments can be replaced with others, with different angulation or gingival height. Special attention must be given to accurately register the implant abutment position. In this respect, a preliminary impression is taken in order to fabricate an acrylic splint and a custom tray. The acrylic splint manufactured in the dental laboratory is sectioned in the area between the implants and then splinted intraorally with acrylic resin. Using this procedure for custom tray impression ensures an accurate tension-free registration of implant abutment position.

Definitive prosthetic design, as the length of dental arch and decision upon using cantilever extensions depends on the site of the most distal implant abutment and patient features, as number of teeth exposed during smile. It is best to use cantilever extension with reduced length, below 6-8 mm in the maxilla and 10 mm in the mandible [25].

Definitive prostheses are screw-retained, the screw-access opening being placed on the occlusal or the lingual side of the prosthesis. Through this method of retention, removal of prosthesis and professional hygiene procedures are easy to perform.

Metal or zirconium-based ceramic, metal-based acrylic or composite, are all options that can be used for manufacturing the definitive prosthesis. In the mandible, metal based acrylic and composite restorations are preferred when opposed by maxillary ceramic prosthesis, as prevention factor of negative complication that may appear in relation to occlusal or parafunctional forces. In order to obtain a natural aspect, pink material is used for replacing the lost hard and soft tissue and for restoring the artificial gingival contour.

Indications. Sky Fast & Fixed treatment concept addresses rehabilitation of complete edentulism, as current or imminent condition, through an immediate fixed-prosthetic implant restoration. It is especially indicated in the cases with severe ridge resorption in the posterior regions of the jaws that prohibit the axial placement of dental implants, in patients for whom extensive bone grafting procedures are not an option. It can be used for either dentate patients that are soon to be edentulous and absolutely refuse interim or definitive removable prosthesis, or for edentulous patients extremely dissatisfied by their conventional or implant removable prosthesis who desire a fixed prosthetic restoration. In some systemic conditions or elderly patients, this treatment option may be more indicated compared to conventional fixed implant restorations (that usually require major grafting procedures), considering that there are fewer and less invasive surgical procedures, that cause less trauma and stress, shorter healing period and a lower risk of developing complications [26, 27].

Contraindications. This treatment alternative basically has the same contraindications as all implant based restorations, mainly in relation to the risks associated to surgical procedures. Even so, there are few absolute contraindications (e.g., recent myocardial infarction, stroke, cardiovascular surgery, and transplant; profound immunosuppression; radiotherapy or bisphosphonate use), the degree of disease-control being far more important than the nature of systemic disorder itself [27,28]. Additionally, there are complications or behavioral aspects that may increase the treatment failure or complication rate, which should be acknowledged (e.g., diabetes, oral hygiene status, smoking, decreased frequency of using the dental services).

Using this specific treatment concept is limited to cases with severe ridge resorption in the anterior region of the jaws, in patients for whom extensive bone grafting procedures are not an option.

Advantages. Sky Fast & Fixed has the general advantages of immediately loaded fixed implant prosthesis, provided through a less invasive treatment compared to the conventional option.

As an immediately-loaded implant-prosthesis, it ensures immediate functional and esthetic rehabilitation, with a positive impact on patient's wellbeing and quality of life. Even more, for the dentate patients it is possible to avoid the edentulism condition treated by removable prosthesis, the imminence of this situation being frequently a major stressor for patients.

Compared to conventional fixed implant prosthesis, Sky Fast & Fixed is considered to be less invasive. The surgical procedure used is simpler, by avoiding extensive bone grafting, placement of fewer implants, using when appropriate a flapless technique, no need for a second stage implant surgery. Also, there is only one-day of surgery. Minor preprosthetic surgery, if required, is done in the same appointment with implant placement, and there is no need of a second stage implant surgery. Correspondently, the less the surgical trauma is, the faster the healing and recovery of the patient is.

Using a reduced number of implants, avoiding some procedures like bone grafting, the possibility of using metal-based acrylic prosthesis, decrease of the number of clinical appointments required, are all factors that may contribute to a decrease of the treatment cost. This may be an important aspect for the edentulous patient that is often aged and has limited financial means.

This treatment concept has advantages also for the dental team. Aspects like the standardized treatment protocol, the reduced number of clinical appointments, the relatively easy way of manufacturing and placement of the interim prosthesis, patient's satisfaction, all have a positive impact.

Complications. This treatment option basically has the same complications with any immediately loaded fixed implant prosthesis. Some aspects, mainly related to Sky Fast & Fixed particularities will be highlighted.

The acrylic interim prosthesis can fracture, this occurring mainly after the ten week period of recommendation of eating soft diet, when patients fell confident to chew harder food. If unmanaged, it can lead to implant failure, due to the alteration of the splinting process. Therefore, the interim prosthesis should not be reinforced, because it may mask the fracture and delay the patient's addressing to the dental office.

If chipping of the ceramic of the definitive prosthesis occurs, this being a relative frequent complication, the interim prosthesis can be used for the time needed for laboratory repairing.

One important risk factor for all implant prosthesis, including this treatment option, that is linked to sometimes severe complications, is the correctness of the registration of maxillo-mandibular relations (respecting the coincidence of maximal intercuspal position and centric relation, and the functional vertical dimension of occlusion). Acknowledging that, in a dentate patient with posterior occluding teeth it is recommended their preservation until after the interim prosthesis is manufactured, in order to ensure a correct registration.

3. Implant overdentures

General presentation. An implant overdenture is a removable dental prosthesis supported or retained by dental implants, through various attachment systems (e.g., ball, locator, magnets, bar). Benefits of overdentures include increased retention and stability of the prosthesis, improved mastication and phonation, decrease of the rate of ridge resorption, all having a positive impact on patients' well-being and quality of life.

An increased usage of this treatment option occurred as a reaction to the relatively frequent retention and stability deficiencies of complete dentures that are addressed at more affordable costs compared to the ones of fixed implant prosthesis [29]. Moreover, nowadays two implant overdentures are considered the minimum standard of care for mandibular edentulism, taking into account performance, patient satisfaction, cost and clinical time [6]. Most probably, overdenture use will increase even more, in relation to its indications, being most appropriate for the aged population segment that is estimated to be increasing.

Implant overdenture treatment concept has the following main features:

- It is designed for complete edentulism, as interim or definitive removable prosthesis, and can be applied in one or both jaws.

- Overdenture has, with regards to their role, three structural elements: the infrastructure (the implants), the mesostructure (the connector between implants and overdentures, the attachment system) and the superstructures (the partial or complete overdentures).

- The use of implants and attachment system aims to improve overdenture retention (1), or retention and stability (2), or retention, stability and support (3).

- Implant overdentures can be supported exclusively by implants (1), by implants and soft tissue (2), or only by the soft tissue (3).

- There are different types of implants that can be used for implant overdentures (e.g., conventional diameter, narrow or mini dental implants; narrow implants with one-piece or two-piece design). These are available in different lengths, diameters and sometimes have different attachment systems (Figure 8).

- The number of dental implants placed in the case of implant overdentures vary between 1 to 4 for mandibular overdenture, and 2 to 6 for maxillary overdenture.

- Selection of the dental implant, as type, diameter and length and establishing their number and position must consider the bone features (ridge width and length; bone density) and treatment objectives (e.g., enhance only overdenture retention, or retention and support). Usually, implant placement without bone grafting can be done anteriorly to the mental foramen in the mandible, and anteriorly to the maxillary sinus in the maxilla. Frequently, for the implants placed in the posterior area of the jaws, bone grafting is required. In order to avoid bone grafting, narrow dental implants can be used in narrow ridges, and short dental implants can be used in reduced ridge height. Bone density, according to Misch classification, should be D1, D2 or D3, not D4 because it is usually accompanied by implant failure [30].

- Depending on patient's features and the material and treatment option chosen, implant placement can be done with or without a flap, using one-stage or two-stage implantation protocol.

- Implants can be unsplinted (e.g., with ball as attachment system) or splinted (e.g., with bar as attachment system). In the first case, implant problems can be more easily addressed by implant replacement or by placing an additional implant. In case of implants splinted by a bar, implant failure may be followed by treatment failure. There is no difference between

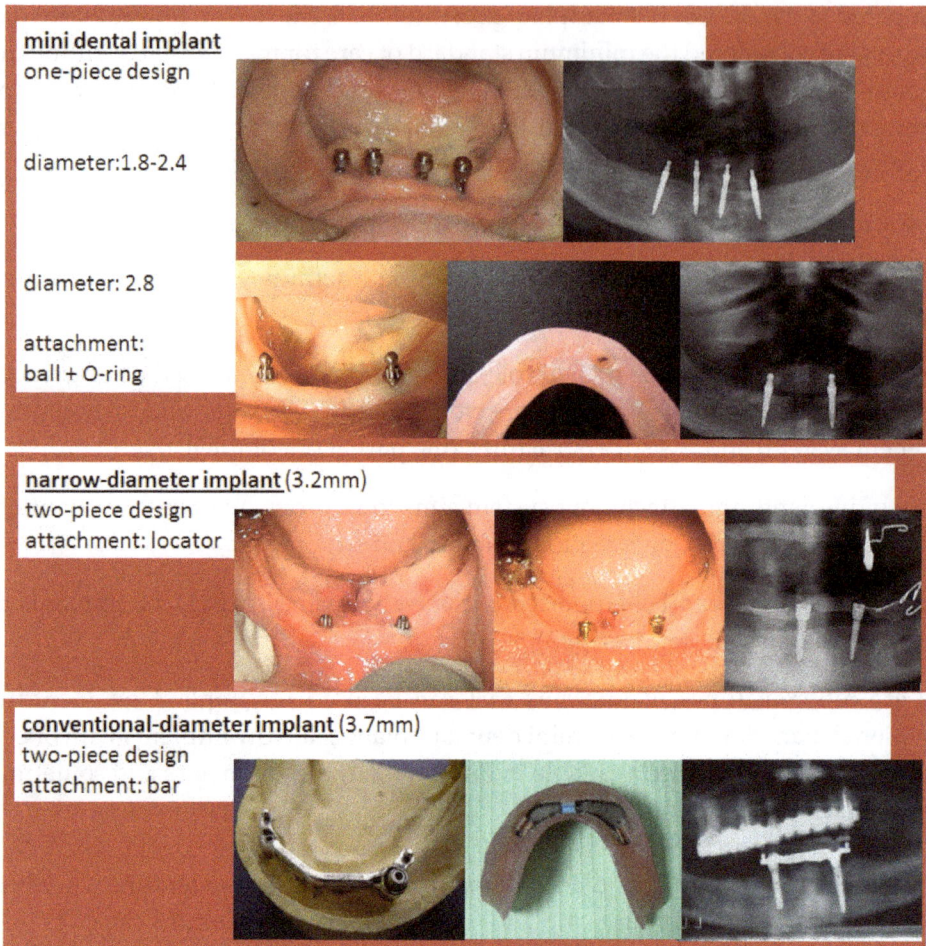

Figure 8. Different type of implants, according to their diameter and attachment system

splinted and unsplinted implant overdentures regarding the peri-implant outcome and patients' satisfaction. Therefore, considering unsplinted implants prostheses have simpler manufacturing and repairing procedure, these may be more indicated for aged edentulous patients [31].

- There are many types of attachment system that can be used for implant overdentures, e.g., ball, bar, locator, magnets, telescope, TiSiSnap. Selecting the attachment system must consider their role, such as only improving overdenture retention (e.g., ball attachment), or retention and stability (e.g., round bar attachment with non-rigid anchorage), or retention, stability and support (e.g., milled bars with rigid anchorage). Aspects related to patient's features (bone resorption, interarch vertical space, patient ability to perform maintenance procedures and expectations), situation of the opposite jaw (dentate or edentulous patient, treated by fixed or removable conventional or implant prosthesis), financial costs, should be all considered.

- The overdenture design is related to the other features of the implant prosthesis. Namely, if ball attachment system are used, that only improve overdenture retention, overdenture is best to be designed as a conventional denture, with complete coverage of the support area, until the anatomical and functional borders, with complete peripheral seal. If an implant-supported overdenture is used, an open palate overdenture can be used, and if desired can be screw-retained, similar to a fixed implant restoration.

- Overdenture reinforcement, in order to prevent its fracture, is mainly indicated when more than two unsplinted implants are used and in bars (considering the costs of the repairing procedure are higher, sometimes being necessary to renew the overdenture).

- In previous denture wearers, sometimes the old denture can be modified and used as the overdenture.

- Oral hygiene maintenance for implant overdentures is relatively easy to perform, considering that by removal of the prosthesis patients can have good access to the peri-implant tissue.

- Usually performing an implant overdenture requires reduced clinical time and number of appointments, additional to those usually required for a complete denture. In immediate loaded implant ball-retained overdentures, implant placement and overdenture adjustment can be done in one day, being accompanied by an immediate functional rehabilitation. In other cases, a delayed loading is required.

- Regular check-ups are most important during the osseointegration phase and in the first year of functioning, considering this is the period when most severe complications usually occur.

There are many treatment planning options when considering treatment of edentulism with implant overdentures, some being more invasive than other. Selection of one of them depends mainly on patient's preferences and needs, and on oral and general health status and particularities.

Among implant overdenture treatment options, those requiring easier and less invasive interventions for execution and maintenance will be detailed further on. There will be addressed mainly the alternatives that require the minimum necessary surgery (mainly implant placement, according to the anatomical limitations), preferably with immediate implant loading (ensures rapid functional reestablishment), and unsplinted implants (give more flexibility in managing future complications, that usually are less severe; maintenance is simpler). These overdentures mainly improve the retention of the prosthesis, and are implemented at moderate biological, financial and time costs.

Clinical phases.

Patient evaluation should comprise the common diagnostic data collection for complete dentures, and implant prosthesis, some of the aspects mentioned below being very important for treatment planning in case of implant overdenture.

Patient's needs, expectations and chief complaints related to the previous prosthetic treatment should be well-acknowledged. Most often, previous complete denture wearers are dissatisfied by its retention, aspect that is usually well addressed by implant overdentures. Dentate patients are often frightened by the idea of removable denture, and have psychological difficulties in accepting it. Therefore, explaining to the patient the main treatment options, with their benefits, limitations and cost, is mandatory.

Considering that often edentulous patients are aged, with multiple comorbidities, less invasive surgery is beneficial. Therefore, bone offer needs to be accurately analyzed, in order to establish implants type, position, diameter and length. Frequently, sufficient natural bone for implant placement is found anteriorly to the mental foramen in the mandible, and anteriorly to the maxillary sinus in the maxilla. In the mandible, bone deficiencies are mostly related to severe ridge resorption and decreased ridge width. In the maxilla, bone deficiencies are mostly related to decreased ridge height and reduced bone density. Consequently, when conventional dental implants cannot be applied without bone grafting, narrow or mini dental implants may be used in the mandible, and an increased number of conventional diameter implants are recommended in the maxilla [32]. In the mandible, two conventional diameter implants (diameter greater than 3.5mm), two narrow diameter implants (diameter below 3.5mm), or four mini dental implants (diameter below 3mm) are usually placed. In the maxilla four conventional diameter implants, four narrow diameter implants or six mini dental implants, of minimum 10 mm length are usually placed.

Thickness of keratinized mucosa should be evaluated in order to properly select the implant and attachment system that are usually designed with alternatives for different gingiva height.

Treatment planning should consider the condition and treatment of the opposite jaw. For example, planning an implant overdenture in the mandible should consider if teeth or fixed restoration, or edentulism treated by conventional denture are found in the maxilla. If teeth or fixed prosthesis are found in the maxilla, it is recommended to increase the number of mandibular implants and special consideration should be given to the vertical prosthetic space that is frequently reduced. If a complete denture is found in the maxilla, signs of combination syndrome may appear due to anterior movement of the masticatory field, favoring the instability of the maxillary denture and the increased bone resorption rate in the anterior maxilla. Consequently, this iatrogenic effect can be managed by using implant overdenture also in the maxilla [33].

Previous denture analysis may offer diagnostic data and further on, depending on their correctness, can be transformed or not into the future overdenture. Aspects like registration of an increased vertical dimension of occlusion or errors in artificial teeth mounting should lead to the decision of manufacturing a new denture, because these may become risk factors for implant overdenture complications.

Surgical procedure includes teeth extractions, preprosthetic interventions and implants placement.

Preprosthetic surgery aims towards obtaining favorable conditions for denture execution and improving the treatment prognosis. It may include intervention on the bone (for exostosis, tori) or the soft tissue (for frenum, hyperplasia). Sometimes, major surgical interventions, such as bone grafting, sinus lift or mental nerve relocation, are needed. Decision regarding the preprosthetic surgical intervention used is linked to patient features and treatment parameters (e.g., using narrow dental implants usually requires less invasive preprosthetic surgical interventions compared to conventional diameter implants). Preprosthetic surgery can be performed before or during implant placement.

Implant placement, as implant number and position, is done according to the treatment plan previously established. In order to obtain the desired implant position and angulation, a surgical guide or template can be used.

Surgical steps of implant placement vary according to patient's features, implant placement protocol and implant type, respecting the manufacturer's instructions.

Case particularities are determinant for choosing a specific treatment conduct. Alveolar ridge width and height, bone density, cortical bone thickness, mucosal resilience and width of keratinized mucosa are decision factors for using flap or flapless technique, one-stage or two-stage implantation protocol with immediate or delayed loading [30].

Implant surgical protocol is achieved using the main following steps, with variation depending on the implant type used (e.g., mini, narrow or conventional diameter implant). Firstly, a surgical exposure of the implant site is done, through flap elevation or mucosal punch, with a flapless technique. Using a flap technique has the advantage of a better assessment of available bone and thickness of the crestal area, information deficiently acknowledged when only clinical examination and panoramic radiographs are used. Flapless technique is mostly used for narrow dental implants (Figure 9). It has the advantage of reduced bleeding and decrease of the clinical time required (avoiding incision and flap elevation in the beginning, and suture in the end), is less invasive compared to the previous therefore promoting a shortened healing period. Afterwards, initial osteotomy is done with the marking or trepan drill, this aiming to pierce the cortical bone and define the implant site. With the same or another drill, usually called pilot drill, the implant osteotomies is initiated, in this stage being important to verify the implant angulation with a parallel pin. Implant placed with an unfavorable divergent angle may associate difficulties related to abutment and attachment system selection and exertion of excessive pressure on the implant during overdenture placement or removal. Osteotomy depth varies according to bone density, being approximately 2/3 of implant length in low bone density (D3) and as implant length in increased bone density (D1, D2). The implant osteotomy is enlarged as necessary using the twist drills. All previous drilling procedures need to be accompanied by irrigation with refrigerated sterile saline. Consequently, implant is placed with the ratchet and handpiece. After that, depending on the implant type and the treatment plan, if the surgical phase is over, placement of cover screw, healing abutment or prosthetic abutment, with suturing flap, are necessary. The surgical appointment usually ends with giving the patient the postoperative instructions regarding care (hygiene, diet and medication), also being scheduled for the next appointment. When needed, a second stage implant surgery is applied for removal of the cover screw and abutment placement [34,35].

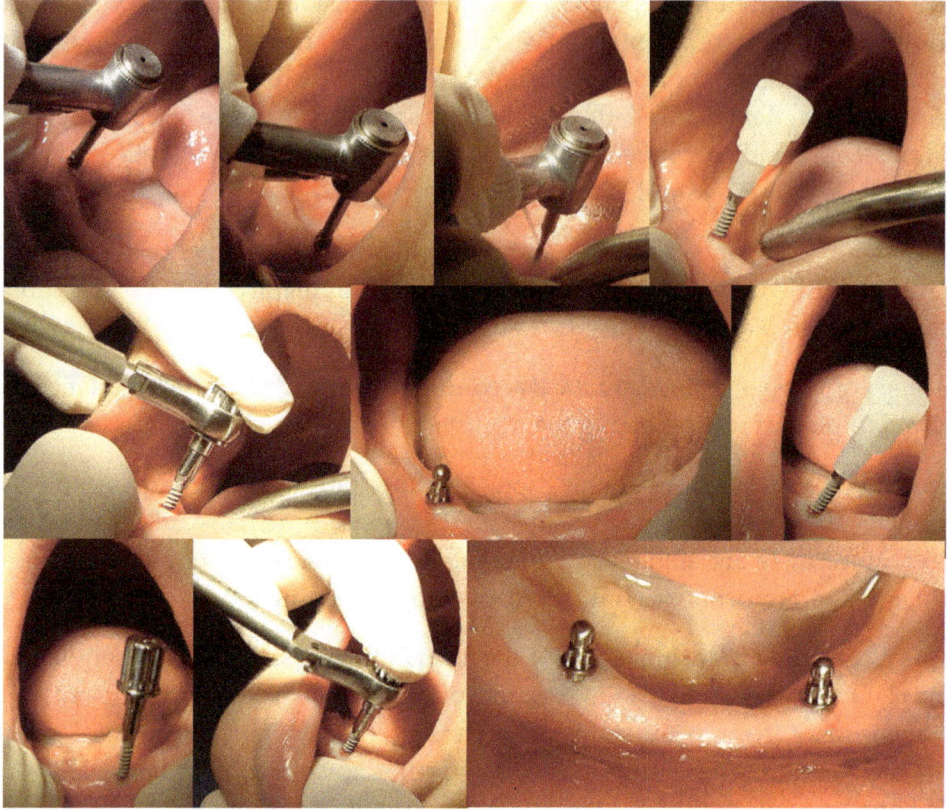

Figure 9. Flapless surgical technique used for placement of mini and narrow dental implants

Considering that generally edentulous patients are aged, with systemic comorbidities and less availability to complex surgical intervention, simpler one-stage surgical interventions are usually preferred [36].Considering that, mini or narrow dental implants may be preferred for increasing the denture retention, due to the simpler and shorter medical intervention [37-39].

The overdenture can be executed before or after implant placement. If applicable, the previous complete denture can be used as interim prosthesis or can be transformed into the new overdenture.

Overdentures that aim only towards improvement of retention, should be designed as a conventional denture, with proper support, retention and stability. If previous dentures are preserved, their correctness should be assessed in order to decide to either keep or replace them.

Using an implant overdenture associates more frequently a less accurate extension of overdenture bearing area, due to the misconception that the attachment system will provide all the retention needed. Overextended flanges dislodge the overdenture during chewing or speaking. Short flanges enhance food and plaque accumulation and retention. Existence of a space between the overdenture and the oral mucosa in the implant site is a risk factor for peri-implantitis or peri-implant mucositis. Therefore, a complete coverage of the overdenture support area, reaching the anatomical and functional borders, with complete peripheral seal should be obtained. For the maxillary denture, complete palatal coverage, with posterior palatal seal is recommended. In order to correctly register the functional limits of the denture bearing area, a mucodynamic functional impression technique can be used.

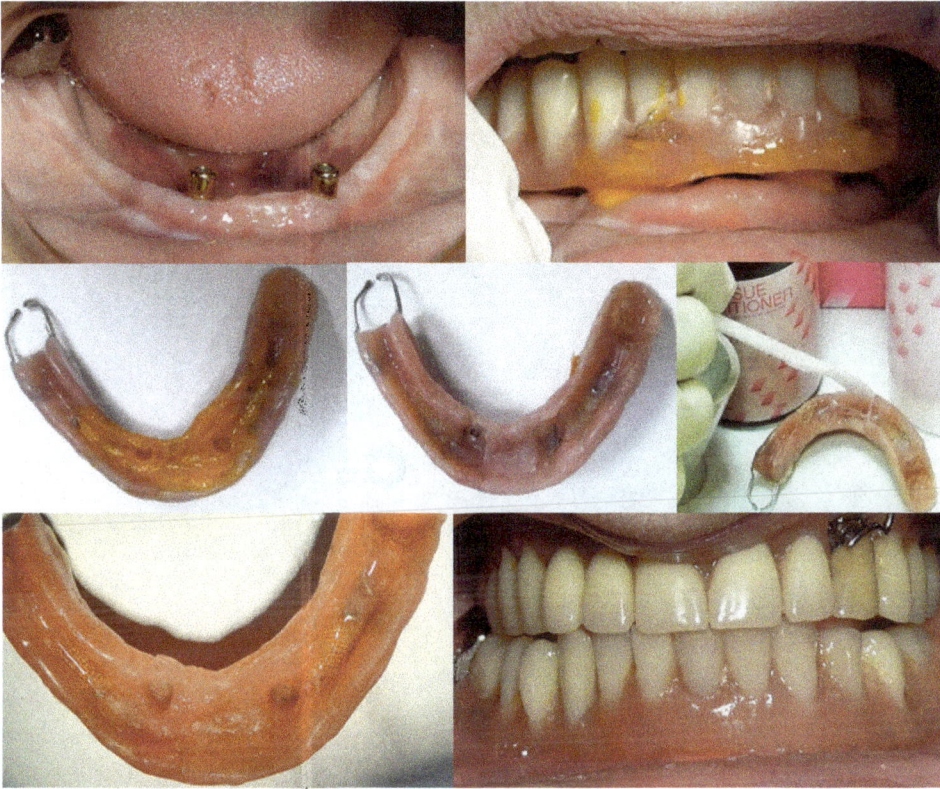

Figure 10. The worn denture was modified as overdenture, and used as an interim prosthesis during the osseointegration period

Registration of maxillomandibular relations aims towards recording the correct functional vertical dimension of occlusion and centric relation. Correctness of this clinical procedure has a major impact of the treatment outcome. Registration of an increased vertical dimension of occlusion can lead to prosthesis intolerance and implant loss, consecutive to the high pressure exerted on them.

In order to obtain a good esthetic outcome, the overdenture can be manufactured first, according to the esthetic principles and patient wishes, followed by implant placement using a surgical template.

For implant overdentures, immediate or delayed implant loading protocols can be used. Delayed implant loading is mainly used for conventional diameter implants. After implant placement, the healing abutments are placed for 10 to 13 weeks; in this period it is important to verify the denture, in order not to exert excessive pressure on implant site and interfere with implant osseointegration. Immediate implant loading is always used for one-piece mini dental implants, and sometimes used for narrow and conventional diameter implants. Using it requires a good primary stability of the implant, linked to a high insertion torque, of 35-40 Ncm. When the value of insertion torque is reduced, immediate implant loading can be done using soft acrylic or silicone materials [40]. In this respect, there are silicone materials especially developed to be used as matrices, such as Retension.Sil (Bredent), that offer three retention levels, i.e., 200, 400, 600 gf (Figure 11).

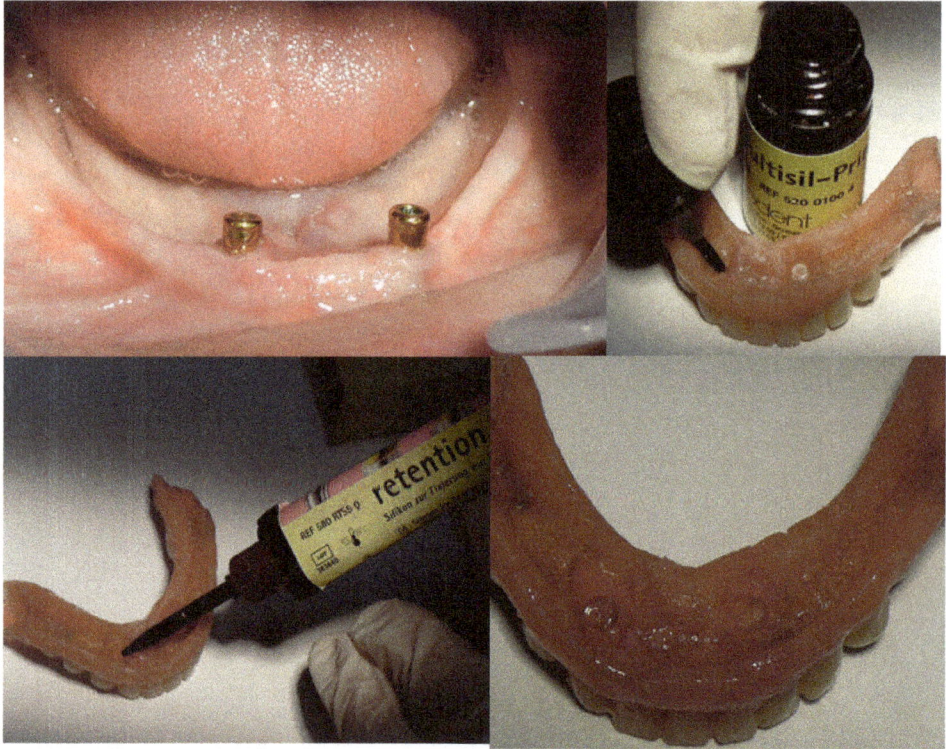

Figure 11. Immediate implant loading with silicone materials.

Attachment systems ensure stable balance (support, retention, stability) of the overdenture. The usual attachment systems used are: round, ovoid or parallel wall shaped bar; ball; Locator; magnets; telescopes. Selection of the attachment system depends on oral and prosthesis features, such as:

- overdenture type (partial or complete) and the role of connection systems (to improve support, stability and/or retention of the prosthesis);

- the implant number, site, angulation and their parallelism (two implant overdenture can be splinted with a bar, or used unsplinted with ball attachment; the selection of the attachment system must take into account the parallelism of the implants, ball attachments can be used up to 30° divergence while Locator allows up to 40° divergence);

- prosthetic conditions: interarch vertical space, resilience of the mucosa, magnitude of occlusal forces, functional particularities, the need for retention;

- patient manual dexterity may be related to selecting a more or less retentive system (dexterity is relevant for denture handling and oral hygiene maintenance, and elderly patients frequently have reduced dexterity);

- biomechanical treatment features (splinting the implants with a bar ensures a more uniform distribution of stress on the implants, but damage to one implant can cause the loss of the entire attachment system; screw of the connection system must be performed at a torque lower than the one used for implant insertion);

- financial and clinical time costs of the treatment (selecting the treatment option should not be based only on finances, but some of them are more expensive than others, e.g., costs of bar attachments are superior to those for ball attachments).

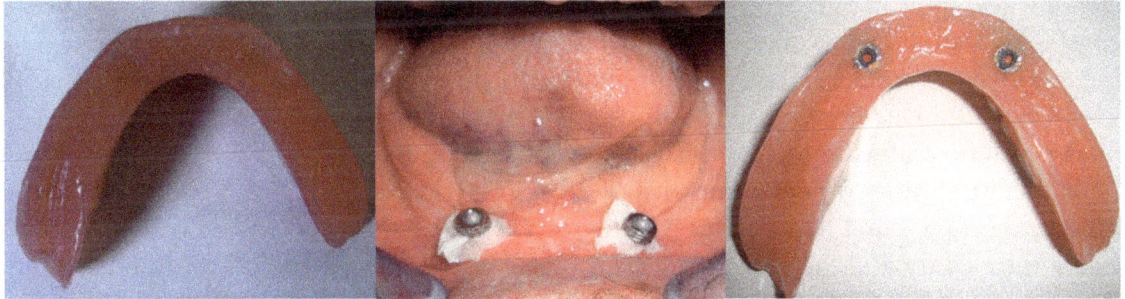

Figure 12. Placement of the metal matrices in the overdenture base

Postoperative instructions usually target the postoperative medications, the adequate plaque control, having a soft diet and wearing the overdentures as little as possible until the next appointment. It is mandatory to schedule the next appointment in the following days, in order to verify if the overdenture is supported only by the oral mucosa and to make occlusal adjustments. During osseointegration phase, pressure exercised on the implants is a major risk factor for implant failure. Additionally, in overdentures with immediate implant loading, patients have difficulties in assessing the cause of a perceived discomfort (implant pain is usually mistaken for trauma related to the prostheses or healing after surgery). Therefore, regular check-ups are recommended and the denture should not be worn overnight.

Indications. Implant overdentures are removable prostheses designed for treatment of edentulism, considered as the minimum standard of care for this condition. They are indicated for unsatisfied complete denture wearers, because by a relative simple intervention patient's complaints can be addressed, usually solving the problem of ill-fitting dentures. Also, they can be used as preventive factor for alveolar ridge resorption in high risk patients (e.g., patients with tooth loss due to periodontitis, with diabetes, during the menopause and postmenopause). Overdenture can be used as palliative treatment in patients with sensitive mucosa or hyposialia. They are particularly recommended in the older completely edentulous patients, which show a more frequent rate of denture intolerance, this way favoring a better adaptability with the prosthesis. Implant overdenture are recommended to be used when there are objective reasons that favor instability of the conventional denture (e.g., mandibular implant overdentures are indicated in skeletal class II patients; maxillary overdentures are indicated in skeletal class III patients). They are also recommended in oral and maxillofacial defects (clefts; after tumors removal, trauma) and in those with poor neuro-muscular coordination.

Contraindications. Implant overdentures have contraindications, mainly in relation to the risks associated to the surgical procedures, even if in some cases in can be regarded as a minimally invasive one. Additionally, using this specific treatment concept is limited to cases with reduced prosthetic vertical space that makes it impossible to apply the attachment systems and also provide adequate prosthesis resistance (e.g., using Locators requires a minimum of 8.5 mm vertical space and 9 mm horizontal space; bar attachments require 10 to 12 mm vertical space) [41]. Implant overdentures are not recommended when there is a decreased D4 bone density, in bruxism and in severe oral hygiene deficiency.

Advantages. Implant overdentures are a viable alternatives to conventional dentures, being considered the optimal solution for the edentulous seniors. Its main advantages are related to the improved retention, stability and support, depending on the attachment system that is used (e.g., improved chewing efficiency, speaking and comfort, with positive consequences on the quality of life). Using it associates a lower bone resorption rate, compared to conventional dentures, due to dental implants and improved denture stability, thus limiting the magnitude of pressures to a biological tolerance level. For the upper arch, if a vomiting reflex exists, the extension of the maxillary base can be reduced. Plaque control for implant overdenture is easier compared to implant fixed prostheses, but more difficult compared to conventional dentures. Considering the relatively easy surgical intervention and the reduced number of implants used, it is better accepted by patients with fear of complex medical interventions. Their execution and maintenance implies lower costs compared to the fixed implant prosthesis, and even if they are not the gold standard treatment, they can be considered as being cost effective due to their obvious benefits.

Complications. The implant overdenture complications occur in relation to patient's features, to surgical procedures or to prosthetic factors, during or after treatment execution. Some of them are considered as being more specific to this treatment option.

The implants' failure, as lack of osseointegration or peri-implantitis, can be linked to factors that affect healing of the bone, such as diabetes, steroids or bisphosphonates treatment, and smoking, to inadequate bone site and poor quality of the bone, to implant trauma exercised by the denture, to poor oral hygiene and decreased patient compliance. Prosthetic complications occur mainly within the first year of functioning [42]. Biomechanical or technical complications of the overdentures or attachment system used can be encountered, such as overdenture fracture, retention loss, aging of the material, teeth wear and attachment system loosening, loss or damage.

Addressing overdenture complications should take into account their nature, etiology and severity. Acknowledgement of patient's general and local features, respecting the removable implant prosthodontic principles, additional to regular check-ups, represent the basis of their prevention and control.

4. Conclusion

Sky Fast & Fixed is one of the less invasive fixed-prosthetic implant restoration for edentulism. It is a relatively simple and quick approach to the patient's medical problem, implemented through a decreased number of appointments, using limited surgery and reduced number of implants. The interim prosthesis is fixed, applied in the same day as implant placement, therefore the removable prosthesis is avoided. This rapid, less invasive, cost-effective fixed implant restoration usually ensures rapid regaining of functionality and resumption of social activities.

The implant overdenture is acknowledged as having a high predictability and numerous advantages compared to the most widely used treatment alternative, namely complete denture. It is important to identify the simpler and less invasive options of implant overdenture when considering the trends of decreasing tooth loss that associate an increasing of the age when edentulism occurs. Elderly patients require prosthetic rehabilitations that ensure good functionality, but considering their multiple systemic comorbidities and reduced availability to complex medical interventions, less invasive treatments with limited surgery, with easy maintenance procedures and that are cost-effective are more realistic and appropriate to their expectations. Therefore, the frequent problem of ill-fitting dentures can be relatively simply approached through placement of a reduced number of conventional diameter, narrow, or even mini implants, this requiring one clinical appointment, a relatively simple medical procedure and moderate costs.

Identifying and presenting to the reluctant edentulous patient the less invasive implant treatment strategies, fixed and removable, with their advantages, disadvantages and limitation, may help overcome their misconceptions and fears towards the implant prosthesis and lead to applying a treatment with a better outcome that promotes higher satisfaction and improved quality of life.

Author details

Elena Preoteasa[1], Laurentiu Iulian Florica[2], Florian Obadan[3], Marina Imre[1] and Cristina Teodora Preoteasa[4*]

*Address all correspondence to: cristina_5013@yahoo.com

1 Department of Prosthodontics, Faculty of Dental Medicine, Carol Davila University of Medicine and Pharmacy, Bucharest, Romania

2 Private Practice, Bucharest, Romania

3 Private Practice, Alexandria, Romania

4 Department of Oral Diagnosis, Ergonomics, Scientific Research Methodology, Faculty of Dental Medicine, Carol Davila University of Medicine and Pharmacy, Bucharest, Romania

References

[1] Felton D, Cooper L, Duqum I, Minsley G, Guckes A, Haug S, Meredith P et al. Evidence-Based Guidelines for the Care and Maintenance of Complete Dentures: a Publication of the American College of Prosthodontists. The Journal of the American Dental Association 2011;142 (Supplement 1):1S-20S.

[2] Douglass CW, Shih A, Ostry L. Will There Be a Need for Complete Dentures in the United States in 2020? Journal of Prosthetic Dentistry 2002;87:5–8.

[3] Carlsson GE1, Omar R. The Future of Complete Dentures in Oral Rehabilitation. A Critical Review. Journal of Oral Rehabilitation 2010;37(2):143-56.

[4] Fitzpatrick AL, Powe NR, Cooper LS, Ives DG, Robbins JA. Barriers to Health Care Access Among the Elderly and Who Perceives Them. American Journal of Public Health 2004; 94(10):1788-94.

[5] Dolan TA, Atchison K, Huynh TN. Access to Dental Care Among Older Adults in the United States. Journal of Dental Education 2005; 69(9): 961-74.

[6] Thomason JM, Kelly SA, Bendkowski A, Ellis JS.Two Implant Retained Overdentures-a Review of the Literature Supporting the McGill and York Consensus Statements. Journal of Dentistry 2012;40(1):22-34.

[7] Nowjack-Raymer RE, Sheiham A. Association of Edentulism and Diet and Nutrition in US Adults. Journal of Dental Research 2003;82(2):123-6.

[8] MacEntee MI, Walton JN.The Economics of Complete Dentures and Implant-Related Services: a Framework for Analysis and Preliminary Outcomes. Journal of Prosthetic Dentistry 1998;79(1):24-30.

[9] Fitzpatrick B. Standard of Care for the Edentulous Mandible: a Systematic Review. Journal of Prosthetic Dentistry 2006;95(1):71-8.

[10] Esposito M, Grusovin MG, Chew YS, Coulthard P, Worthington HV. One-stage versus two-stage implant placement. A Cochrane Systematic Review of Randomised Controlled Clinical Trials. European Journal of Oral Implantology 2009;2(2):91-9.

[11] Visser A, de Baat C, Hoeksema AR, Vissink A. Oral Implants in Dependent Elderly Persons: Blessing or Burden? Gerodontology 2011;28(1):76-80.

[12] Brennan M, Houston F, O'Sullivan M, O'Connell B. Patient Satisfaction and Oral Health-Related Quality of Life Outcomes of Implant Overdentures and Fixed Com-

plete Dentures. The International Journal of Oral & Maxillofacial Implants 2010;25(4): 791-800.

[13] Carr AB, Choi YG, Eckert SE, Desjardins RP. Retrospective Cohort Study of the Clinical Performance of 1-Stage Dental Implants. The International Journal of Oral & Maxillofacial Implants 2003;18(3):399-405.

[14] Preoteasa E, Marin M, Imre M, Lerner H, Preoteasa CT. Patients' Satisfaction With Conventional Dentures and Mini Implant Anchored Overdentures. Revista Medico-Chirurgicala a Societatii de Medici si Naturisti din Iasi 2012;116(1): 310-16.

[15] Malo P, Rangert B, Nobre M. All-on-4 Immediate-Function Concept with Branemark System Implants for Completely Edentulous Maxillae: a 1-year Retrospective Clinical Study. Clinical Implant Dentistry and Related Research 2005;7(Supplement 1):S88-94.

[16] Lopes A, Malo P, de Araujo Nobre M, Sanchez-Fernández E. The NobelGuide® All-on-4® Treatment Concept for Rehabilitation of Edentulous Jaws: A Prospective Report on Medium-and Long-Term Outcomes. Clinical Implant Dentistry and Related Research 2014. doi: 10.1111/cid.12260.

[17] Malo P, de Araujo Nobre M, Lopes A, Moss SM, Molina GJ. A Longitudinal Study of the Survival of All-on-4 Implants in the Mandible with up to 10 Years of Follow-up. The Journal of the American Dental Association 2011;142(3):310-20.

[18] Kistler F, Kistler S. All-on-four, Neue Philosophie Bei der Implantologischen Versorgung im Zahnlosen Kiefer. Bayerisches Zahnärzteblatt 2005. www.bzb-online.de/apr05/46.pdf (accesed 20 September 2014).

[19] Ata-Ali J, Peñarrocha-Oltra D, Candel-Marti E, Peñarrocha-Diago M. Oral Rehabilitation with Tilted Dental Implants: a Metaanalysis. Medicina Oral Patologia Oral y Cirugia Bucal 2012;17(4):e582-7.

[20] Jivraj S, Zarrinkelk H. Graftless Solutions in Implant Dentistry: Part 2. Diagnosis, Treatment Planning and Delivery of the Immediate Load Prosthesis. Dental Tribune 2012; 4:6-14.

[21] Jivraj S, Zarrinkelk H. Graftless Solutions in Implant Dentistry: Part 1. Diagnosis, Treatment Planning and Delivery of the Immediate Load Prosthesis. Dental Tribune 2012; 3:8-19.

[22] Choi BH, Jcong SM, Kim J, Engelke W. Flapless Implantology. Hanover Park: Quintessence Pub Co; 2010.

[23] Spinelli D, Ottria L, DE Vico G, Bollero R, Barlattani A, Bollero P. Full Rehabilitation with Nobel Clinician(®) and Procera Implant Bridge(®): Case Report. Oral & Implantology 2013;6(2):25-36.

[24] Bergkvist G. Immediate Loading of Implants in the Edentulous Maxilla. Swedish Dental Journal. Supplement 2008;(196):10-75.

[25] Armellini D, von Fraunhofer JA. The Shortened Dental Arch: a Review of the Literature. Journal of Prosthetic Dentistry 2004;92(6):531-5.

[26] Preoteasa E, Imre M, Preoteasa CT. A 3-Year Follow-up Study of Overdentures Retained by Mini–Dental Implants. The International Journal of Oral & Maxillofacial Implants 2014; 29(5): 1034-41.

[27] Diz P, Scully C, Sanz M. Dental Implants in the Medically Compromised Patient. Journal of Dentistry 2013;41(3):195-206.

[28] Gomez-de Diego R, Mang-de la Rosa M, Romero-Pérez MJ, Cutando-Soriano A, Lopez-Valverde-Centeno A. Indications and Contraindications of Dental Implants in Medically Compromised Patients: Update. Medicina Oral Patologia Oral y Cirugia Bucal 2014;19(5):e483-9.

[29] Attard NJ, Zarb GA, Laporte A. Long-Term Treatment Costs Associated with Implant-Supported Mandibular Prostheses in Edentulous Patients. The International Journal of Prosthodontics 2005;18(2):117-23.

[30] Misch CE. Contemporary Implant Dentistry 2nd edition. St. Louis: Mosby Inc; 1999.

[31] Al-Ansari A. No Difference Between Splinted and Unsplinted Implants to Support Overdentures. Journal of Evidence Based Dental Practice 2012;13(2):54-5.

[32] Preoteasa E, Meleşcanu-Imre M, Preoteasa CT, Marin M, Lerner H. Aspects of Oral Morphology as Decision Factors in Mini-Implant Supported Overdenture. Romanian Journal of Morphoogy and Embryology 2010;51(2): 309-14.

[33] Kreisler M, Behneke N, Behneke A, d'Hoedt B. Residual Ridge Resorption in the Edentulous Maxila in Patients With Implant-Supported Mandibular Overdentures: An 8-Years Retrospective Study. International Journal of Prosthodontics 2003;16(3): 265-300.

[34] Al-Faraje L. Oral Implantology Surgical Procedures-Quintessence Checklist Series. Quintessence Publishing Co; 2013.

[35] Al-Faraje L. Surgical Complications in Oral Implantology Etiology, Prevention, and Management. Quintessence Publishing Co, 2011.

[36] Esposito M, Grusovin MG, Chew YS, Coulthard P, Worthington HV. One-Stage versus Two-Stage Implant Placement. A Cochrane Systematic Review of Randomised Controlled Clinical Trials. European Journal of Oral Implantology 2009;2(2):91-9.

[37] Elsyad MA, Gebreel AA, Fouad MM, Elshoukouki AH. The Clinical and Radiographic Outcome of Immediately Loaded Mini Implants Supporting a Mandibular Overdenture. A 3-year Prospective Study. Journal of Oral Rehabilitation 2011;38(11): 827-34.

[38] Tadić A, Mirković S, Petronijević B, Knezević MJ. Stabilisation of Lower Denture Using Mini Dental Implants. Medicinski pregled 2012;65(9-10):405-8.

[39] Scepanovic M, Calvo-Guirado JL, Markovic A, Delgardo-Ruiz R, Todorovic A, Milicic B, Misic T. A 1-year Prospective Cohort Study on Mandibular Overdentures Retained by Mini Dental implants. European Journal of Oral Implantology 2012;5(4): 367-79.

[40] Preoteasa CT, Nabil Sultan A, Popa L, Ionescu E, Iosif, L, Ghica, MV, Preoteasa E. Wettability of Some Dental Materials. Optoelectronics and Advanced Materials – Rapid Communications 2011; 5(8): 874-8.

[41] Massad JJ1, Ahuja S, Cagna D. Implant Overdentures: Selections for Attachment Systems. Dentistry Today 2013;32(2):128, 130-2.

[42] Walton JN, MacEntee MI. Problems with Prostheses on Implants: a Retrospective Study. Journal of Prosthetic Dentistry 1994;71(3):283-8.

7

Role of Implants in Maxillofacial Prosthodontic Rehabilitation

Derek D'Souza

1. Introduction

Maxillofacial prostheses play a vital role in comprehensive rehabilitation by restoring physical and psychological well-being in patients with missing or disfigured anatomical structures due to congenital abnormalities, trauma, or disease [1]. It is possible to restore esthetics, function and re-establish the self confidence of the patient by providing a well designed prosthesis such as a prosthetic ear, eye, nose, cranial plate or a combination of these.

The last few decades have witnessed a significant increase in extensive malignancies of the head and neck region [2]. This has resulted in increasing number of patients with extensive post-surgical defects. Many of them need to be suitably rehabilitated to minimize long-term physical, functional and psychological consequences and ensure early return to normal life. In addition, these patients could be more willing to accept large surgical resections, if counseled about prosthetic reconstruction, prior to definitive surgery. It is crucial that all such patients receive a pre-operative referral to a maxillofacial prosthodontist prior to surgery [3].

When these patients report to the maxillofacial prosthetic clinic they report with complex defects and their general health status is also compromised. Achieving adequate retention of the prosthesis, especially when the defect is extensive, is a big challenge and requires a multi-disciplinary approach. With the advent of predictable osseointegration, a new era dawned in the field of prosthodontic rehabilitation of the head and neck region. Cases that were earlier condemned as "hopeless" were suddenly given a new range of options and the chance to be comprehensively restored to form and function. This chapter discusses the role of implants in comprehensive maxillofacial rehabilitation.

2. Retention of maxillofacial prostheses

Historically the means of achieving retention of facial prostheses has been primarily by use of medical adhesives or by means of anatomical or mechanical retention using various devices such as spectacles, springs, studs, clips or magnets [3]. An ideal adhesive should be one that provides firm functional retention under flexure or extension during speech, facial expressions, and moisture or perspiration contact, however such an adhesive is not yet available. Facial prostheses may additionally be retained by judicious use of anatomic tissue undercuts, thereby minimizing the displacement potential caused by other external forces. There is a potential for tissue irritation with use of this technique and due care and regular follow up is a must. Special care is warranted where tissues have been previously irradiated.

2.1. Cellular level changes of osseointegration

It is necessary to have a clear concept about the science of implantation and the healing of bone following a successful implant placement. Osseous healing along an implant follows a similar process to fracture healing but is subjective to the nature of the surface of the implant [4]. As soon as blood comes into contact with the surface of the implant, proteins adsorb to it, platelets get activated and bind to the adsorbed protein which results in the formation of a clot. This coagulum at the implant surface supports the deposition of proteins, releases inflammatory mediators and initiates new tissue formation. The release of numerous signaling molecules influence the migration of monocytes, neutrophils (both involved in inflammation), and mesenchymal cells (cells that can differentiate into osteoblasts) towards the implant surface [4]. Following the aggregation of neutrophils and macrophages from nearby capillary beds to the implant site there is further release of inflammatory mediators which are necessary for the initiation of osteogenesis. Components of tissue growth factor β (TGF-β) super-family are also expressed within 24 hours of implantation, including bone morphogenetic proteins (BMPs) and growth & differentiation factors (GDFs). These signaling molecules result in the collection, migration, and differentiation of mesenchymal cells, which take part in the formation of woven bone. Woven bone subsequently undergoes a sequence of remodeling, resulting in the formation of mature bone which is the desired end result [5].

2.2. Implant surface modifications

Various surface modifications are being commercially marketed since the days of the first Brånemark implants [6]. Grit-blasting and acid etching still remain the most commonly employed surface modification techniques in use today. Sand blasting increases the surface area of the implant as compared to machined surfaces. The resultant increase in surface area has been shown to improve cell attachment and proliferation which results in increased implant stability [7 – 10]. Electrochemical anodization is another chemical surface modification method that has been employed. This process increases surface micro-texture and also modifies the chemistry of the implant coating resulting in a titanium oxide layer that is several orders of magnitude thicker than a passivated surface [11, 12]. The addition of a ceramic coating to the roughened surface is another method of improving osseoconductivity. Here a plasma sprayed hydroxyapatite (HA) coating is used to create an irregular surface for osseointegration. The process involves blasting the implant surface with HA particles at a high temperature. The result is a coating that develops cracks as it rapidly cools. These coatings show enhanced bone-to-implant contact initially, in vivo, however the mechanical properties of the bone-coating interface has exhibited non-uniform degradation in the long term [13-16].

In other alternatives, crystalline deposition of nano-sized calcium phosphate and addition of a fluoride treatment to roughened titanium surfaces have also been tried with varying success [17-19]. While several advances in surface modification have been made in order to improve implant osseointegration, no treatment addresses the issue of reducing infection. While some manufacturers claim to be bacteria-proof due to their tight interlocking, the implant itself does not prevent bacterial attachment which can lead to formation of biofilms and subsequent implant failure [20, 21].

2.3. Craniofacial implants

In order to obtain predictable craniofacial osseointegration, different protocols had to be developed. It was necessary to have certain modifications as compared to the oral implants. These implants were made from titanium alloys and were generally shorter i.e. 3 – 5 mm long, threaded and with the same machined surface as the oral implants. It was further found important to attach a flange in the coronal part of the fixture [Figure 1]. The reason for this was the idea that even if the implant was subjected to a longitudinally directed trauma, the flange would prevent it to from being pushed into the deeper structures. This has also proved to be a safe and secure measure, as several trauma cases have occurred, but only a minority have caused fractures of the skull bone, and none have caused severe damage [22].

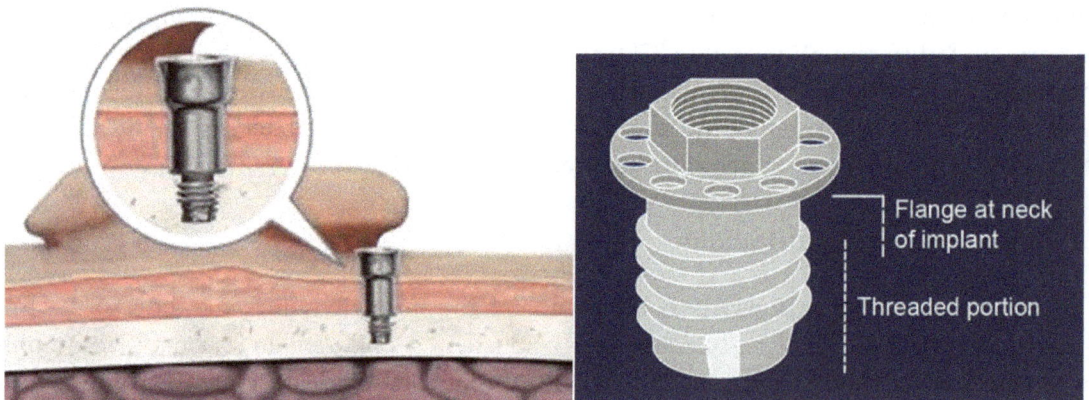

Figure 1. Design of craniofacial implants

The first abutment that was originally used was also of an intraoral type, but with time, extra-oral abutments of different types were developed. These include abutments for the bone-anchored hearing aid (BAHA) and abutments for bone-anchored epistheses (BAE). The length of the fixtures to be used is determined by the thickness of the cranial bones. In a normal adult the temporal bone has a thickness of approximately 4 mm. This is also the length of the most commonly available implants. It may be possible to install longer fixtures in the frontal bone, zygoma and maxilla. The skin over the abutments has to be reduced to a minimum. This is to prevent constant discomfort or trauma experienced by the patient when the prosthesis will move. Patients who have split skin grafts around the implant abutment show the least skin penetration problems [22, 23].

In pediatric cases the skull bone is much thinner, sometimes barely 1–3 mm thick. In these cases a different approach is necessitated. A simple technique is by the utilization of a semi-permeable membrane at the first stage surgery [24]. By utilizing this technique, 1–2 mm bone can be gained during a 6-month healing period, thus making it possible to install a 4-mm long fixture also in children. The semi-permeable membrane is then removed at the second stage surgery.

Osseointegration in irradiated bone was early believed to be contraindicated. Patients who are recovering from various forms of cancer need comprehensive rehabilitation and can benefit a lot from the use of osseointegrated implants. Clinically though there were higher failure rates along with certain other problems such as dehiscence of the soft tissue as well as osteoradio-necrosis [25]. Taking into consideration that the irradiated bone will take longer to heal it is advisable to first delay the placement of the implant and also to allow 4 to 8 months for osseointegration. Another approach is to expose the patients to adjunctive hyperbaric oxygen therapy (HBO). HBO has been shown to accelerate healing and also prevent osteoradionecrosis [26, 27]. In 2013, de Oliveira, Abrahão and Dib [28] however found that there is no difference in implant success between irradiated and normal bone. Keeping all things constant and knowing the risk factors involved it seems to be better to ensure all precautions are maintained in case selection, implant placement and also to ensure that the patient receives HBO therapy to reduce failures in patients who have received some form of radiotherapy and/or chemo-therapy.

2.4. Factors of importance for predictable osseointegration

There are six factors of importance that must be carefully monitored to ensure predictable osseointegration [29-31].

Material of the fixture-Titanium alloys are the most commonly used as these are known to integrate in the bone without causing adverse effects. It can remain incorporated into the bone for many decades, and be used as anchorage for different prostheses.

Macrostructure of the implant-A screw-shaped implant ensures better primary stability as compared to a conical shaped implant. This may be due to micro-movements of the conical shape and reduced osseointegration.

Microstructure of the implant-Original Brånemark implants had a smooth surface as they were manufactured by machining. Clinically however it has been observed that very smooth surfaces have lesser degree of osseointegration, along with minor amount of resorption. On the other hand a highly roughened surface shows rapid integration; but later secondary inflammation and secondary resorption is noticed that can endanger the long-term survival of the implant.

Osseous bed into which the implant is placed-Geriatric patients with bone that is osteoporotic will show lesser degree of osseointegration. Similar is the case of patients who have had radiotherapy or who have sustained severe burns that alter the osseous quality and reduce its capacity for osseointegration.

Surgical technique – The surgical intervention should be carefully monitored with slow speed, high torque and copious irrigation with cold water. The temperature should never be allowed to rise as the osteoblasts are extremely heat labile and get damaged easily. The implant itself should never be touched by gloves or gauze. It is vital that the surgical bed be free from fibers, powder and any other foreign matter that might hinder osseointegration.

Loading the implant – The implant should be loaded along its long axis as far as feasible. Lateral, torsional or cantilever forces are least tolerated and should be minimized by efficient planning and design.

2.5. Retention of maxillofacial prostheses and craniofacial implants

With the increased use of osseointegrated implants, dependence on adhesive and anatomic methods of retention has diminished. Magnets or clips can be used to effectively retain the prostheses [Figure 2] and will also minimize force transfer to the implant and supporting bone. The resultant decrease in dependence on chemical (adhesives) and anatomic (tissue undercuts) retention is beneficial to both the patient and the prosthodontist [31 – 35].

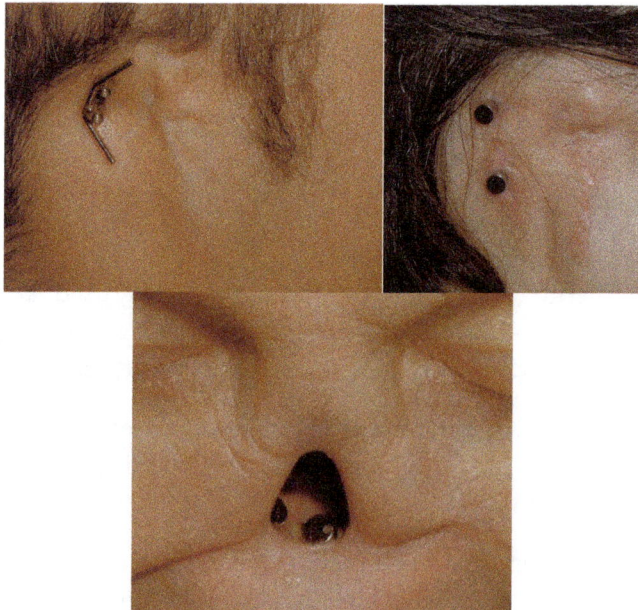

Figure 2. Different retention options for attachment of craniofacial prostheses

Craniofacial implants require adequate osseous thickness of the bone on the temporal and mastoid regions, for example in the rehabilitation of a case of congenital microtia. Thus, implant placement may not be as ideal in normal situations or with acquired defects from accidents. Other designs may also be provided if the distance between the two implants is too close or too far apart. Other crucial factors in rehabilitating this type of defect are marginal fit, good retention, and acceptable esthetics. Various studies have shown that retention using craniofacial implants has improved the satisfaction of patients with craniofacial prostheses. However, the actual level of satisfaction depends, to a large extent, on the location or type of defect, sex, and age of the patient [36 – 38].

3. Orbital prosthesis

In order to address the area of rehabilitation of the orbit it is vital to understand the different types of surgical techniques used in ophthalmic surgeries. Evisceration, enucleation, and exenteration are the three main surgical techniques by which all or parts of the orbital contents are removed [39]. Evisceration is the removal of the contents of the globe while leaving the sclera and extra-ocular muscles intact. Enucleation is the removal of the eye from the orbit while preserving all other orbital structures. Exenteration is the most radical of the three procedures and involves removal of the eye, adnexa, and part of the bony orbit.

Evisceration is usually indicated in cases of endophthalmitis unresponsive to antibiotics and for improvement of esthetics in an eye that is damaged and has lost its vision. Enucleation is indicated for the above two conditions as well as for painful eyes with no useful vision, malignant intraocular tumors, in ocular trauma to avoid sympathetic ophthalmia in the second eye, in phthisis with degeneration, and in congenital anophthalmia or severe microphthalmia to enhance development of the bony orbit. Exenteration is indicated mainly for large orbital tumors or orbital extension of intraocular tumors [39].

The first two namely evisceration and enucleation can be easily rehabilitated with excellent cosmetic results using custom made ocular prostheses [1, 3]. These are fabricated after custom made impressions using silicone impression materials and can be retained fairly well if the eyelids and ocular muscles are intact [Figure 3 – 5]. If required then additional soft tissue components may be fabricated using silicone elastomers which can be shaded and colour matched to the skin of the subject. They may be retained with suitable eye-frames or by use of local undercuts and adhesives [1, 3].

Exenteration surgical procedures are far more extensive and need expert and multi-specialty approach for rehabilitation. Post operatively when the patient reports for rehabilitation it may be necessary to advise the patient to undergo an additional surgical procedure to deepen the existing socket or for thinning of the skin flaps used for the initial wound closure. This will ensure better cosmetic outcome as there will be adequate space to accommodate the retentive framework, ocular component as well as the bulk of silicone elastomer. These large prostheses do not function well with adhesives or eye glasses alone [Figure 6 – 8]. Application of implants in these large orbital defects reduces the need for adhesives and enables easy insertion and

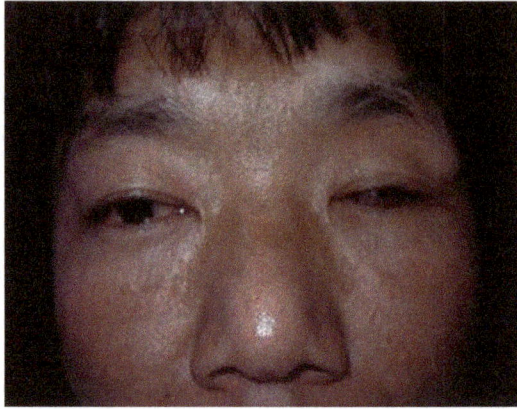

Figure 3. Ocular Defect Left eye

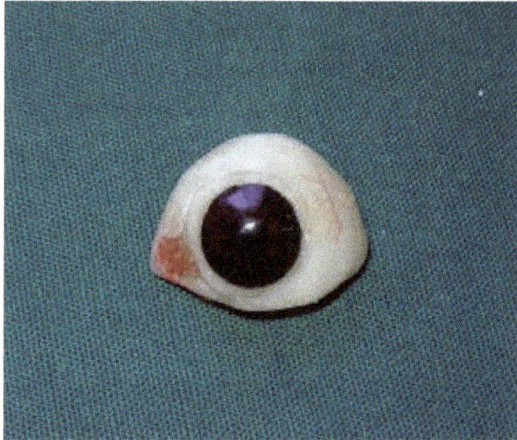

Figure 4. Custom-made ocular prosthesis

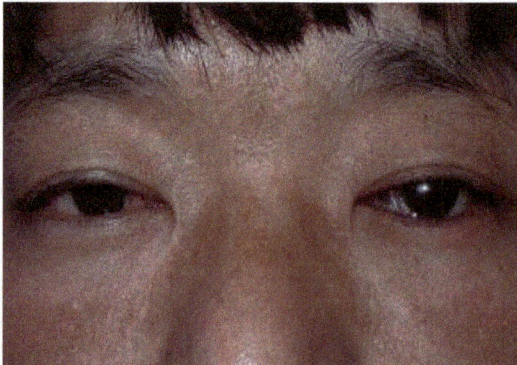

Figure 5. Customised orbital prosthesis *in situ*

removal of the prosthesis. Patients can easily remove the prosthesis when not in use and also replace it quickly and effortlessly [39 – 41].

The ideal locations where craniofacial implants may be placed are the supero-lateral rim and the infero-lateral rim. The implants are placed in such a manner that they project into the defect space. The advantage of this is that the boundaries of the prosthesis can conceal the retentive mechanism effectively. It is advisable to place at least three implants both in the upper and the lower orbital rims. This ensures adequate retention even if one or more implants fail. In case the patient has received irradiation as part of the onco-therapeutic process they need to be advised hyperbaric oxygen therapy as described earlier [25 – 27]. The bony architecture in this region is mostly cortical and therefore shorter implants may be are used. It is advisable to wait for 6-8 months for complete osseointegration before the implants are uncovered. The eye prostheses gain maximum retention by use of Neodymium magnets housed in a carrier superstructure within the orbit. Due to the natural shape of the orbit being oval, the abutments, once placed on the implants, will converge toward the center of the orbit. It is therefore important to allow for adequate space of at least 1cm apart between the implants during the surgical phase so that the abutments do not contact thereby interfering with the superstructure.

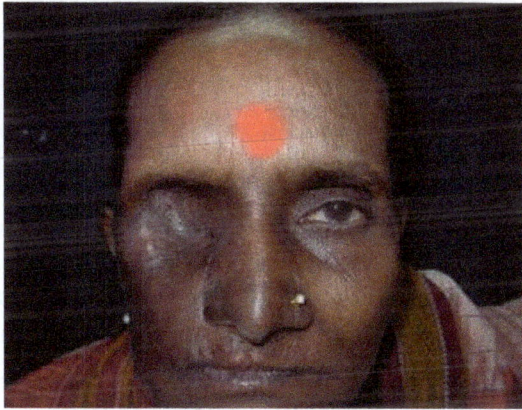

Figure 6. Post-exenteration orbital defect

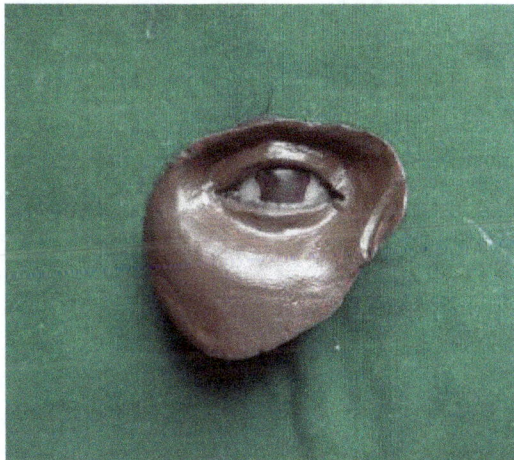

Figure 7. Custom-made orbital prosthesis

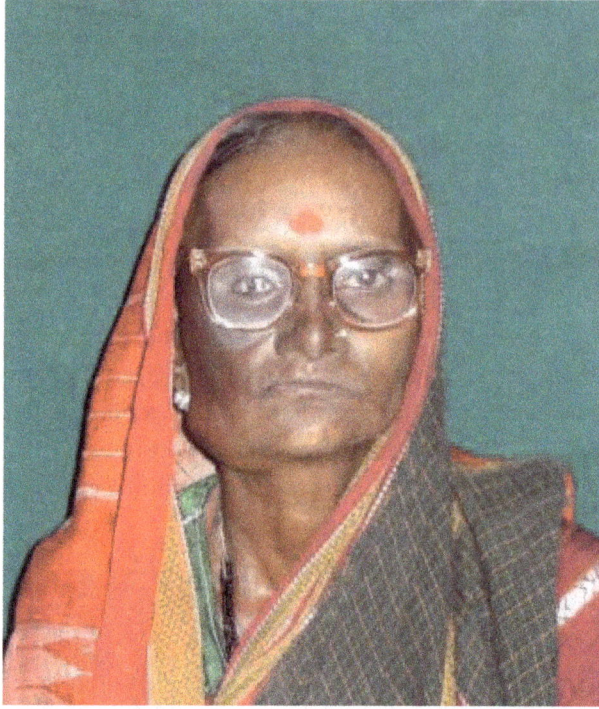

Figure 8. Orbital prosthesis retained with spectacles

After the abutments are attached the fabrication of the prosthesis may be carried out by the maxillofacial prosthodontic team. The margins of the prosthesis may be thinned to ensure better esthetic outcome. Simple frames may also be used so that the borders are concealed [Figure 8]. Patients need to be kept on regular follow-up protocol for any changes in the implants, skin or colour changes in the prosthesis itself [39, 41].

4. Nasal prosthesis

The nose and its adjacent structures play a vital role in facial esthetics. Unlike other facial structures it cannot be easily hidden or camouflaged and hence any person with a congenital or acquired defect looks for early rehabilitation. Small defects are best reconstructed by the plastic surgeon but when both bone and soft tissue have been lost as a result of malignancy related surgeries or due to severe mid-face trauma, then other alternatives are required [1, 42]. Retention using less invasive methods such as the use of tissue or bony undercuts or mechanical with spectacles has been tried with limited success. Even though it may be a challenge, the use of osseointegrated fixtures will ensure excellent retention and esthetic outcome. Ideally three implants need to be placed for adequate retention. It is recommended that a triangular placement around the residual nasal aperture be used. Two implants should be placed at the area of alar base in a vertical line drawn downward from the medial canthus of each eye. One additional implant is placed at the nasal bridge in the midline inferior to the frontal sinus to complete an isosceles triangle [Figure 9]. The implants at the alar base should project out at 90° to surface. The implant at the midline of the nasal bridge should project downward 30° or at the same angle as the nasal bones project from frontal bone [43].

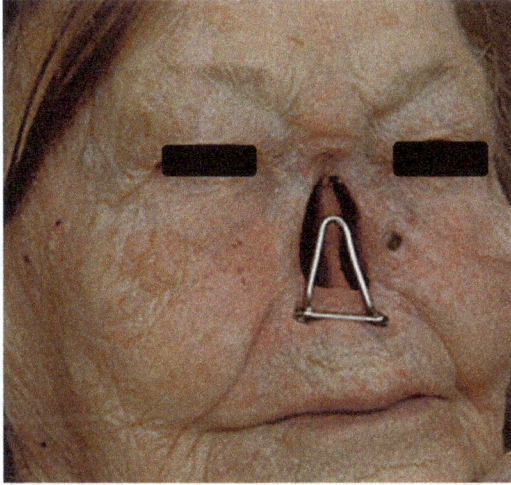

Figure 9. Nasal defect with bar attachment on three implants

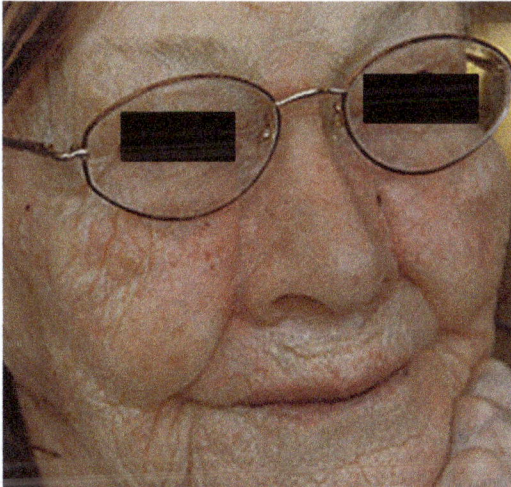

Figure 10. Nasal prosthesis in situ

The prosthetic superstructure is fabricated in silicone and retained with the help of clips or magnets [Figure 10] within the prosthesis that engage a metal bar connecting the implants [1, 3]. The connector framework ensures even force distribution over all the three fixtures. In certain cases where there is complete or partial loss of the maxilla and associated midfacial structures, the nasal component may be magnetically connected to the intraoral obturator [Figure 11] thus providing mutual retention to each other [44 – 46]. The use of spectacles once again distracts the observer's vision from the borders between the skin and the prosthesis and ensures better esthetic outcome [1, 3].

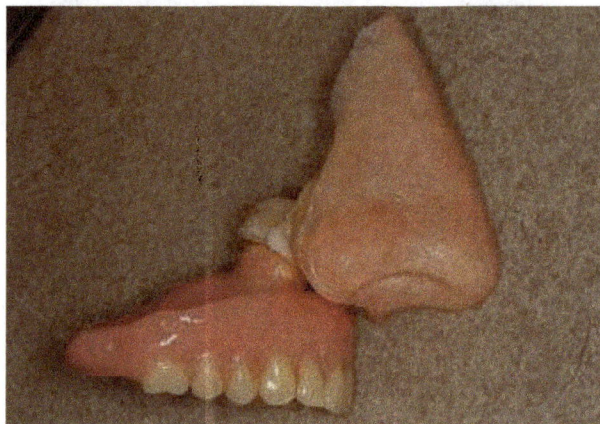

Figure 11. Nasal and maxillary obturator prosthesis connected with magnets

5. Auricular defects

The auricle may be congenitally malformed as in microtia or may be disfigured as a result of trauma following road traffic accidents, burns, acid attacks, or animal or human bites. Surgically they may be removed due to local malignancies. Plastic surgeons may attempt an autogenous reconstruction of the external ear but it is extremely challenging and technically demanding. In contrast an esthetically pleasing and excellent shade matched auricular prosthesis may be fabricated from acrylic polymers or from silicone elastomers [Figure 12 – 15]. The main problem with these prostheses has been their retention. Traditionally tissue undercuts, mechanical retention with springs, clips, hairpieces and adhesives have been used to hold them in place [3]. These have serious limitations as retention is not very strong and can be dislodged by daily activities of life [47 – 50].

Once again osseointegrated implants have proven to be a boon and are presently the method of choice. In these cases two or three implants placed external to the external auditory meatus in the temporo-mastoid region are sufficient [Figure 16]. Implants placed to retain a prosthetic ear are limited in length by the thickness of the mastoid and temporal bones as well as the mastoid air cells. Positioning of implants in the temporal bone is critical to the overall esthetic result and so the use of a surgical guide is mandatory. In cases of microtia or where there are

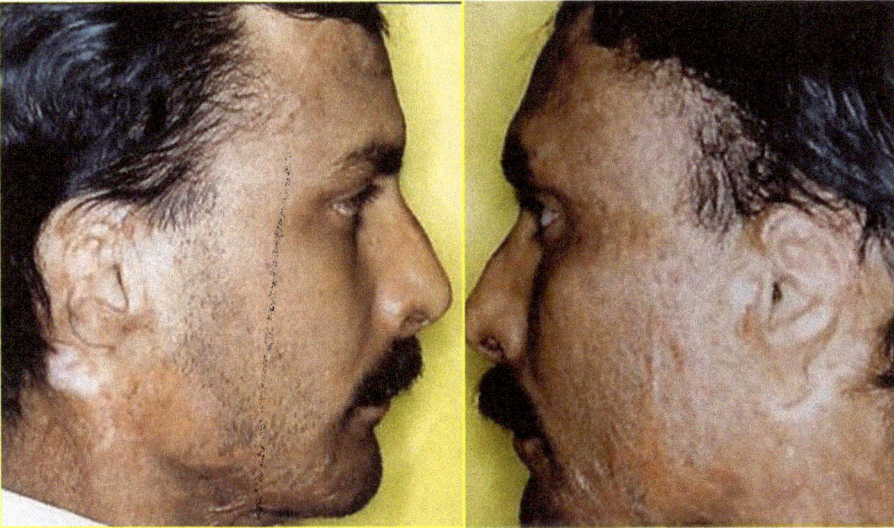

Figure 12. Bilateral auricular defect following severe burns

a malformed tissue tags it may be beneficial to have them surgically removed prior to the start of the rehabilitation process [48, 51].

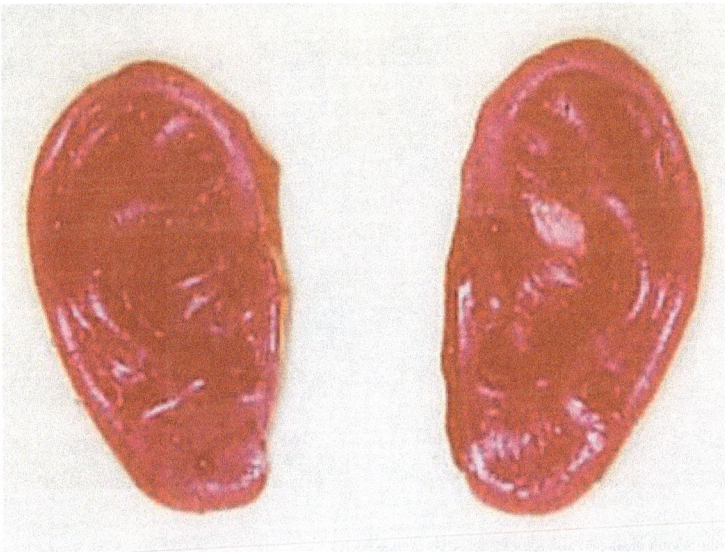

Figure 13. Wax patterns of ear prosthesis

The maxillofacial prosthodontist should fabricate a diagnostic wax-up of the proposed prosthesis replicating the anatomic features of contra-lateral ear and properly positioned to provide facial symmetry [51]. Using the wax pattern a surgical guide is then replicated with acrylic resin or vinyl acetate. The guide should indicate the most optimal location for implant placement. The implants are usually related to the anti helix of the external ear. In this position

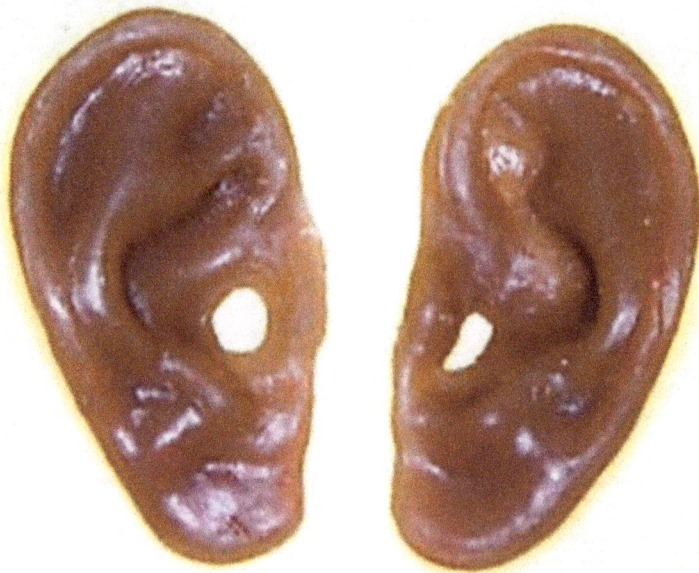

Figure 14. Finished and polished silicone ear prostheses

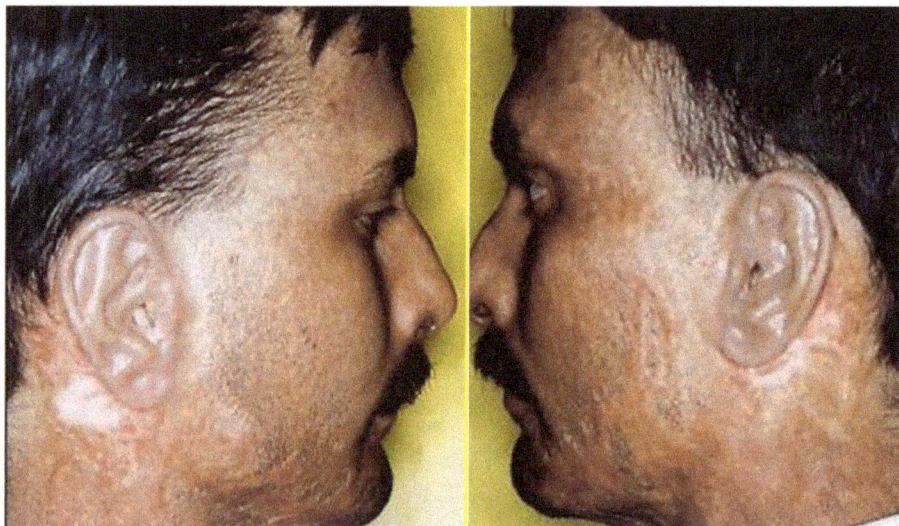

Figure 15. Bilateral auricular prosthesis (mechanically retained)

the exposed implants and the retention system have the best opportunity to be hidden from view. Two retention systems using either metal bars of 2 mm diameter soldered to metallic cylinders or retention clips may be used separately or in combination [Figure 17, 18]. The fabrication steps of the silicone prosthesis follow the routine steps as for other external prostheses. The advantage of having long hair to hide the margins is an added advantage. Cleanliness and proper maintenance is a must and should be ensured at follow-up [51 – 54].

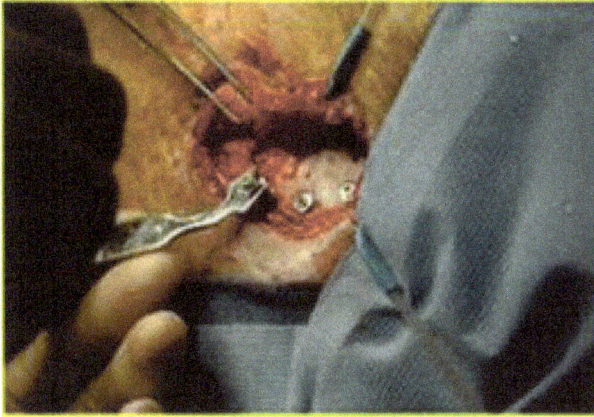

Figure 16. Craniofacial implants placed for ear prosthesis

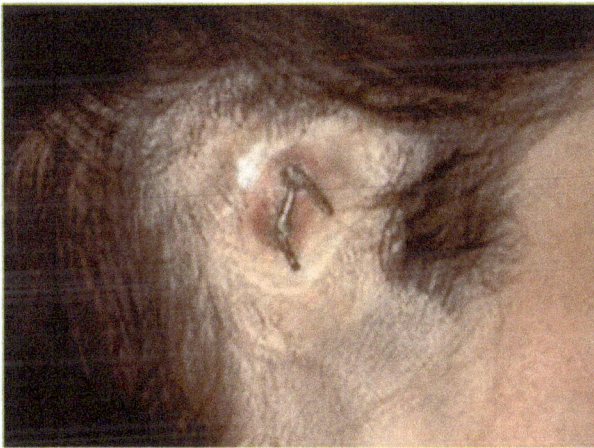

Figure 17. Bar retainer connected to the abutments

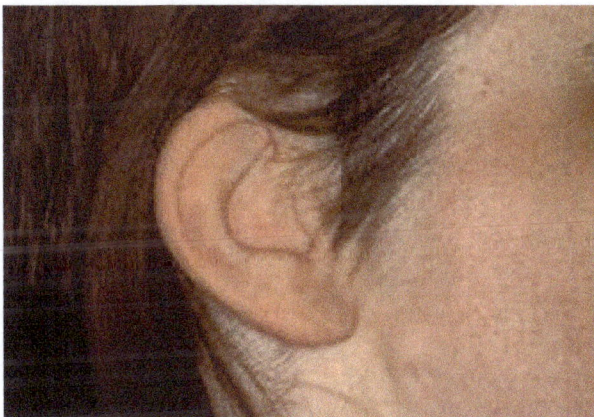

Figure 18. Implant retained ear prosthesis in situ

6. Management of the dentate maxillectomy patient

The dental health status of the patient is the first consideration when planning for prosthetic implantation. Preservation of all possible teeth and vigorous dental hygiene are important in the preoperative period to reduce problems in the postoperative period, when cleaning will be difficult if not impossible. The decision to remove maxillary teeth may come into question if the patient may receive pre and post-operative radiation. It is felt by most prosthodontists that the potential risk of osteoradionecrosis resulting from dental treatment in the maxilla is minimal. Each tooth that can be saved has tremendous potential value as an abutment for the obturator prosthesis. Therefore, all teeth should be retained except those that are grossly carious and cannot be restored by any means [55]. In addition to assessment and preservation of teeth, it important to obtain maxillary and mandibular casts in the pre-operative period. Two maxillary casts should be obtained; one to be used as a permanent record, and the other for reproduction of the anticipated surgical defect to be used as a guide for fabrication of the prosthesis. One copy of the pre-operative cast should be kept at all times and further duplication done if so required.

Various designs of intra-oral prostheses are possible keeping in mind the principles as applicable for removable cast framework partial dentures. Where required other forms of additional retention are possible using the myriad commercially available intra-coronal or extra-coronal precision attachments. These should suffice to provide a prosthesis that is functionally stable and acceptable to the patient [55 – 58].

6.1. Obturators

Various types and designs of obturators may be planned. Based on the time of placement they can be classified as: surgical, interim and definitive. Surgical obturators are those that are placed immediately after surgery. Although there has been some disagreement about the value of surgical obturators, they do offer distinct advantages for the surgeon and the patient.

Design of the surgical obturator is a challenge, and involves communication between the surgeon and the prosthodontist. The preoperative plan should be discussed, and actual anticipated defects should be clearly marked on the preoperative cast. Areas that will definitively be resected should be outlined, as well as areas that may be involved. The type of retention method that the surgeon prefers should be communicated prior to surgery [56, 59]. Retention holes in the acrylic plate should be created on the defect side so that the edges can be sutured immediately after surgery to the cheek to support the surgical pack *in situ* [Figure 19, 20].

Interim obturators are those prostheses which are placed immediately after removal of the surgical packing and should be used until tissue contracture is minimal [Figure 21 – 24]. Time between removal of the pack and obturator placement should be minimal, as tissue contraction and edema will quickly alter the shape of the defect, making it difficult to insert an obturator. For this reason, it is important to have a post-surgical obturator made prior to removal of packing. It is also important that the prosthodontist be present with the surgeon when packing is removed so the prosthesis can be inserted immediately after inspection of the surgical site by the surgeon [59].

The definitive obturator is designed when the surgical defect has stabilized, approximately 3 to 12 months after definitive surgery [Figure 25]. The bulb portion that extends into the defect area must be kept hollow in order to lessen the weight of the prosthesis [Figure 26]. The design of the prosthesis should allow maximal distribution of forces to all available teeth, remaining hard palate, walls of the defect, and areas of remaining alveolus. In addition, occlusion must be restored to the best extent possible so that the prosthesis can be functional and not just cosmetic. Regular follow-up is mandatory and modifications should be carried out as required. The prosthodontist must be careful to note signs that the obturator is no longer functioning, such as fluid reflux into the nasal cavity, change in voice quality or TMJ problems [56, 59].

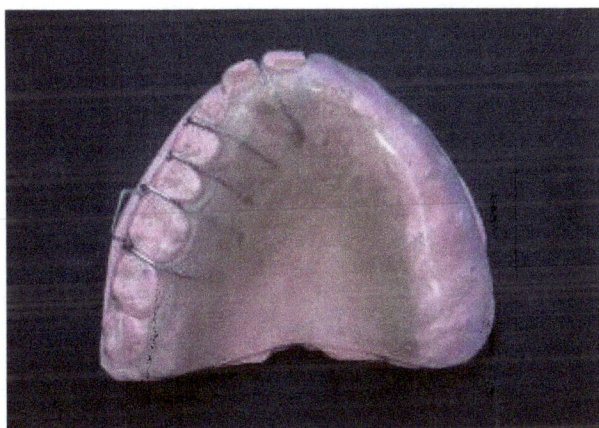

Figure 19. Surgical obturator with retentive holes on surgical side (left)

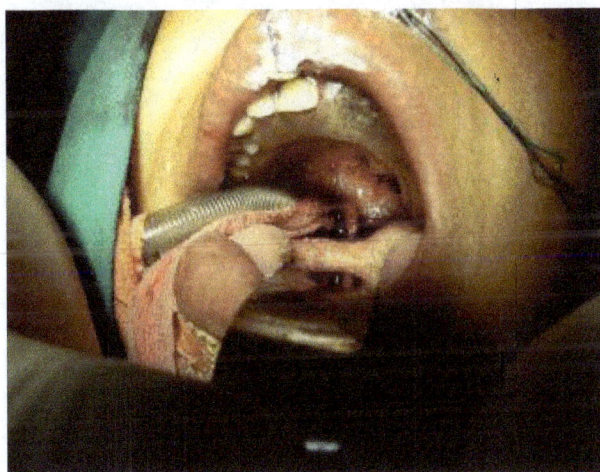

Figure 20. Surgical obturator fixed in situ immediately following surgery

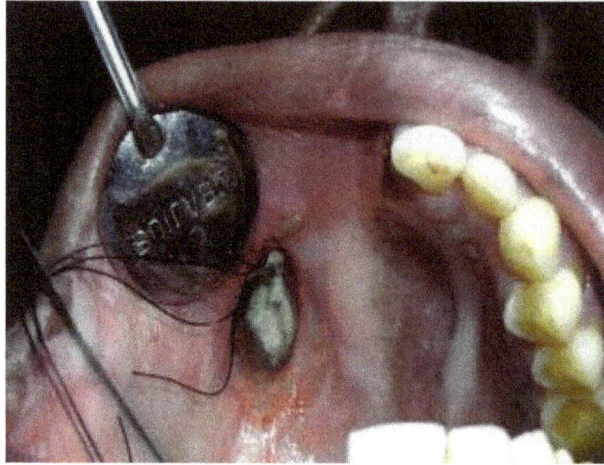

Figure 21. Healed maxillary defect (mirror image)

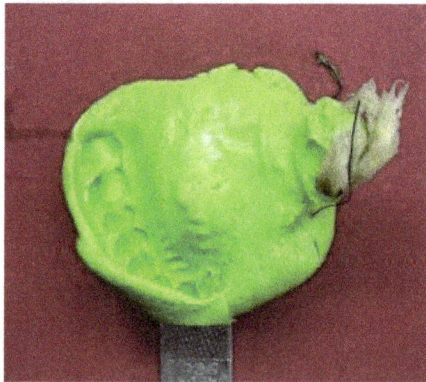

Figure 22. Impression made in irreversible hydrocolloid

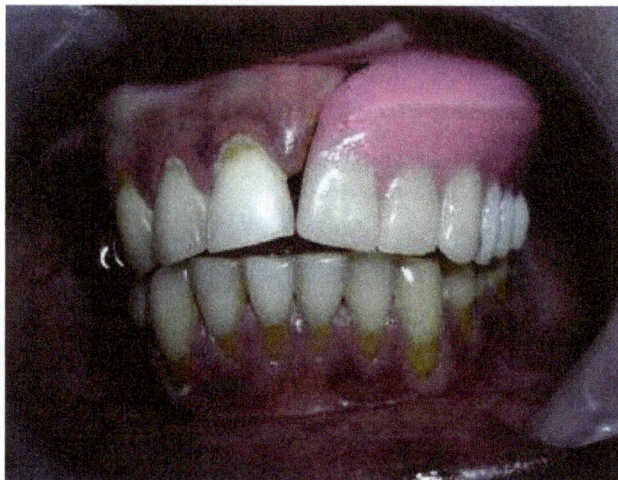

Figure 23. Try-in of maxillary obturator prosthesis

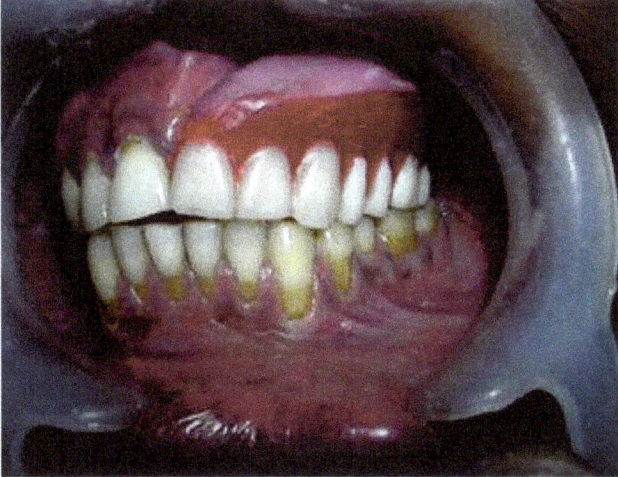

Figure 24. Interim obturator prosthesis in situ

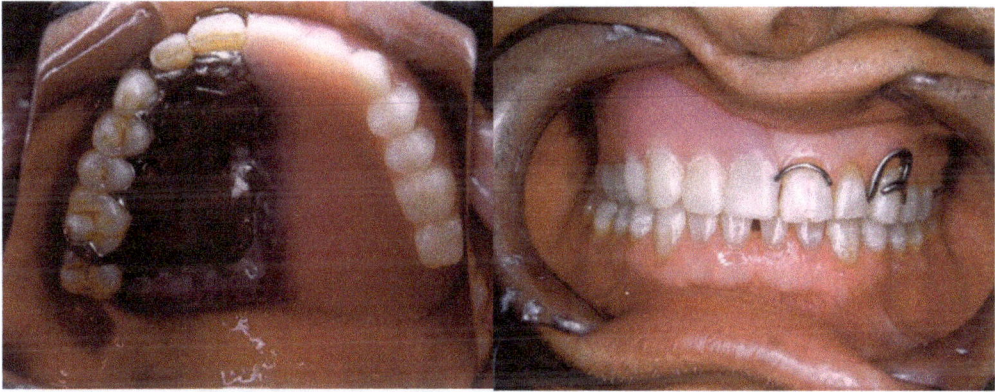

Figure 25. Definitive obturator prosthesis in situ

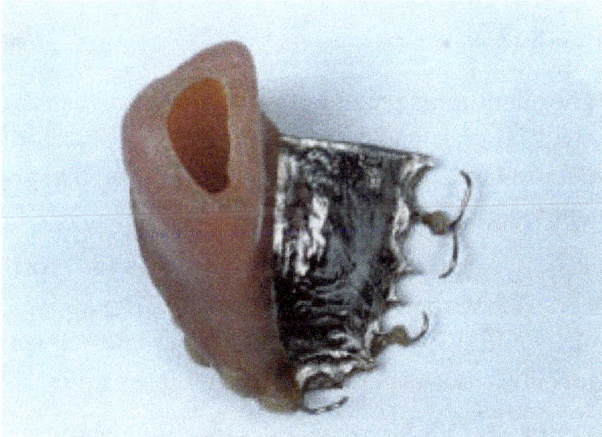

Figure 26. Definitive obturator prosthesis showing hollow bulb

6.2. Management of the edentulous maxillectomy patient

Edentulous maxillectomy patients are always a challenge for the maxillofacial team due to the complexity of postoperative rehabilitation. Retention of the obturator is a problem since there is a lack of support of adjacent teeth for stabilization. In addition, the reduced volume of residual ridge of the edentulous patient demands that stress be distributed to all available portions of the palate.

Some of the important guidelines to be informed to the maxillofacial surgeon or oncosurgeon at the time of resection are as follows:-[59-62].

Maintain as much hard palate as possible. Since the edentulous patient must rely on remnants of the hard palate for primary retention, support and stability, the prosthodontist should advise the surgeon to resect only that portion of the hard palate that is mandatory to allow for clean margins [Figure 27]. It is vital to ensure that the ipsilateral palate is preserved which will allow a tripoding effect. If the anterior alveolus can be maintained, the patient will have better facial esthetics and less contracture postoperatively.

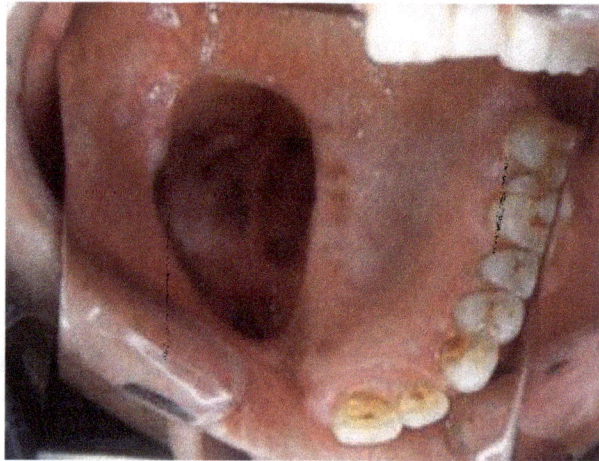

Figure 27. Maximum retention of hard palate (mirror image)

Skin graft the cheek flap The edentulous patient requires maximal distribution of forces, and the mucosa on the cheek will be an area of contact with the obturator. The thick squamous epithelium of a split-thickness skin graft will resist the wear and tear applied by the obturator as compared to the friable oral tissues.

Remove the inferior turbinate. By removing the inferior turbinate, the prosthesis can be contoured to fit into the nasal cavity. This vertical height will resist the rotational forces applied during mastication. In addition, by adding an extension into the nasal cavity, a larger surface of bone may be utilized to balance the stresses generated during mastication.

Skin graft the maxillary sinus walls This is necessary as the movements of the obturator bulb will transmit greater force to the sinus walls in the edentulous patient. These walls can be prepared during surgery to allow the bony undercuts to serve for retention or for vertical support to

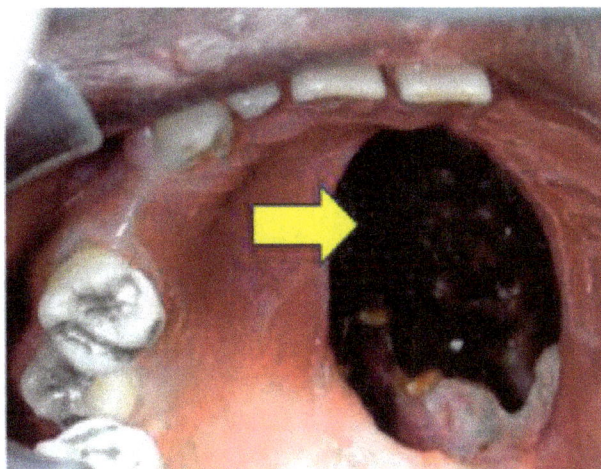

Figure 28. Skin graft on lateral wall of maxillary post-surgical defect

keep the prosthesis from rotating into the defect during mastication. The sinus walls are covered with respiratory mucosa, which must be denuded and covered with a split-thickness skin graft. Grafting the sinus walls stops formation of polypoid tissue and mucus generation within the sinus and allows the walls to become load-bearing areas [Figure 28].

With the increased use of osseointegrated implants, dependence on mechanical and anatomic methods of retention has diminished. Osseointegrated implants provide excellent retention to the definitive obturator. Retentive magnets and various designs of clips are available to minimize force transfer to the implant and supporting bone [3, 63, 64].

For a long time it was considered taboo to place implants in irradiated bone. However numerous studies have shown that use of hyperbaric oxygen chambers can be of immense value in such patients and allow for successful osseointegration as discussed earlier [25 – 27].

6.3. Zygomatic implants

Remote bone anchorage using zygoma implants for extensive maxillofacial defects is another option. Effective axial loading of the zygoma implant is accomplished by cross-arch stabilization with a rigid splint framework using at least 4 implants with adequate anterior – posterior spread [Figure 29]. When patients present with maxillary defects that do not have ideal residual anatomy, it is may be possible to place zygoma implants in areas that will enhance the desired splinting effect of the bar assembly. The most significant and immediate benefit of this approach is the ability to extend the prosthesis anchorage points into defect areas, thus minimizing the cantilever forces on teeth and implants in residual ridge tissue. Maxillectomy and severely resorbed maxilla are challenging to restore with provision of removable prostheses. Dental implants are essential to restore aesthetics and function and subsequently quality of life in such group of patients. Zygomatic implants reduce the complications associated with bone grafting procedures and simplify the rehabilitation of atrophic maxilla and maxillectomy [65, 66].

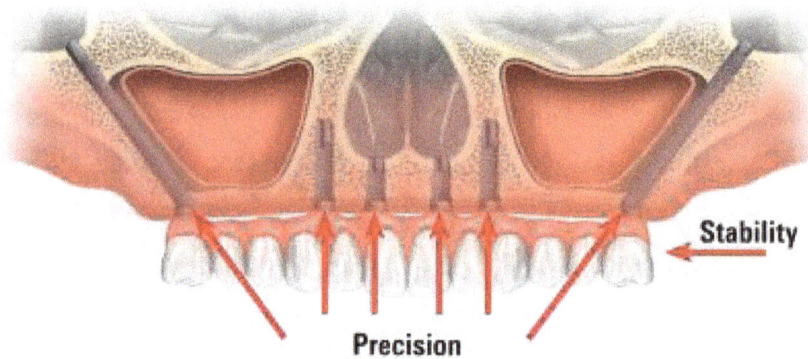

Figure 29. Diagrammatic representation of zygomatic implants

Studies using three-dimensional finite element analysis were carried out to study the impact of different levels of zygomatic bone support (10, 15, and 20 mm) on the biomechanics of zygomatic implants. Results indicated maximum stresses within the fixture were increased by three times, when bone support decreased from 20 to 10 mm, and concentrated at fixture/bone interface. However, stresses within the abutment screw and abutment itself were not significantly different regardless of the bone support level. Supporting bone of 10 mm showed double the stress as compared to levels of 15 and 20 mm. The deflection of the fixtures was decreased by two to three times as the level of bone support increased to 15 mm and 20 mm respectively. Therefore, it important that the zygomatic bone support should not be kept at less than 15 mm. This will reduce the amount of deflection of the fixture and ensure long-term success of the implants [67, 68].

Placement of zygomatic implants lateral to the maxillary sinus, according to the extra-sinus protocol, is one of the treatment options in the rehabilitation of severely atrophic maxilla or following maxillectomy surgery in the head and neck cancer patients. Studies on a full-arch fixed-prosthesis supported by four zygomatic implants in the atrophic maxilla under occlusal loading have shown that maximum von Mises stresses were significantly higher under lateral loading compared with vertical loading within the prosthesis and its supporting implants. Peak stresses was found to be concentrated at the interface between the prosthesis and the fixtures when subjected to vertical load and also at the internal line angles of the prosthesis when subjected to lateral load. The zygomatic bone exhibited much lower stress levels as compared to the alveolar bone especially under lateral load. The zygomatic bone overall showed less values of stress than the alveolar bone and the prosthesis-implant complex under both types of loading [67]. Further research and long-term studies needs to be carried out on these types of implants so that the rehabilitation of the atrophied or missing maxilla can be successfully carried out.

7. Microimplants and maxillofacial rehabilitation

Patients with craniofacial birth defects present with extreme skeletal deformities and often require a multi-pronged approach for achieving acceptable esthetic results. Vachiramon et. al. [69], have described a series of cases in which orthodontic microimplants were used to better the surgical outcome of such patients. Use of these microimplants for support helped in distraction osteogenesis procedures involving the mandible, maxilla, or midface. The microimplants were additionally used to stabilize the dentition for orthodontic tooth movement or for resisting change from long-term use of inter-arch elastics. They concluded that microimplants appear to have good potential in the approach to treat patients with craniofacial anomalies. They can also be useful to present an alternative treatment plan in patients who refuse orthognathic surgery. Microimplants may be of great utility for the rehabilitation of craniofacial patients with congenitally missing permanent teeth; malformed teeth or patients with ectodermal dysplasia with reduced dentition that makes reciprocal orthodontic anchorage difficult [69].

8. Future trends in maxillofacial rehabilitation

The use of Computed Tomography (CT) and Magnetic Resonance Imaging (MRI) in conjunction with Rapid Prototyping (RP) have revolutionized the methods of old-fashioned impressions using various types of dental materials and sculpting of the prosthesis by hand in wax or clay [Figure 30, 31]. Recently advances in 3D optical imaging using 3D whole field profilometer based on the projection of incoherent light and 3D laser eye-safe scanners have been utilized [70, 71]. The advantages of such a system are that they are non-invasive, have a higher speed of data acquisition, and the scanners are more rugged and portable than the CT or MRI scanners [70].

Once the data has been acquired the virtual 3D models are obtained and the final prosthesis can be designed virtually. Two models one with the defect and another with the built up prosthesis are generated using epoxy photo-polymerising resins in a 3D printer [Figure 32, 33]. The final prosthesis is then fabricated from silicone rubber using these moulds [70 – 72].

In order to minimize the harmful effects of the metallic implants and their by-products, several newer materials are being tried. New alloys like tantalum, niobium, zirconium, and magnesium are receiving attention given their satisfying mechanical and biological properties. Non-oxide ceramics like silicon nitride and silicon carbide are being currently developed as a promising implant material possessing a combination of properties such as good wear and corrosion resistance, increased ductility, good fracture and creep resistance, and relatively high hardness in comparison to alumina. Polymer/magnesium composites are being developed to improve mechanical properties as well as retain polymer's property of degradation [73].

Nanotechnology and tissue engineering along with the concepts of stem cell technology are poised to dramatically define the next quantum leap in the field of maxillofacial reconstruction.

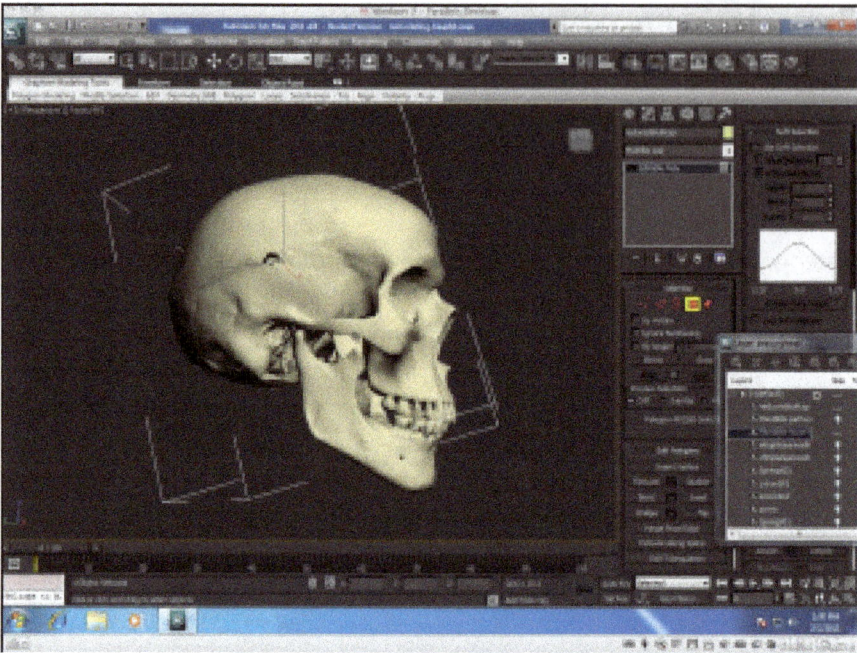

Figure 30. 3D virtual reconstruction and planning

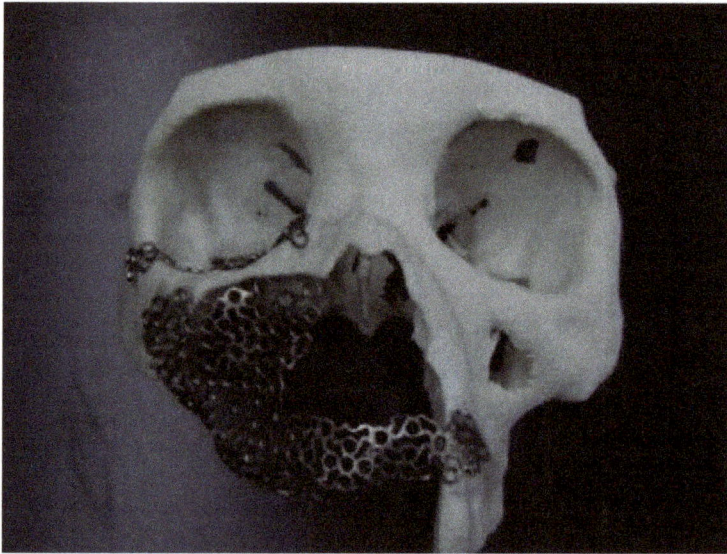

Figure 31. Rapid prototype modelling of maxillofacial prosthesis

Whether it is regeneration of new osseous tissue *in vivo* for placement of implants or even the regeneration of a complete ear or nose literally 'grown' from the stem cells of the person or a suitable donor-the possibilities are endless [74, 75]. It seems to be just a matter of time before the dream of autologous reconstruction of defective or missing anatomical structures soon becomes a reality.

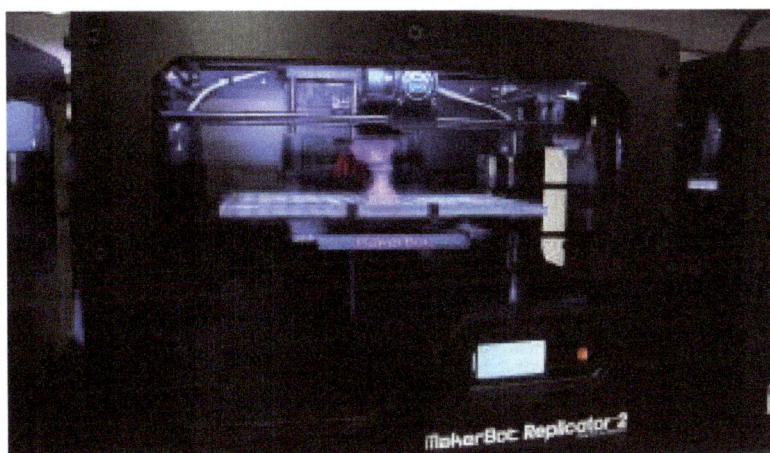

Figure 32. 3D printer

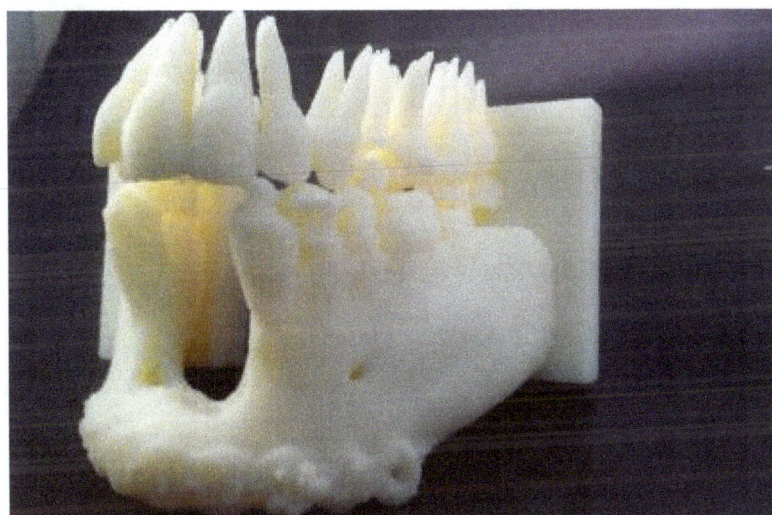

Figure 33. 3D printed model of mandibular defect

9. Conclusion

The discovery of osseointegration has been arguably one of the most beneficial medical breakthroughs especially in the head and neck region. The number of successful implants being placed is increasing rapidly as better implants, more efficient investigative techniques and superior armamentarium is readily available. These implants have also revolutionized the scope and the efficacy of rehabilitation of the entire craniofacial region [76].

Despite the rise in cancers of the head and neck region there is also a deeper understanding of the changes at cellular level and better treatment options and targeted medication. It is hoped that with each passing day there will be continued dedicated research to fight and eradicate all these killer diseases. Until then the science of craniofacial implantology will ensure that the patients receive the most comprehensive rehabilitation that can be offered and ensure that their early return to form and function.

In future it is hoped that technological advances in allied fields such as radio-diagnosis and imaging, CAD-CAM manufacturing, tissue engineering, laser scanning, 3D-printing, development of newer nano-based materials and robotic placement of implants will work in tandem to ensure that larger numbers of patients can be treated early, economically and effectively [77-79]. Then alone will the dream of health for all be truly a reality.

Acknowledgements

I gratefully acknowledge all my respected teachers, enthusiastic students and tolerant patients who have taught me that I know so little and shown me that there is so much more learn.

Author details

Derek D'Souza*

Address all correspondence to: dsjdsouza@gmail.com

Consultant Prosthodontist, Pune, India

References

[1] Brecht LE. Craniofacial and maxillofacial prosthetics. In: Thorne CH et al. (eds.) Grabb and Smith's Plastic Surgery. 6th edn. Philadelphia: Lippincott Williams & Wilkins; 2007: 350 –7.

[2] Semple C, Parahoo K, Norman A, McCaughan E, Humphris G, Mills M. Psychosocial interventions for patients with head and neck cancer. Cochrane Database of Systematic Reviews 2013, 7: CD009441.

[3] Mantri S and Khan Z. Prosthodontic Rehabilitation of Acquired Maxillofacial Defects. In: Agulnik M (ed.) Head and Neck Cancer Rijeka: InTech; 2012: 315 – 36.

[4] Villar CC, Huynh-Ba G, Mills MP, Cochran DL. Wound healing around dental implants. Endodontic Topics 2011; 25: 44–62.

[5] Kuzyk PR, Schemitsch EH. The basic science of peri-implant bone healing. Indian J Orthop 2011; 45:108-15.

[6] Coelho PG, Granjeiro JM, Romanos GE, Suzuki M, Silva NR, Cardaropoli G, et al. Basic research methods and current trends of dental implant surfaces. J Biomed Mater Res B Appl Biomater 2009; 88:579-96.

[7] Actis L, Gaviria L Ong JL. Antimicrobial surfaces for craniofacial implants: state of the art. J Korean Assoc Oral Maxillofac Surg. 2013; 39(2): 43–54.

[8] Ramaswamy Y, Wu C, Zreiqat H. Orthopedic coating materials: considerations and applications. Expert Rev Med Devices 2009; 6:423-30.

[9] Özcan M, Hämmerle C. Titanium as a reconstruction and implant material in dentistry: Advantages and Pitfalls. Materials 2012; 5:1528-45.

[10] Stanford CM. Surface modifications of dental implants. Aust Dent J 2008; 53(Suppl 1): S26–S33

[11] Lin YH, Peng PW, Ou KL. The effect of titanium with electrochemical anodization on the response of the adherent osteoblast-like cell. Implant Dent 2012; 21(4): 344-9.

[12] Kim MH, Lee SY, Kim MJ, Kim SK, Heo SJ, Koak JY. Effect of biomimetic deposition on anodized titanium surfaces. J Dental Res 2011; 90(6):711-16.

[13] Hanawa T. Degradation of dental implants. In: Eliaz N (ed) Degradation of Implant Materials. Springer: New York; 2012: 57-78.

[14] Iezzi G, Malchiodi L, Quaranta A, Ghensi P, Piattelli A. Peri-implant bone response around a human hydroxyapatite-coated implant retrieved after a 10-year loading period: A case report. Int J Oral Maxillofac Implants 2012; 28(4): 190-4.

[15] Baker MI, Eberhardt AW, Martin DM, McGwin G, Lemons JE. Bone properties surrounding hydroxyapatite-coated custom osseous integrated dental implants. J. Biomed. Mater. Res 2010; 95B: 218–24.

[16] van Oirschot BAJA, Bronkhorst EM, van den Beucken JJJP, Meijer GJ, Jansen JA, Junker R. Long-term survival of calcium phosphate-coated dental implants: a meta-analytical approach to the clinical literature. Clin. Oral Impl. Res. 24, 2013, 355–62.

[17] Jimbo R, Coelho PG, Vandeweghe S, Schwartz-Filho HO, Hayashi M, Ono D, Wennerberg, A. Histological and three-dimensional evaluation of osseointegration to nanostructured calcium phosphate-coated implants. Acta Biomaterialia 2011; 7(12): 4229-34.

[18] Goené RJ, Testori T, Trisi P. Influence of a nanometer-scale surface enhancement on de novo bone formation on titanium implants: a histomorphometric study in human maxillae. Int J Periodontics Restorative Dent 2007; 27: 211-9.

[19] Hong YS, Kim MJ, Han JS, Yeo IS. Effects of hydrophilicity and fluoride surface modifications to titanium dental implants on early osseointegration: An in vivo study. Implant Dent 2014; 23(5): 529-33.

[20] Monjo M, Petzold C, Ramis JM, Lyngstadaas SP, Ellingsen JE. In vitro osteogenic properties of two dental implant surfaces. Int J Biomater 2012; 181024: 1-14.

[21] Abraham CM. A brief historical perspective on dental implants, their surface coatings and treatments. Open Dent J 2014; 8: 50-5.

[22] Granström, G. Craniofacial osseointegration. In: Oral Diseases 2007; 13: 261–9.

[23] Rocke DJ, Tucci DL, Marcus J, McClennen J, Kaylie D. Osseointegrated implants for auricular defects: Operative techniques and complication management. Otol Neurotol 2014; 35(9): 1609-14.

[24] Kelly JA. Craniofacial and Maxillofacial Implants. In: Devlin H, Nishimura I (eds.) Oral and Cranial Implants Springer-Verlag; 2013: 28 – 37.

[25] Chrcanovic BR, Albrektsson T, Wennerberg A. Dental implants in irradiated versus non-irradiated patients: A meta-analysis. Head Neck 2014; doi: 10.1002/hed.23875.

[26] Anderson L, Meraw S, Al-Hezaimi K, Wang HL. The influence of radiation therapy on dental implantology. Implant Dent 2013; 22(1): 31–8.

[27] Javed F, Al-Hezaimi K, Al-Rasheed A, Almas K, Romanos, GE. Implant survival rate after oral cancer therapy: A review. Oral Oncol 2010; 46(12): 854-9.

[28] de Oliveira JAP, Abrahão M, Dib LL Extraoral implants in irradiated patients Braz J Otorhinolaryngol 2013; 79(2):185-9.

[29] Wennerberg A, Albrektsson T. On implant surfaces: a review of current knowledge and opinions. Int J Oral Maxillofac Implants 2010; 25 (1): 63-74.

[30] Ramazanoglu M, Oshida Y. Osseointegration and bioscience of implant surfaces-Current concepts at bone-implant interface In: Implant Dentistry-A Rapidly Evolving Practice, Turkyilmaz I (ed) Rijeka; InTech; 2011; 57 – 82.

[31] Thimmappa B, Girod SC. Principles of implant-based reconstruction and rehabilitation of craniofacial defects. Craniomaxillofac Trauma Reconstr. 2010; 3(1): 33–40.

[32] Goiato, MC, dos Santos DM, de Carvalho DSF, Pellizzer EP, Santiago Jr JF, Moreno A. Craniofacial implants success in facial rehabilitation. J Craniofac Surg 2011; 22(1): 241-2.

[33] Pekkan G, Tuna SH, Oghan F. Extraoral prostheses using extraoral implants. Int J Oral Maxillofac Surg 2011; 40(4): 378-83.

[34] Nemli SK, Aydin C, Yilmaz H, Bal BT, Arici YK, Quality of life of patients with implant-retained maxillofacial prostheses: A prospective and retrospective study. J Prosthet Dent 2013;109(1): 44–52.

[35] Ariani N, Visser A, van Oort RP, Kusdhany L, Rahardjo TB, Krom BP et al. Current state of craniofacial prosthetic rehabilitation. Int J Prosthodont 2012: 26(1): 57-67.

[36] Curi MM, Oliveira MF, Molina G, Cardoso CL, De Groot OL, Branemark PI, de Cássia BRK. Extraoral implants in the rehabilitation of craniofacial defects: implant and prosthesis survival rates and peri-implant soft tissue evaluation. J Oral Maxillofac Surg 2012; 70(7): 1551-7.

[37] Cohen M. Craniofacial surgery: the first 25 years. Where do we come from? Who are we? Where are we going? J Craniofac Surg 2014; 25(1): 14-6.

[38] Smolarz-Wojnowska A, Raithel F, Gellrich NC, Klein C. Quality of implant anchored craniofacial and intraoral prostheses: Patients evaluation. J Craniofac Surg 2014; 25(2): 202-7.

[39] Alford M. Enucleation, evisceration, and exenteration techniques In: Duane's Clinical Ophthalmology [CD ROM] Lippincott Williams & Wilkins. 2006; (5) Chapter 82.

[40] Ozcelik TB, Yilmaz B Two-piece impression procedure for implant-retained orbital prostheses. Int J Oral Maxillofac Implants. 2012; 27(5): 93-5.

[41] Karakoca-Nemli, S, Aydin, C, Yilmaz H and Bal BT. A method for fabricating an implant-retained orbital prosthesis using the existing prosthesis. J Prosthodont 2011; 20: 583–6.

[42] Ethunandan M, Downie I, Flood T. Implant-retained nasal prosthesis for reconstruction of large rhinectomy defects: the Salisbury experience. Int J Oral Maxillofac Surg. 2010; 39 (4): 343-9.

[43] Bedrossian E, Brånemark PI. Systematic treatment planning protocol for patients with maxillofacial defects: avoiding living a life of seclusion and depression. Atlas Oral Maxillofac Surg Clin North Am 2012; 20(1): 135-58.

[44] Banerjee S, Kumar S, Bera A, Gupta T, Banerjee A. Magnet retained intraoral-extra oral combination prosthesis: a case report. J Adv Prosthodont 2012; 4(4): 235-8.

[45] Goyal S, Goyal MK, Kallingan P. Magnetically retained extra oral prosthesis and maxillary interim obturator. Eur J Prosthodont 2014; 2: 37-40.

[46] Dholam KP, Shetty KG, Bhirangi PP. Restoration of nasal defect with implant-retained nose prosthesis. J Indian Prosthodont Soc; 2007; 7 (4): 196-9

[47] Lovely M, Dathan PC, Gopal D, George BT, Nair KC. Implant retained auricular prosthesis with a modified Hader bar: A case report J Indian Prosthodont Soc 2014; 14(2): 187-190.

[48] Aydin C, Karakoca S, Yilmaz H, Yilmaz C. Implant retained auricular prosthesis: An assessment of implant success and prosthetic complications. Int J Prosthodont 2008; 21: 241-4.

[49] Guo G, Schwedtner O, Klein M. A retrospective study of implant-retained auricular prosthesis. Int J Oral Maxillofac Implants 2008; 23: 539-43.

[50] Nanda A, Jain V, Kumar R, Kabra K. Implant-supported auricular prosthesis. Indian J Dent Res 2011; 22:152-6.

[51] Wright RF, Zemnick C, Wazen JJ, Asher E. Osseointegrated implants and auricular defects: a case series study. J Prosthodont 2008; 17(6): 468-75

[52] Federspil, PA. Auricular Prostheses In: Staudenmaier R (ed) Aesthetics and functionality in ear reconstruction. Basel, Karger; 2010; 68: 65-80.

[53] Dilber E, Koc O, Ozturk AN, and Karamese M Craniofacial implant-retained auricular prosthesis: A case report. J Oral Implant 2013; 39 (4): 479-82.

[54] Kievit, H, Verhage-Damen GW, Ingels KJ, Mylanus EA, Hol MK. Long-term quality of life assessment in patients with auricular prostheses. J Craniofac Surg 2013; 24(2): 392-7.

[55] Kim DR, Lim YJ, Kim MJ, Kwon HB. The importance of remaining teeth reconstruction in the definite obturator for a hemimaxillectomy patient. J Craniofac Surg 2011; 22(6): 2359-61.

[56] Lethaus B, Lie N, de Beer F, Kessler P, de Baat C, Verdonck HW. Surgical and prosthetic reconsiderations in patients with maxillectomy. J Oral Rehab 2010; 37(2): 138-42.

[57] Shirota T, Shimodaira O, Matsui Y, Hatori M, Shintani S. Zygoma implant-supported prosthetic rehabilitation of a patient with a maxillary defect. Int J Oral Maxillofac Surg 2011; 40(1): 113-7.

[58] Murat S, Gurbuz A, Isayev A, Dokmez B, Cetin U. Enhanced retention of a maxillofacial prosthetic obturator using precision attachments: Two case reports. Eur J Dent 2012; 6(2): 212-7.

[59] Jacob RF. Clinical management of the edentulous maxillectomy patient In: Taylor TD (ed) Clinical Maxillofacial Prosthetics Quintessence 2000: 85 – 102.

[60] Kumar P, Alvi HA, Rao J, Singh BP, Jurel SK, Kumar L, Aggarwal H. Assessment of the quality of life in maxillectomy patients: A longitudinal study J Adv Prosthodont 2013; 5: 29-35

[61] Pace-Balzan A, Shaw RJ, Butterworth C. Oral rehabilitation following treatment for oral cancer. Periodontol 2000. 2011; 57: 102–17.

[62] Sharma AB, Buemer J III. Reconstruction of maxillary defects: the case for prosthetic rehabilitation. J Oral Maxillofac Surg 2005; 63: 1770-3.

[63] Parr GA, Tharp GE, Rahn AO. Prosthodontic principles in the framework design of maxillary obturator prosthesis. J Prosthet Dent 2005; 93: 405-11.

[64] Padmanabhan TV, Kumar VA, Mohamed KK, Unnikrishnan N. Prosthetic rehabilitation of a maxillectomy with a two-piece hollow bulb obturator. A clinical report. J Prosthodont 2011; 20: 397–401.

[65] Sharma A, Rahul GR. Zygomatic implants/fixture: a systematic review. J Oral Implantol 2013; 39(2): 215-24.

[66] Gonçalves, LM, Gonçalves TMSV, Rodrigues AHC, Lanza MD, Nascimento PRG, Girundi FMS. Intra-and extra-oral prostheses retained by zygoma implants following resection of the upper lip and nose. J Prosthodont 2014; doi: 10.1111/jopr.12178.

[67] Romeed SA, Malik R, Dunne SM. Zygomatic implants: the impact of zygoma bone support on biomechanics. J Oral Implantol. 2014; 40(3): 231-7.

[68] Pasquale P, Ferrari F, Trevisiol L, Francesco NP. Zygoma implant-supported prosthetic rehabilitation of a patient after subtotal bilateral maxillectomy. J Craniofac Surg 2013; 24(2): 159-62.

[69] Vachiramon A, Urata M, Kyung HM, Yamashita DD, Yen SLK, Cleft Palate Craniofac J; 2009, 46 (2):136-46.

[70] Cavagnini G, Sansoni G, Vertuan A, Docchio F. 3D optical body scanning: application to forensic medicine and to maxillofacial reconstruction. In: International Conference on 3D Body Scanning Technologies 2010: 167-78.

[71] Qiu J, Gu X, Xiong Y, Zhang F. Nasal prosthesis rehabilitation using CAD-CAM technology after total rhinectomy: A pilot study. In: Supportive Care in Cancer 2011; 19 (7): 1055-9.

[72] Subburaj K, Nair C, Rajesh C, Meshram SM, Ravi B. Rapid development of auricular prosthesis using CAD and rapid prototyping technologies. Int. J. Oral Maxillofac Surg 2007; 36: 938–43.

[73] Jakobsen C, Sørensen JA, Kassem M, and Thygesen TH. Mesenchymal stem cells in oral reconstructive surgery: A systematic review of the literature. J Oral Rehabil 2013; 40: 693–706.

[74] Mantripragada VP, Lecka-Czernik B, Ebraheim NA, Jayasuriya AC. An overview of recent advances in designing orthopedic and craniofacial implants. J Biomed Mater Res 2013; 101A: 3349–64.

[75] Nayyer L, Patel KH, Esmaeili A, Rippel RA, Birchall M, O'toole G, Butler PE, Seifalian AM. Tissue engineering: revolution and challenge in auricular cartilage reconstruction. Plast Reconstr Surg. 2012; 129(5):1123-37.

[76] Roumanas ED, Freymiller EG, Chang TL, Aghaloo T, Buemer J III. Implant retained prosthesis for facial defects: An up to 14-year follow-up report on the survival rates of implants at UCLA. Int J Prosthodont 2002; 15: 325-32.

[77] Olszewski, R. Surgical engineering in cranio-maxillofacial surgery: a literature re-
      view. J Healthc Eng 2012; 3(1): 53-86

[78] Watson D, Reuther MS. Advancing the art of rhinoplasty with tissue engineering. In
      Shiffman MA, Giuseppe AD (Eds) Advanced Aesthetic Rhinoplasty. Springer Berlin
      Heidelberg 2013; 1107-18.

[79] Davis BK, Emert R. The role of technology in the maxillofacial prosthetic setting. In:
      Printed Biomaterials Biological and Medical Physics, Biomedical Engineering 2010;
      111-20.

8

Rationale for Dental Implants

Ilser Turkyilmaz and Gokce Soganci

1. Introduction

The loss of just one tooth will eventually have a global impact on the entire stomatognathic system. Bone loss, shifting of teeth, occlusal changes, decreased bite force and many more effects are felt throughout the entire system [1-3]. In attempt to prevent the progression of these effects, dentistry has continually searched for the ideal tooth replacement. With the advent of dental implants, clinicians can now restore patients higher levels of health and function than ever before [4-8].

The deleterious effects of tooth loss have been well know for centuries. As early as 600AD we have evidence of early Honduran civilizations attempting to implant seashells as replacements of a missing tooth and root complex [9]. As an alternative to replacing the entire tooth complex, the profession of dentistry has also created innovations targeted at replacing just the coronal aspect of the deficient site. An example of this would be the classic three unit fixed dental prosthesis to replace an extracted maxillary molar. This modality of treatment presents many attractive features. The time involved to restore only the coronal deficiency is minimal, often times being accomplished in as little as one hour. Commonly, this will involve alteration of existing, and sometimes virgin, teeth to support a tooth borne, fixed dental prostheses. The unfortunate side effect of this treatment lies in the eventual development of future complications on those abutment teeth. [10]. Whether it be recurrent decay, material failure, or a different ailment, at some point the prosthesis will start to breakdown and the next restoration will be more invasive, costly and time consuming to both the patient and the practitioner [11]. More importantly, entire system will still experience negative effects because the root was never replaced. Both hard and soft tissues underneath the pontic site are still subjected to the cycle of breakdown as if the tooth was never replaced. Even with known future flaws in this design, the speed and affordability of these restorations have kept them as a popular method to replace missing teeth.

The patient driven treatment plan classically places emphasis on speed of restoration and direct cost to the consumer. Until recently, implant dentistry has performed poorly in those two categories when compared to tooth borne restorations. Continued development in both macroscopic and microscopic elements in implant design have ushered in the era of speedier implant treatment. Traditional dental implant protocols were known to prescribe long time periods of healing. Patient and doctor demand have recently placed a high value to shortening the time period involved in implant dentistry. From dual stage, to single stage to immediate loading, the trend is consistent in shortening the treatment times to allow for immediate results [12-14]. Further, the increase in the number of companies in the industry, and improved methods of manufacturing have helped keep the cost of implant treatment attainable to the vast majority of patients. Contemporary implant dentistry has not only started to rival classic tooth borne care, but it is becoming the clear choice for tooth replacement. This has caused the number of implants being sold and surgically placed to grow exponentially [15]. With the advent of immediate placement and loading, this industry is poised to command the lion's share of the tooth replacement market as it will be satisfying all the demands of both the patients and practitioners with regard to speed, cost and healthy replacement of the all the missing components in the system.

Historically, there have been many valuable contributions from clinicians that helped implant dentistry evolve. Implant dentistry main consistent feature has been constant evolution in design, materials and protocols. The list of contributors is a different topic of discussion than what is targeted in this book. However Dr. Per-Ingvar Branemark is deserving of special attention.

In the 1950's Dr. Branemark was involved with in-vivo blood flow experiments on rabbits [16]. Initially, titanium chambers were being embedded in the ears of rabbits to record data for their investigations. When Dr. Branemark moved those chambers into the femurs of rabbits he later discovered he could not remove the chambers from the bone into which he had placed the chambers. He found the bone to have grown around the chambers and thus integrated to the titanium surface. Following this discovery, Dr. Branemark performed additional studies that verified the phenomenon of osseointegration [17]. His collaborative efforts verified pure titanium to be the material of choice. His efforts from that point on were largely targeted to the development of dental implants and improving the quality of life in the edentulous population or those suffering from maxillofacial defects [17,18].

2. Tooth loss and edentulism

Although the profession of dentistry is developing osteoinductive, osseoconductive and regenerative products. The native alveolar bone is still the ideal support apparatus for teeth and dental implants. The lack of osseous stimulation from the tooth complex results in bone loss. This loss is manifested in both density and volume. Once the tooth and periodontal ligament are no longer in place, the body initiates changes to remove the alveolar bony support it had once provided. Osteoclastic activity increases and the alveolar bone is eroded away. If the loss of a tooth is followed by placement of a dental implant, the loss of hard and soft tissue in the patient will be greatly reduced. If this process is not intercepted in a timely manner there will be a number of negative consequences dealt to the patient. Severe resorption of the bony processes harms both the quality of life and the quality of dental restorations that are able to be offered to the patients. The patient that waits to replace their teeth will often be informed that extensive grafting is needed to support dental implants. This results in increased cost and complexity. Whereas patients that are proactive in the transition from the dentate to edentate phases afford the clinician a better scenario to design for optimum results. Procedures such as "All on 4" have been designed to take an unhealthy, failing dentition to a healthy and fully restored state in as little as one day [19-21].

3. Expansion of the market

Currently, global populations are living longer. At the time when Dr Branemark discovered osseointegration, the worlds life expectancy was 52. Currently, the life expectancy worldwide is 69.2 years. As our populations continue to live longer, there will be an increased demand on the dental profession's ability to both maintain oral health and effectively treat the edentulous population. Although there is speculation that the edentulous rate is dropping, the increased number of people entering the elderly population counters that number to yield an increase in the number of patients entering edentulism [15]. In fact, the total number of edentulous arches will climb to 37.9 million by the year 2020. This translates into a rise in the number of patients requiring at least one full arch of tooth replacement. Current evidence suggest that the restoration of the edentulous mandible with a conventional denture is no longer the most appropriate first choice of prosthodontic treatment [22,23].

While this demographic evolution may place strain on the worlds medical model, it serves as an ideal situation for the dental practitioner. Opportunistic clinicians are recognizing this trend and learning the skills to provide the great services that can be offered using dental implants.

Modern society has placed a high value on appearances. In the midst of an economic recession in 2009 the United States of America's population spent 10.5 billion dollars on cosmetic surgery. Patients exert a demand upon the dental practitioner to provide esthetics and function. The days of patients succumbing to edentulism and alteration of lifestyle are over. Through various forms of marketing, the modern population is aware of our ability to restore lost function and esthetics. The global market for dental implants is currently 3.4 billion dollars, with expected growth in the coming years.

Contemporary dental practices are in an ideal position to provide implant dentistry to patients. Through marketing and patient to patient interactions, the public is becoming aware of what implant dentistry can provide to the world. Improvements in surgical protocols and implant designs have enabled the clinician to immediately restore missing pieces of the stomatognathic system. However, it is up to the clinician to take the time and learn the techniques and protocols if they wish to capitalize on this market.

4. Surface technologies

Through the initial experiments of Dr. Branemark and coworkers in 1977 [17] and recent researchers [24-26], the dental profession adopted commercially pure grade 4 (high oxygen content) titanium as the material of choice for the implant body. Recently, the alloy form of Ti-6Al-4V has also been adopted into the dental implant industry to improve strength, corrosion resistance and density [27-29]. While the use of an alloy gives added strength to an implant, the lower grade titanium will give an increased osseointegration. Research by Johansson and coworkers showed only slight differences in removal torque values after periods of healing when placing implants of various grades in rabbits [30]. These authors concluded that the level of integration was sufficient in the alloy group and an argument can be made to use the alloys which give improved strength characteristics. Current dental research has allowed for further modifications to both microscopic and macroscopic aspects of dental implants that have improved success rates and healing times.

Surgical integration in combination with healing and loading dynamics are the main factors of whether or not an implant is integrated successfully. The general purpose of surface technologies is targeted to specific goals. Increasing bioacceptance, speeding up the healing of the surgical site and osseiointegration of the implant. Previous improvements on the micron level have been helpful, but the control of tissue response at the nano technological level is the current goal of researchers [31-33]. The implant itself will fall into one or a combination of the three possible categories. Metal, ceramic, or polymer are the three broad chemical classifications of the materials.

Metals have enjoyed a long successful history in various areas of medical and dental implant practice. Biomechanical properties and suitability to sterilization are two advantages to this type of material. One must always remember that when the implant, abutment, or connecting screw are of dissimilar chemical composition, the risk of galvanic interactions exists [34-36]. Further, a galvanic reaction can yield corrosion, oxidation and even the production of pain in the host. This sort of complication is rarely reported, but the whenever we use dissimilar metals in our treatment plans we should be aware of this potential.

Ceramics can be seen as the entire implant or as a surface modification to the metal implant body. Common forms of coatings are hydroxyapatite, tricalcium phosphate or a form of bioglass [37-39]. The possibility of surface degradation, especially with hydroxyapatite, has been an area of contention with many pointing to this element when adverse implant to bone interactions occur.

Polymers were once thought to have advantageous qualities to be incorporated into implant design. Specifically, the shock absorbing capability was once thought to counteract the lack of periodontal ligaments with regards to occlusion. However, research and clinical reports have shown this material to be inferior to those previously discussed and is seldom incorporated today.

Surfaces are generally going to be further classified by the biodynamic response they illicit from the body [40]. No material is completely accepted by the body, but to optimize the implant's performance emphasis is placed on minimizing biologic response while allowing adequate function. Bioinert, bioactive or biotolerant are the current terms used in this area of investigation [41,42]. All three of these descriptive adjectives imply biocompatibility to the host.

A biotolerant material is one that is not rejected by the host but, rather is surrounded by a fibrous layer. Bioinert materials are described as allowing close apposition of bone to the surface, lending itself to contact osteogenesis. Bioactive refers to allowing formation of new bone onto the surface but ion exchange with host tissue leading to formation of chemical bonds along the interface.

When the implant is inserted into the osteotomy site it will have an effect on the bone and blood clot that it is in intimate contact with. Osseoconductive and osseoinductive are common terms to describe the body's response to dental materials. Bioinert and bioactive materials are grouped into the osseoconductive category [41,42]. This refers to the ability to act as a scaffold, or allowing bone formation on their surface. Osseoinductive refers to a materials ability to induce bone formation de novo. An example of this is seen in recombinant human bone morphogenetic protein 2 [43,44].

A number of microscopic surface coating changes have been shown to provide improved healing to the implant surface. Generally, surface coatings are sprayed onto the implant. One must realize that surface coatings rely on adhesive qualities to remain on the implant during insertion. Bond strengths are currently reported to be in the range of 15-30 MPa. This low strength brings into question how practical a surface coating may be in the clinical environment. Speculation exists whether or not the coating is maintained during the placement of the implant into a osteotomy. However, many manufacturers are using this technology on their implants which suggests positive feedback from the clinical results.

Turned surfaces, sandblasted, plasma sprayed, acid etched, anodized, HA, zirconia, and more have been heavily advertised as additions to the to pure titanium body. This list will continue to grow as implant companies position themselves to achieve faster healing times and thus allow for immediate loading. The common theme advertised from all the manufacturers is increasing bone to implant contact in both volume and speed. Examples of popular surfaces will be discussed. Currently there is over 80 companies producing over 250 different types of dental implants. Caution is recommended to the dentist with regards to this aspect of implant dentistry. As this field is rapidly changing. It is up to the clinician to use professional judgement on whether or not to adopt a new surface into their implant practice. Food and Drug Administration (FDA) clearance is often a good sign of whether or not a manufacturer's claim has undergone any actual scientific investigation.

4.1. Microscopic topography

Currently, most all manufacturers have made the shift from smooth implant surfaces to a rough surface [5,24,45,46]. Recently, even the smooth collar model that was promoted for increased hygiene has seen reduced promotion and use. This signals that most contemporary research points to rough surfaces functioning better in the role of promoting the mechanical interlocking of the surrounding tissues. On the microscopic level of this element lies cell differentiation responses to different microscopic topographies. The appositional response of the extracellular matrices in the bone to implant environment have shown potential for providing improvement in implant performance [47,48]. Similar to the computer industry, the major advances in this area are found in nanotechnological engineering [32,33]. The word nano-lithography may be the next buzz word in advertisements from implant manufacturers. As a profession we will get there, but as technologically advanced as this sounds, the reality of current manufacturing is a surface is being textured by some sort of grit blasting process.

TiUnite is the current surface advertised by NobelBiocare. This adds an osseoconductive element to implants manufactured by NobelBiocare. It is a highly crystalline and phosphate enriched titanium oxide characterized by a micro structured surface with open pores in the low micrometer range. The surface is generated by spark anodization and consists of titanium oxide [49,50]. The following ptohos show an implant with TiUnite surface, and scanning electron microscopic (SEM) images of TiUnite surface during osseointegration (Figures 1-4).

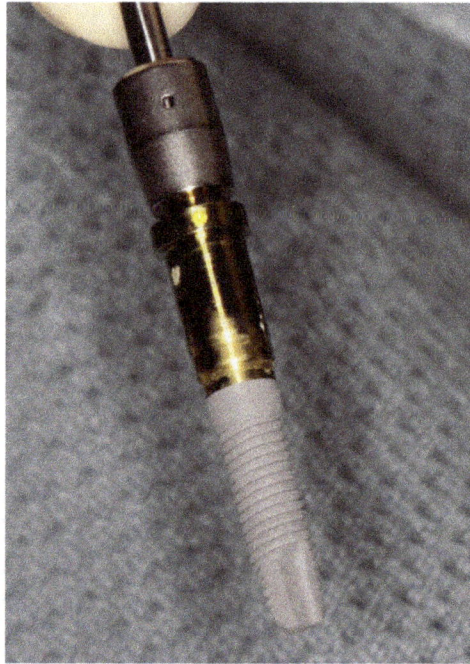

Figure 1. NobelReplace Straight Groovy Implant with TiUnite surface.

Strauman currently promotes a surface by the name of SLActive [51-53]. This title denotes how the implant is conditioned for optimizations. Sandblasting with Large grit followed by Acid etching is how the manufacturer achieves the surface topography. To create the 'active' surface, the implant is conditioned with nitrogen and preserved in an isotonic saline solution.

Astratech dental implants are currently promoting a TiOblast and Osseospeed surface [54,55]. Essentially the surface of the implant is grit blasted with titanium dioxide particles to achieve

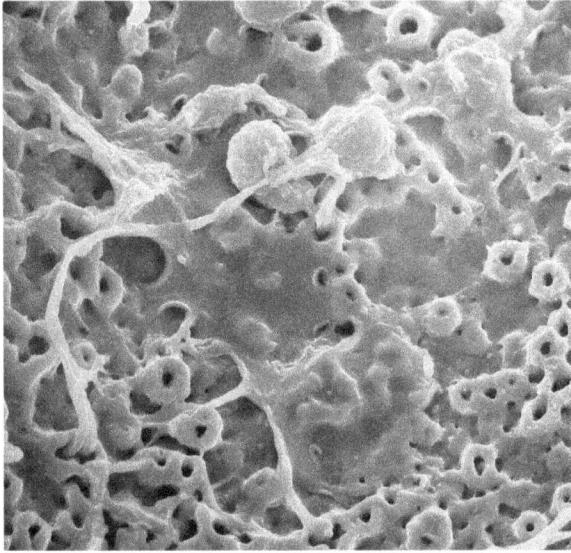

Figure 2. SEM view of TiUnite surface during osteoblasts are attaching on it.

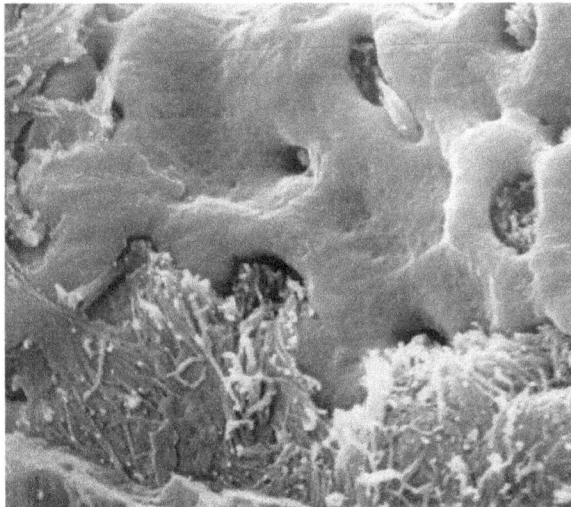

Figure 3. SEM view of TiUnite surface when osteoblasts have filled pores on the implant surface.

an isotropic, moderately roughened surface. Later the implant is chemically conditioned with fluoride to gain slight topographical changes.

Zimmer contemporary surface is called MTX [56,57]. This acronym denotes 'micro-texturing' the implant surface. The implant is Grit blasted with hydroxyapatite particles and then conditioned a non-etching environment to remove residual blasting material.

3i, or implant innovations Inc, uses surface technology termed nano-tite [58,59]. After micro-texturing like the companies previously listed, the implant is then conditioned into a calcium phosphate solution.

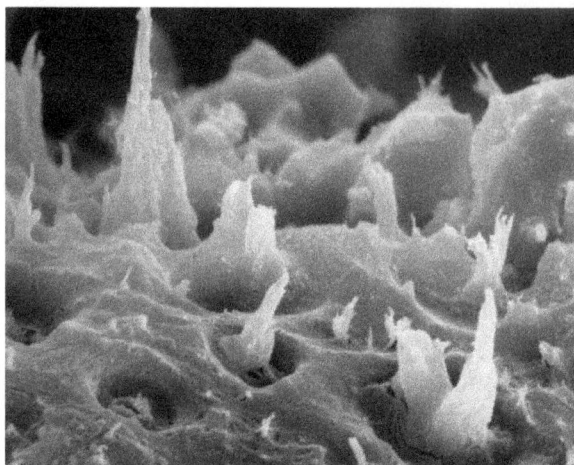

Figure 4. Another SEM view of TiUnite surface when osteoblasts have filled pores.

If all five of these surfaces from the five major manufacturers are compared, not much difference exists. Currently, a textured surface is created which is then followed by some element of conditioning thought to improve bioactivity.

An additional step to spraying on coatings or roughening the surface of implants is seen in the chemical treatment of the implant surface. The overriding goal in this treatment modality is to improve the wettability of the implant surface itself, or otherwise, to make the implant surface more hydrophilic [60]. Clinicians are advised that the contact angle of pre-existing surfaces was never poor and may be sufficient without additional modification. Early experiments have been promising in showing improvements in this area. However, it is not know to what extent this actually plays in implant success.

It is impossible to predict what the next big thing in implant dentistry will be. In fact, dentistry as a profession is changing so rapidly, it is a challenge for the practicing clinician to remain current with what the research world can produce. An over-riding principle must always be to be critical of what is advertised.

5. Macroscopic design

Dental implants have assumed a variety of shapes through the years. From frames to baskets and cylinders to tapered screw threaded forms, the macroscopic design has seen numerous functional advances. Currently the threaded implant body enjoys the majority share of the market. Experiments have shown that screw type implants maintain a higher bone to implant contact through years of function [9]. With this body shape dominating the market, a discussion in the elements of the screw shape is deserving.

There are four basic types of threads seen in a screw shape [9]. V-thread, buttress thread, reverse buttress thread and square threads. All of these designs will exert different forces on the surrounding tissues when subjected to various load patterns. The thread pitch denotes the distance between adjacent threads. Thread depth will refer to the distance between the major and minor diameter of the implant. In addition to load distribution, the geometry of the thread will impact the surgical behavior of the implant during placement.

Implant bodies are commonly available as tapered or parallel. With regard to immediate load, clinicians are often looking for immediate stability. The tapered design imparts the ability to place an implant into an underprepared osteotomy site resulting in higher insertional torque values [61]. Controversy exists over what is the maximum torque that results in negative effects on the supporting tissues. Modern implants are being designed to withstand the high torquing forces on the implant body itself. However, some argue these high forces placed on the surrounding bone have the ability to cause compression necrosis. This is a current point of contention amongst various researchers. With regards to implant length, some manufacturers/ researchers are promoting the use of shorter length implants [62,63]. However, caution is advised to the clinicians in this area, especially for implants shorter than 10mm.

When considering force distribution in the final prosthesis it is imperative to consider both biomechanics and limitations of biology [64]. By using longer and wider implants, the surface area of a load is increased. This in-turn lowers the force on the overall system (F=M/A). In contrast, if a wide platform implant is chosen for a given osteotomy site, one must be careful not to exceed the biologic parameters of the patient. For example, if a wide implant results in insufficient buccal bone, the gain in force distribution will be negated by the decrease of vascularity to the buccal bone in that site and potential implant complications.

The design of the implant to abutment connection is another aspect of treatment that the clinician must decide upon prior to treatment [65,66]. Whether to use external or internal hex, trilobe, conical, morse taper, platform switching are all decisions that must be made by the dentist (Figures 5,6). As in other areas of dentistry, there is a blend of art and science. Some clinicians use what works best in their hands or make decisions based on feel. Hopefully, as evidence based dentistry matures and actually starts to produce tangible recommendations, the decision making tree will become more research based.

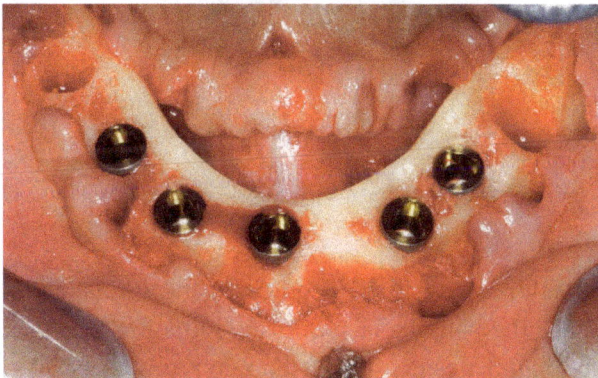

Figure 5. Immediate implant placement with NobelReplace implants with internal trilobe connection.

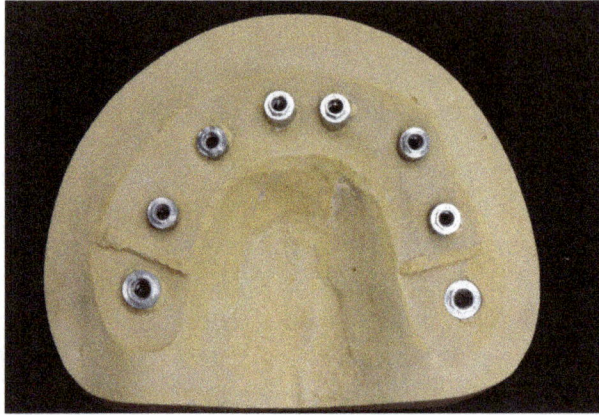

Figure 6. Cast with Branemark implant replicas with external hex connection.

In 1982, Dr. Gerald Niznick introduced the internal hex connection [67]. The purpose of this design was to create an implant to abutment connection that shifted the force from the implant screw to the platform connection. Prior to this innovation, screw fractures were a common complication [10]. Numerous studies have shown this to be a structural improvement with regards to reducing the stress placed upon the abutment screw [68,69]. Most clinicians prescribe implants with internal connections. Even with this said, the external hex remains a viable option and is still used by many dentists. After the decision of making your connection internal or external (Figures 7-9), the next choice is whether or not to use a platform shift.

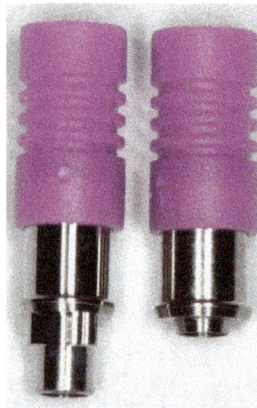

Figure 7. Engaging and non-engaging UCLA abutments for NobelBiocare Replace implants with internal trilobe connection.

The term platform shift refers to a mismatched fit of the implant platform and that of the abutment. In the late 1980s the benefits of platform switching was unforeseen by the practitioners using this mismatched design. Wide diameter implants did not have a matching platform for the abutments so a regular platform was used. Upon follow up examination, the crestal bone levels were thought to be equal or better than platform matched connections [70,

71]. Current research suggests the medial movement of the implant / abutment junction is beneficial in reducing crestal bone loss. The marginal gap is thought to exert a sphere of influence on the biological reaction from the bone and soft tissues. A mismatched connection of.4 mm or greater appears to result in statistically significant less bone loss [72].

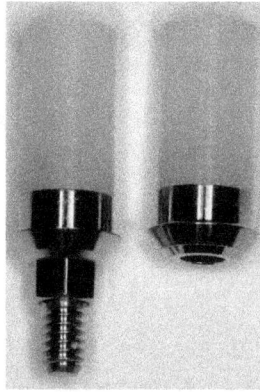

Figure 8. Engaging and non-engaging UCLA abutments for Zimmer implants with internal hex connection.

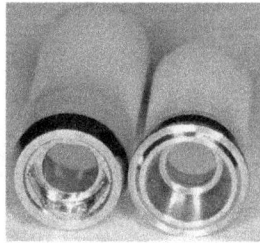

Figure 9. Engaging and non-engaging UCLA abutments for implants with external hex connection.

In implant dentistry, current paradigms for treatment success are based not only on true clinical outcomes such as implant survival, restoration survival, and patient satisfaction but also on surrogate clinical outcomes such as dentogingival esthetics and health of surrounding soft tissues [73]. This is especially important for implant therapy in maxillary and mandibular anterior regions, where esthetics play a predominant role in treatment success. A variety of abutments, and restorations differing in design and biomaterials have been introduced to achieve optimal mechanical, biological, and esthetic treatment outcomes. As an abutment material, traditionally titanium is selected due to its mechanical properties. However, the color of underlying titanium abutments negatively affected the appearance of peri-implant mucosa. To provide more predictable results regarding esthetic aspects, all-ceramic abutments made out of alumina and zirconia were introduced about 10 years ago. In vitro and in vivo studies [74,75] demonstrated superior fracture resistance of zirconia abutments with esthetic outcomes (Figures 10-13).

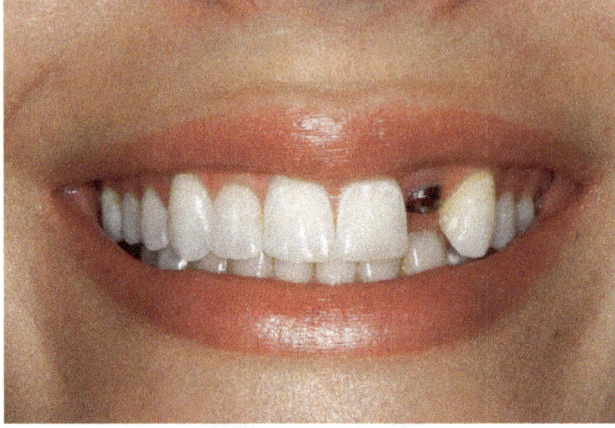

Figure 10. Implant is placed to restore maxillary left lateral tooth.

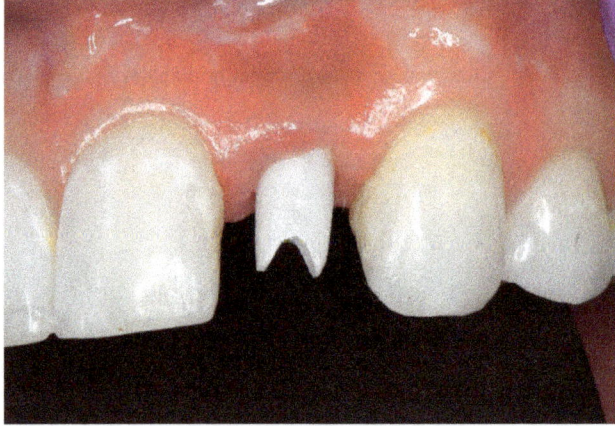

Figure 11. Zirconia abutment is screwed on the implant.

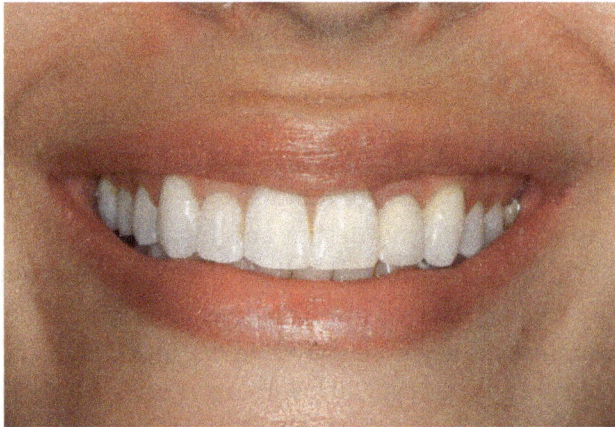

Figure 12. All-ceramic crown is cemented on zirconia abutment.

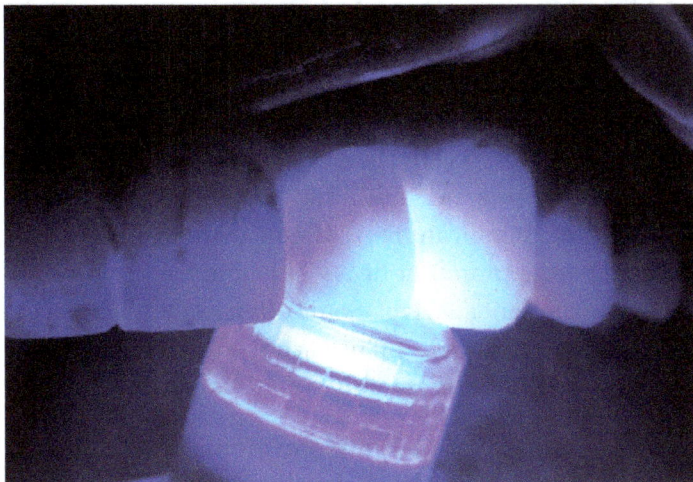

Figure 13. Translucency of natural teeth and all-ceramic restorations is similar, giving more esthetic outcomes.

6. Risk factors for implant candidates

Many attempts to use the phrase contraindications to dental implants have been made [76]. However those lists are often subject to controversy as the severity of a disease or patient condition exists on a sliding scale. For example, one diabetic patient may be at a higher risk than another [77,78]. Or one could ask, at what point does tobacco smoking effect implant survival? Case reports may exist for complications related to various patient conditions, but the doctor is reminded that those reports fall very low on the scale of strength of evidence the clinician can use and apply to their patient pool. Recently, the focus has fallen away from indications and contraindications and more emphasis is placed on risk factors. Risk factors are characteristics statistically associated with, although not necessarily causally related to, an increased risk of morbidity or mortality.

Multiple consensus review groups have recommended that risk factors be divided into two groups [76,79]. Systemic factors and local factors are the groups usually recommended and the latter is further subdivided into very high risk and significant risk. A noteworthy statement that resulted from these reports was in regard to the many attempts from other authors to create a list of relative and absolute contraindications to dental implant placement. This idea is discredited by this group because for many topics weak evidence exists in placing different conditions into an absolute contraindication. A case report of limited sample size is simply not enough evidence to create an absolute contraindication.

The chapter classified very high risk patients as those who could be attributed to having serious systemic disease, immunocompromised health status, drug abusers, and non-compliant patients [76]. A systemic disease can interfere with dental implant therapy at the level of local healing by altering tissue responses to implant placement and surgical treatments. Further, the medications that a patient may be taking for the systemic disease can interfere with normal cellular functions and thereby affect healing and osseointegration. The American Society of Anesthesiology (ASA) has a well known publication to help classify a patient's risk to anesthesia leading into a surgical procedure [76]. Although many dental implants are not placed under general anesthesia, this classification system is an effective way to gauge the patients status for receiving any surgical treatment. For patients that fall into categories, dental treatment is not generally recommended until the patients health status improves and they are placed in a lower category. Significant risk patients were those who had prior irradiation, severe diabetes, bleeding disorders and/ or heavy smoking habits. Local factors are of particular concern with regard to implant survival. Some often highlighted factors are interdental / interimplant space, infected implant sites, soft tissue thickness, width of keratinized soft tissue, bone density, bone volume and implant stability.

In the era of immediate loading of dental implants, initial stability is of primary concern [46,80,81]. Reports have concluded through clinical research that initial stability is related to success with implant survival. There are a number of ways to measure the initial stability of an implant. The most common method of that is to measure the insertion torque of the implant during the final stage of placement using a torque wrench. Resonance frequency has recently been examined and verified to provide useful intrapatient information [80] (Figures 14, 15). Specifically, values of multiple implants in the same patient are useful gauges on implant stability throughout the life of the implant. A correlation between preoperative CBCT scans and resonance frequency values at the time of placement has shown that primary implant stability may be able to be calculated preoperatively [81,82].

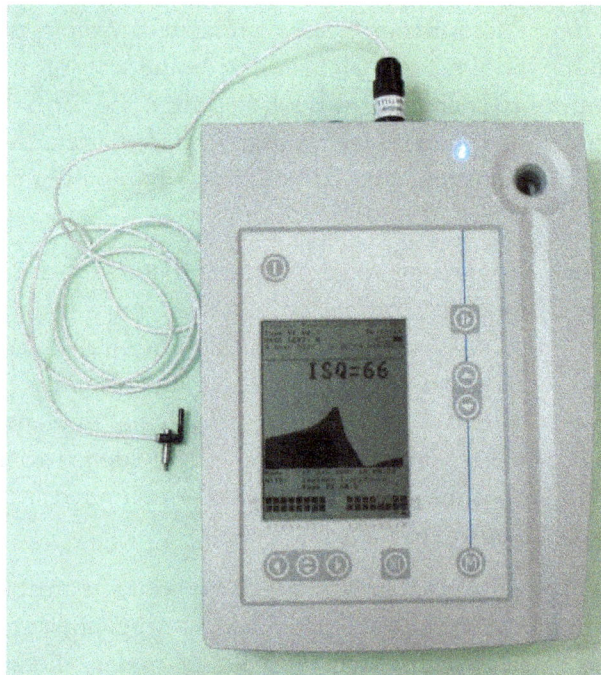

Figure 14. Osstell instrument used to determine implant stability.

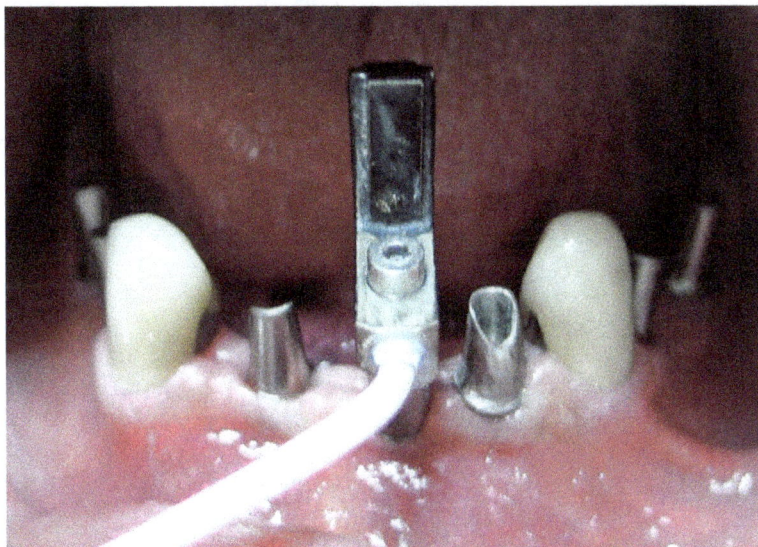

Figure 15. Transducer of Osstell instrument attached to implant for measurement.

It is questioned if an adequate amount of interdental space needs to exist between an implant and an adjacent tooth [83,84]. Studies have shown that interdental spaces of less than 3mm were associated with increased bone loss around the implants. In this particular study, cases where this space was compromised seemed to especially result in bone loss around maxillary lateral incisors.

An infected tooth site is generally defined as one that exhibits signs or symptoms of pain, periapical radiolucency, fistula, suppuration, or a combination of these. The clinical scenario whereby an infected tooth is to be extracted and subsequently followed by implant placement in that site is commonplace in many practices. Whether or not placement of an implant in that site immediately is a key decision the dentist must face. Several clinical reports have been published on this topic, all with varying degrees of success [85,86]. However, studies like that of Villa have shown success in the placement of dental implants and immediate loading into previously infected sites. This idea is relatively new to dentistry, but the preliminary results do appear promising.

The subject of bone density and volume is of particular concern to the implant clinician. While bone density is often a topic of discussion, there exists little data on the relationship of bone density and implant success. With regard to bone volume, it is generally accepted that there are critical parameters in bone volume to support the success of a dental implant. An implant must be surrounded by bone that has adequate vascularity. If the surrounding bone does not have adequate thickness and therefore compromised vascularity, the implant has a higher chance of experiencing both soft and hard tissue attachment loss.

In addition to local and systemic biologic factors previously listed, a patient having a positive history to periodontitis and/or use of smoking tobacco should be noted and considered by the implant clinician. Drs. Heitz-Mayfield and Huynh-Ba performed a comprehensive review of the literature on this subject in 2009 [87]. They found numerous studies have targeted at success rates in patients that fit this demographic of past periodontal disease and tobacco use. With regards to patients that had a history of treated periodontal disease they were able to identify patterns and make following useful conclusions;

a.   implant survival in patients with a histoy of treated periodontitis ranged from 59% to 100%,

b.   the majority of studies reported high implant survival rates >90% for implants with turned or moderately rough surfaces,

c.   all studies reported regular supportive periodontal therapy.

When discussing the issue of a positive history to tobacco smoking they found results that enabled them to make the following conclusions;

a.   Implant outcomes in 45 patients who were rehabilitated following an immediate loading protocol in the mandible were evaluated following 1 year of loading. The results showed there was no statistically significant difference in the smokers and non-smokers with regards to immediate loading protocol.

b.   The majority of studies showed implant survival rates in smokers of 80% to 96%.

c.   Overall there is limited data on the survival and success rates of implants in former smokers.

d.   There are studies that show an increased risk of peri-implantitis for patients that smoke.

The take away message from these reviews for the clinician should be; patients with a history of treated periodontitis and or smoking have an increased risk of implant failure and peri-implantitis. However, neither of these risk factors are absolute contraindications to implant therapy.

7. Conclusion

Implant dentistry has come a long way since the discovery of osseointegration of dental implants. In the last 40 years, the use of dental implants has dramatically increased. Initially, very few specialists were trained in surgical placement and subsequent restoration. As the treatment became more predictable, the benefits of therapy became evident. The tremendous demand for implants has fueled a rapid expansion of the market. Presently, general dentists and multiple specialists offer implant treatments. The field is evolving and expanding, from surgical techniques to types of restorations available.

In this chapter, general information regarding the need for dental implants, implant types and designs, and possible risks factors for patients who are looking for implant treatments have been provided. In the following chapters, more detailed information about several topics will be covered.

Author details

Ilser Turkyilmaz[1*] and Gokce Soganci[2]

*Address all correspondence to: ilserturkyilmaz@yahoo.com

1 Department of Comprehensive Dentistry, University of Texas Health Science Center at San Antonio, Texas, USA

2 Department of Prosthodontics, Oral and Dental Health Center, Ankara, Turkey

References

[1] Craddock HL, Youngson CC, Manogue M, Blance A. Occlusal changes following posterior tooth loss in adults. Part 2. Clinical parameters associated with movement of teeth adjacent to the site of posterior tooth loss. Journal of Prosthodontics. 2007;16(6):495-501.

[2] Gibbs CH, Anusavice KJ, Young HM, Jones JS, Esquivel-Upshaw JF. Maximum clenching force of patients with moderate loss of posterior tooth support: a pilot study. The Journal of Prosthetic Dentistry. 2002;88(5):498-502.

[3] Petridis HP, Tsiggos N, Michail A, Kafantaris SN, Hatzikyriakos A, Kafantaris NM. Three-dimensional positional changes of teeth adjacent to posterior edentulous spaces in relation to age at time of tooth loss and elapsed time. The European Journal of Prosthodontics and Restorative dentistry. 201;18(2):78-83.

[4] Rocci A, Rocci M, Rocci C, Scoccia A, Gargari M, Martignoni M, Gottlow J, Sennerby L. Immediate loading of Brånemark system TiUnite and machined-surface implants in the posterior mandible, part II: a randomized open-ended 9-year follow-up clinical trial. International Journal of Oral and Maxillofacial Implants. 2013;28(3):891-5.

[5] Turkyilmaz I. 26-year follow-up of screw-retained fixed dental prostheses supported by machined-surface Brånemark implants: a case report. Texas Dental Journal. 2011;128(1):15-9.

[6] Turkyilmaz I, Aksoy U, McGlumphy EA. Two alternative surgical techniques for enhancing primary implant stability in the posterior maxilla: a clinical study including bone density, insertion torque, and resonance frequency analysis data. Clinical Implant Dentistry and Related Research. 2008;10(4):231-7

[7] Turkyilmaz I, Tozum TF, Fuhrmann DM, Tumer C. Seven-year follow-up results of TiUnite implants supporting mandibular overdentures: early versus delayed loading. Clinical Implant Dentistry and Related Research. 2012;14(Suppl 1):e83-90.

[8] Berberi AN, Sabbagh JM, Aboushelib MN, Noujeim ZF, Salameh ZA. A 5-year comparison of marginal bone level following immediate loading of single-tooth implants placed in healed alveolar ridges and extraction sockets in the maxilla. Frontiers in Physiology. 2014;31(5):29.

[9] Misch CE, Strong JT, Bidez MW. Scientific Rationale for Dental Implant Design. In: Contemporary Implant Dentistry, (Misch CE) 3rd ed. Mosby Elsevier, St. Louis, Missouri; 2008; pp.200-229.

[10] Goodacre CJ, Bernal G, Rungcharassaeng K, Kan JY. Clinical complications in fixed prosthodontics. The Journal of Prosthetic Dentistry. 2003;90(1):31-41.

[11] Owall B, Cronstrom R. First two-year complications of fixed partial dentures, eight units or more. Swedish Guarantee Insurance claims. Acta Odontologica Scandinavica. 2000;58(2):72-6.

[12] Turkyilmaz I. Alternative method to fabricating an immediately loaded mandibular hybrid prosthesis without impressions: a clinical report. The International Journal of Periodontics and Restorative Dentistry. 2012;32(3):339-45.

[13] Rungcharassaeng K, Kan JY, Yoshino S, Morimoto T, Zimmerman G. Immediate implant placement and provisionalization with and without a connective tissue graft: an analysis of facial gingival tissue thickness. The International Journal of Periodontics and Restorative Dentistry. 2012;32(6):657-63.

[14] Abboud M, Wahl G, Guirado JL, Orentlicher G. Application and success of two stereolithographic surgical guide systems for implant placement with immediate loading. International Journal of Oral and Maxillofacial Implants. 2012;27(3):634-43.

[15] Turkyilmaz I, Company AM, McGlumphy EA. Should edentulous patients be constrained to removable complete dentures? The use of dental implants to improve the quality of life for edentulous patients. Gerodontology. 2010;27(1):3-10.

[16] Branemark PI. Vital microscopy of bone marrow in rabbit. Scandinavian Journal of Clinical and Laboratory Investigation. 1959;11(Suppl 38):1-82.

[17] Branemark PI, Hansson BO, Adell R, Breine U, Lindstrom J, Hallen O, Ohman A. Osseointegrated implants in the treatment of the edentulous jaw. Experience from a 10-year period. Scandinavian Journal of Plastic and Reconstructive Surgery. Supplementum. 1977;16:1-132.

[18] Tjellstrom A, Lindstrom J, Hallen O, Albrektsson T, Branemark PI. Osseointegrated titanium implants in the temporal bone. A clinical study on bone-anchored hearing aids. The American Journal of Otology. 1981;2(4):304-10.

[19] Butura CC, Galindo DF. Combined immediate loading of zygomatic and mandibular implants: a preliminary 2-year report of 19 patients. International Journal of Oral and Maxillofacial Implants. 2014;29(1):e22-9.

[20] Crespi R, Vinci R, Cappare P, Romanos GE, Gherlone E. A clinical study of edentulous patients rehabilitated according to the "all on four" immediate function protocol. International Journal of Oral and Maxillofacial Implants. 2012;27(2):428-34.

[21] Butura CC, Galindo DF, Jensen OT. Mandibular all-on-four therapy using angled implants: a three-year clinical study of 857 implants in 219 jaws. Dental Clinics of North America. 2011;55(4):795-811.

[22] Kuoppala R, Napankangas R, Raustia A. Outcome of implant-supported overdenture treatment--a survey of 58 patients. Gerodontology. 2012;.29(2):e577-84.

[23] Jabbour Z, Emami E, de Grandmont P, Rompre PH, Feine JS. Is oral health-related quality of life stable following rehabilitation with mandibular two-implant overdentures? Clinical Oral Implants Research. 2012;.23(10):1205-9.

[24] Polizzi G, Gualini F, Friberg B. A two-center retrospective analysis of long-term clinical and radiologic data of TiUnite and turned implants placed in the same mouth. The International Journal of Prosthodontics. 2013;26(4):350-8.

[25] Sayardoust S, Grondahl K, Johansson E, Thomsen P, Slotte C. Implant survival and marginal bone loss at turned and oxidized implants in periodontitis-susceptible smokers and never-smokers: a retrospective, clinical, radiographic case-control study. Journal of Periodontology. 2013;84(12):1775-82.

[26] Ravald N, Dahlgren S, Teiwik A, Grondahl K. Long-term evaluation of Astra Tech and Branemark implants in patients treated with full-arch bridges. Results after 12-15 years. Clinical Oral Implants Research. 2013;24(10):1144-51.

[27] Milosev I, Kapun B, Selih VS. The effect of fluoride ions on the corrosion behaviour of Ti metal, and Ti6-Al-7Nb and Ti-6Al-4V alloys in artificial saliva. Acta Chimica Slovenica. 2013;60(3):543-55.

[28] Liu YJ, Cui SM, He C, Li JK, Wang QY. High cycle fatigue behavior of implant Ti-6Al-4V in air and simulated body fluid. Biomedical Materials and Engineering. 2014;24(1):263-9.

[29] Joshi GV, Duan Y, Neidigh J, Koike M, Chahine G, Kovacevic R, Okabe T, Griggs JA. Fatigue testing of electron beam-melted Ti-6Al-4V ELI alloy for dental implants. Journal of Biomedical Materials Research. Part B, Applied Biomaterials. 2013;101(1): 124-30.

[30] Johansson CB, Han CH, Wennerberg A, Albrektsson T. A quantitative comparison of machined commercially pure titanium and titanium-aluminum-vanadium implants in rabbit bone. International Journal of Oral and Maxillofacial Implants. 1998;13(3): 315-21.

[31] Guida L, Oliva A, Basile MA, Giordano M, Nastri L, Annunziata, M. Human gingival fibroblast functions are stimulated by oxidized nano-structured titanium surfaces. Journal of Dentistry. 2013;41(10):900-7.

[32] Bryington MS, Hayashi M, Kozai Y, Vandeweghe S, Andersson M, Wennerberg A, Jimbo R. The influence of nano hydroxyapatite coating on osseointegration after extended healing periods. Dental Materials. 2013;29(5):514-20.

[33] Zhang W, Wang G, Liu Y, Zhao X, Zou D, Zhu C, Jin Y, Huang Q, Sun J, Liu X, Jiang X, Zreiqat H. The synergistic effect of hierarchical micro/nano-topography and bioactive ions for enhanced osseointegration. Biomaterials. 2013;34(13):3184-95.

[34] Ozkomur A, Erbil M, Akova T. Diamondlike carbon coating as a galvanic corrosion barrier between dental implant abutments and nickel-chromium superstructures. International Journal of Oral and Maxillofacial Implants. 2013;28(4):1037-47.

[35] Cortada M, Giner L, Costa S, Gil FJ, Rodríguez D, Planell JA. Galvanic corrosion behavior of titanium implants coupled to dental alloys. Journal of Materials Science. Materials in Medicine. 2000;11(5):287-93.

[36] Taher NM, Al Jabab AS. Galvanic corrosion behavior of implant suprastructure dental alloys. Dental Materials. 2003;19(1):54-9.

[37] Wu CL, Ou SF, Huang TS, Yang TS, Wang MS, Ou KL. Cellular response of calcium phosphate bone substitute containing hydroxyapatite and tricalcium phosphate. Implant Dentistry. 2014;23(1):74-8.

[38] Vidigal GM Jr, Groisman M, de Sena LA, Soares Gde A. Surface characterization of dental implants coated with hydroxyapatite by plasma spray and biomimetic process. Implant Dentistry. 2009;18(4):353-61.

[39] Kim YK, Ahn KJ, Yun PY, Kim M, Yang HS, Yi YJ, Bae JH. Effect of loading time on marginal bone loss around hydroxyapatite-coated implants. Journal of the Korean Association of Oral and Maxillofacial Surgeons. 2013;39(4):161-7.

[40] Sykaras N, Iacopino AM, Marker VA, Triplett RG, Woody RD. Implant materials, designs, and surface topographies: their effect on osseointegration. A literature review. International Journal of Oral and Maxillofacial Implants. 2000;15(5):675-90.

[41] Jayaswal GP, Dange SP, Khalikar AN. Bioceramic in dental implants: A review. Journal of Indian Prosthodontic Society. 2010;10(1):8-12.

[42] Choi JY, Lee HJ, Jang JU, Yeo IS. Comparison between bioactive fluoride modified and bioinert anodically oxidized implant surfaces in early bone response using rabbit tibia model. Implant Dentistry. 2012;21(2):124-8.

[43] Lee JH, Ryu MY, Baek HR, Lee HK, Seo JH, Lee KM, Lee AY, Zheng GB, Chang BS, Lee CK. The effects of recombinant human bone morphogenetic protein-2-loaded tricalcium phosphate microsphere-hydrogel composite on the osseointegration of dental implants in minipigs. Artificial Organs. 2014;38(2):149-58.

[44] Coomes AM, Mealey BL, Huynh-Ba G, Barboza-Arguello C, Moore WS, Cochran DL. Buccal bone formation after flapless extraction: a randomized, controlled clinical trial comparing recombinant human bone morphogenetic protein 2/absorbable collagen carrier and collagen sponge alone. Journal of Periodontology. 2014;85(4):525-35

[45] Friberg B, Jemt T. Rehabilitation of edentulous mandibles by means of four TiUnite implants after one-stage surgery: a 1-year retrospective study of 75 patients. Clinical Implant Dentistry and Related Research. 2010;12(Suppl 1):e56-62.

[46] Kokovic V, Jung R, Feloutzis A, Todorovic VS, Jurisic M, Hammerle CH. Immediate vs. early loading of SLA implants in the posterior mandible: 5-year results of randomized controlled clinical trial. Clinical Oral Implants Research. 2014;25(2):e114-9.

[47] Pecora GE, Ceccarelli R, Bonelli M, Alexander H, Ricci JL. Clinical evaluation of laser microtexturing for soft tissue and bone attachment to dental implants. Implant Dentistry. 2009;18(1):57-66.

[48] Weiner S, Simon J, Ehrenberg DS, Zweig B, Ricci JL. The effects of laser microtextured collars upon crestal bone levels of dental implants. Implant Dentistry. 2008;17(2):217-28.

[49] Yamamoto A, Tanabe T. Treatment of peri-implantitis around TiUnite-surface implants using Er:YAG laser microexplosions. The International Journal of Periodontics and Restorative Dentistry. 2013;33(1):21-30.

[50] Degidi M, Nardi D, Piattelli A. 10-year follow-up of immediately loaded implants with TiUnite porous anodized surface. Clinical Implant Dentistry and Related Research. 2012;14(6):828-38.

[51] Filippi A, Higginbottom FL, Lambrecht T, Levin BP, Meier JL, Rosen PS, Wallkamm B, Will C, Roccuzzo M. A prospective noninterventional study to document implant success and survival of the Straumann Bone Level SLActive dental implant in daily dental practice. Quintessence International. 2013;44(7):499-512.

[52] Gomes JB, Campos FE, Marin C, Teixeira HS, Bonfante EA, Suzuki M, Witek L, Zanetta-Barbosa D, Coelho PG. Implant biomechanical stability variation at early implantation times in vivo: an experimental study in dogs. International Journal of Oral and Maxillofacial Implants. 2013;28(3):e128-34.

[53] Guler AU, Sumer M, Duran I, Sandikci EO, Telcioglu NT. Resonance frequency analysis of 208 Straumann dental implants during the healing period. The Journal of Oral Implantology. 2013;39(2):161-7.

[54] Yoon WJ, Jeong KI, You JS, Oh JS, Kim SG. Survival rate of Astra Tech implants with maxillary sinus lift. Journal of the Korean Association of Oral and Maxillofacial Surgeons. 2014;40(1):17-20.

[55] Fermergard R, Astrand P. Osteotome sinus floor elevation without bone grafts--a 3-year retrospective study with Astra Tech implants. Clinical Implant Dentistry and Related Research. 2012;14(2):198-205.

[56] Ormianer Z, Piek D, Livne S, Lavi D, Zafrir G, Palti A, Harel, N. Retrospective clinical evaluation of tapered implants: 10-year follow-up of delayed and immediate placement of maxillary implants. Implant Dentistry. 2012;21(4):350-6.

[57] Kim YK, Lee JH, Lee JY, Yi YJ. A randomized controlled clinical trial of two types of tapered implants on immediate loading in the posterior maxilla and mandible. International Journal of Oral and Maxillofacial Implants. 2013;28(6):1602-11.

[58] Martens F, Vandeweghe S, Browaeys H, De Bruyn H. Peri-implant outcome of immediately loaded implants with a full-arch implant fixed denture: a 5-year prospective case series. The International Journal of Periodontics and Restorative Dentistry. 2014;34(2):189-97.

[59] Alves CC, Correia AR, Neves M. Immediate implants and immediate loading in periodontally compromised patients-a 3-year prospective clinical study. The International Journal of Periodontics and Restorative Dentistry. 2010;30(5):447-55.

[60] Liao J, Ning C, Yin Z, Tan G, Huang S, Zhou Z, Chen J, Pan H. Nanostructured conducting polymers as intelligent implant surface: fabricated on biomedical titanium

with a potential-induced reversible switch in wettability. Chemphyschem. 2013;14(17):3891-4.

[61] Barikani H, Rashtak S, Akbari S, Fard MK, Rokn A. The effect of shape, length and diameter of implants on primary stability based on resonance frequency analysis. Dental Research Journal (Isfahan). 2014;11(1):87-91.

[62] Al-Hashedi AA, Ali TB, Yunus N. Short dental implants: An emerging concept in implant treatment. Quintessence International. 2014;45(6):499-514.

[63] Tawil G, Younan R. Clinical evaluation of short, machined-surface implants followed for 12 to 92 months. International Journal of Oral and Maxillofacial Implants. 2003;18(6):894-901.

[64] Bidez MW, Misch CE.. Clinical Biomechanics in Implant dentistry. In: Contemporary Implant Dentistry, (Misch CE) 3rd ed. Mosby Elsevier, St. Louis, Missouri; 2008. pp. 543-556.

[65] Pita MS, Anchieta RB, Barao VA, Garcia IR Jr, Pedrazzi V, Assuncao WG. Prosthetic platforms in implant dentistry. The Journal of Craniofacial Surgery. 2011;22(6): 2327-31.

[66] Schmitt CM, Nogueira-Filho G, Tenenbaum HC, Lai JY, Brito C, Doring H, Nonhoff J. Performance of conical abutment (Morse Taper) connection implants: a systematic review. Journal of Biomedical Materials Research. Part A. 2014;102(2):552-74.

[67] Niznick GA. The Core-Vent implant system. The Journal of Oral Implantology. 1982;10(3):379-418.

[68] Raoofi S, Khademi M, Amid R, Kadkhodazadeh M, Movahhedi MR. Comparison of the Effect of Three Abutment-implant Connections on Stress Distribution at the Internal Surface of Dental Implants: A Finite Element Analysis. Journal of Dental Research, Dental Clinics, Dental Prospects. 2013;7(3):132-9.

[69] Covani U, Ricci M, Tonelli P, Barone A. An evaluation of new designs in implant-abutment connections: a finite element method assessment. Implant Dentistry. 2013;22(3):263-7.

[70] Singh R, Singh SV, Arora V. Platform switching: a narrative review. Implant Dentistry. 2013;22(5):453-9.

[71] Cumbo C, Marigo L, Somma F, La Torre G, Minciacchi I, D'Addona A. Implant platform switching concept: a literature review. European Review for Medical and Pharmacological Sciences. 2013;17(3):392-7.

[72] Atieh MA, Ibrahim HM, Atieh AH. Platform switching for marginal bone preservation around dental implants: a systematic review and meta-analysis. Journal of Periodontology. 2010;81(10):1350-66.

[73] Bidra AS, Rungruanganunt P. Clinical outcomes of implant abutments in the anterior region: a systematic review. Journal of Esthetic and Restorative Dentistry. 2013;25(3): 159-76.

[74] Muhlemann S, Truninger TC, Stawarczyk B, Hammerle CH, Sailer I. Bending moments of zirconia and titanium implant abutments supporting all-ceramic crowns after aging. Clinical Oral Implants Research. 2014;25(1):74-81.

[75] Lops D, Bressan E, Chiapasco M, Rossi A, Romeo E. Zirconia and titanium implant abutments for single-tooth implant prostheses after 5 years of function in posterior regions. International Journal of Oral and Maxillofacial Implants. 2013;28(1):281-7.

[76] Misch CE, Resnik RR. Medical Evaluation of the Dental Implant Patient. In: Contemporary Implant Dentistry, (Misch CE) 3rd ed. Mosby Elsevier, St. Louis, Missouri; 2008. pp. 421-466.

[77] Dubey RK, Gupta DK, Singh AK. Dental implant survival in diabetic patients; review and recommendations. National Journal of Maxillofacial Surgery. 2013;4(2):142-50.

[78] Michaeli E, Weinberg I, Nahlieli O. Dental implants in the diabetic patient: systemic and rehabilitative considerations. Quintessence International. 2009;40(8):639-45.

[79] Clementini M, Rossetti PH, Penarrocha D, Micarelli C, Bonachela WC, Canullo L. Systemic risk factors for peri-implant bone loss: a systematic review and meta-analysis. International Journal of Oral and Maxillofacial Surgery. 2014;43(3):323-34.

[80] Kahraman S, Bal BT, Asar NV, Turkyilmaz I, Tozum TF. Clinical study on the insertion torque and wireless resonance frequency analysis in the assessment of torque capacity and stability of self-tapping dental implants. Journal of Oral Rehabilitation. 2009;36(10):755-61.

[81] Turkyilmaz I, McGlumphy EA. Influence of bone density on implant stability parameters and implant success: a retrospective clinical study. BMC Oral Health. 2008;24(8):32.

[82] Turkyilmaz I, Tumer C, Ozbek EN, Tozum TF. Relations between the bone density values from computerized tomography, and implant stability parameters: a clinical study of 230 regular platform implants. Journal of Clinical Periodontology. 2007;34(8):716-22.

[83] Lazzara RJ. Criteria for implant selection: surgical and prosthetic considerations. Practical Periodontics and Aesthetic Dentistry. 1994;6(9):55-62.

[84] Chu SJ, Tarnow DP. Managing esthetic challenges with anterior implants. Part 1: midfacial recession defects from etiology to resolution. The Compendium of Continuing Education in Dentistry. 2013;34(7):26-31.

[85] Palmer R. Evidence for survival of implants placed into infected sites is limited. Journal of Evidence Based Dental Practice. 2012;12(3 Suppl):187-8.

[86] Meltzer AM. Immediate implant placement and restoration in infected sites. The International Journal of Periodontics and Restorative Dentistry. 2012;32(5):e169-73.

[87] Heitz-Mayfield LJ, Huynh-Ba G. History of treated periodontitis and smoking as risks for implant therapy. International Journal of Oral and Maxillofacial Implants. 2009;24(Suppl):39-68.

9

Biotechnology of Tissues and Materials in Dentistry — Future Prospects

Andréa Cristina Barbosa da Silva,
Diego Romário da Silva, Rafael Grotta Grempel,
Manuel Antonio Gordón-Núñez and
Gustavo Gomes Agripino

1. Introduction

Long ago, humanity has sought alternatives to replacing living tissue, mainly due to birth defects, disease and accidents, using synthetic or natural substances as substitutes, best known as biomaterials. Thus, tissue engineering has emerged, a new and challenging field of modern medicine, which aims at recreating tissues and/or healthy organs to replace missing or diseased body parts [1].

Regenerative medicine which used medical devices and grafts underwent some changes in recent years, changing to a more biological approach, with use of specific biodegradable bioactive and supports (scaffolds) with cells and / or biological molecules to create a functional tissue repair in a diseased or damaged site. Thus, some newer and inter-related strategies are being used for the regeneration of tissues such as cell injection, cell induction and cells seeded in scaffolds (cell seeded scaffold) (detailed later in this chapter) [2]. These approaches depend on the use of one or more key elements, such as cells, growth factors and matrix for guiding tissue regeneration [3].

The technique used to obtain tissues (tissue engineering) is the regeneration of organs and living tissues, through recruitment of the patient's own tissue, which are dissociated into cells and cultured on synthetic or biological carriers, known as scaffolds (scaffolds, three-dimensional matrices, structures, etc.) and then being reinserted into the patient. As a multidisciplinary science, the work involves knowledge of the areas of biology, health sciences and engineering and materials science [4, 5].

Thus, one important step for reconstruction of an organ or tissue is the scaffold selection to the cells, which must take into consideration the type, location and extent of injury. The scaffold structure provides mechanical support to the cell growth and allows transport of nutrients, metabolites, growth factors, and other regulatory molecules, both towards the extracellular environment to the cells, as in the opposite direction [6]. When prepared with bioresorbable polymeris, scaffolds, the scaffolds have specific implementation strategies [7].

After a degradable polymer is identified as a possible candidate for applications in tissue engineering, it must be used for manufacturing a porous scaffold [8, 9, 10, 11]. In this case, two methods are required for proper material manufacture: 1) a method that forms the polymer into a bulk material; 2) a method to make porous such material [12]. The optimal method of manufacturing depends in part on the chemical nature of the polymer. Long, saturated and linear polymers such as PLG are typically formed into bulk materials by entangling the individual polymer chains to form a loosely bound polymer network. Polymer chain entanglement is often achieved by casting the polymer within a mold. The advantage to these methods is that they are relatively simple. However, since the material is elastic solid only because of entangled polymer chains, the material is generally lacking significant mechanical strength. This disadvantage is difficult to overcome without altering the chemical structure of the polymer [12].

Another method to form a bulk material from a linear polymer involves forming chemical bonds between polymer chains, known as polymer cross linking [13, 14]. Cross linking is most often performed between unsaturated carbon-carbon double bonds, and thus this moiety, or a similarly reactive one, is required to exist on somewhere along the polymer chain. An initiation system, typically either radical or ionic, is also needed to promote cross-linking. The initiator system is combined with the polymer and, in response to a signal such as heat, light, a chemical accelerant, or simply time, the initiator forms species that propagate cross-linking. As these polymers are formed into bulk materials by covalent cross-linking, they typically posses significant mechanical strength. Furthermore, their ability to cure in response to an applied signal allows these materials to be injected into the defect site and cure in situ. The major disadvantage of crosslinked materials is that the growing complexity of the material, in terms of the number of components and presence of a chemical reaction, often leads to problems with cytotoxicity and biocompatibility [12].

In this context, biomaterials are extremely important for tissue regeneration process, and can be defined as any substance constructed in such a way that, alone or as part of a complex system, is used for driving, through the control of interactions with components a living system, the course of a diagnostic or therapeutic procedure, whether in humans or animals [15].

In recent decades, biomaterials have been used to repair tissue function, such as metal implants, without concern for its effect on local tissues or on the cells. Thus, polymers and other synthetic materials with biological properties were then developed. More recently, degradable and natural scaffolds, considered a breakthrough for regenerative medicine have been used. Thus, there was an evolution of the use of biomaterials that simply replaced the damaged tissue, to others more specific, allowing the development in three dimensions of a tissue regenerated in full operation and structurally acceptable [2].

To use a material with the purpose of replacing a part of the body or induce the formation of a given tissue, a range of tests and assessments are necessary to establish the potential benefits and possible adverse effects that the material may have. Thus, biomaterials should have the following characteristics: not inducing thrombus formation as a result of contact between the blood and the biomaterial, not inducing adverse immune response, not being toxic or carcinogenic, not disturbing the blood flow, and not producing chronic or acute inflammatory response that prevents the proper differentiation of adjacent tissues [16].

In other words, the biomaterial must be fully biocompatible, that is, must have the ability to perform its desired function with respect to a medical therapy without inducing any undesirable local or systemic effect to the body; but generating cellular and tissue responses beneficial in that specific situation, and optimizing the clinically relevant responses of that therapy [15]. However, it is worth noting that despite the material having been considered inert for a considerable time, it was suggested that they may induce physical and chemical changes after deployment. Thus, before a biological perspective, no material can be considered in fact inert.

2. Strategies for formation and development of tissues

The strategies employed for tissue engineering can be classified into three main classes: conductive or inductive approaches and cell transplantation.

The conductor/conductive approaches using biomaterials in a passive manner to facilitate the growth or regeneration capacity of existing tissue such as, for example, use of membranes or barriers for applied regeneration, adhesion molecules, growth factors, etc. in cases of periodontal diseases [1, 17, 18] or dental implant itself, which is a relatively simple implementation because the apparatus used does not include the use of living cells or other diffusible biological signals [19]. In the conductive techniques is usually accomplished the neoformation of periodontal complex structures, including cementum and periodontal ligament fibers [1]. The periodontium regeneration is the first engineering technology for dental tissue [17].

In 1965, Urist [20] demonstrated for the first time that the new bone formation could occur in a non-mineralized site after implantation of powder bone. This discovery led to the isolation of the active ingredients (specific growth factors - proteins) from bone powder, and the cloning of the genes encoding these proteins. These concepts have been used by many companies for production and expansion of these factors on a large scale [21]. Another method employed is the induction type or inductive approach, which involves the activation of cells near the defect site with specific biological signals that stimulate proliferation and assist in regeneration and repair of tissues by use of materials such bone morphogenetic proteins (BMPs) [20, 22] with promising results for supplementation therapies and the regeneration and bone repair in cases of fractures and periodontal disease [1].

In other words, an alternative approach is the use of diffusible growth factors, and consists of placing specific extracellular matrix molecules on a scaffold to allow the tissue growth. These molecules have the ability to direct or induce the function of cells already present in this location, and in consequence, promoting the formation of a tissue type or a particular desired structure at the location [23].

For the tissue induction can be clinically successful, it is necessary that the biologically active factors are delivered properly to the desired location and in the correct dose for the time period necessary. Typically, many such proteins have a short half-life in the body, but must be present for a long time to be effective. Doctors and researchers have shown these concerns so far by offering large doses of protein at the sites of interest [19]. The most recent research involves the development of a controlled release system of these proteins (inducing factors) [24] and, with the advent of genetic engineering in current biotechnology, a somewhat similar approach involves transfection of a gene encoding the inducing factor, instead of delivering the protein itself [19].

Cell transplantation is the third method, which consists of the direct transplantation of cells grown in the laboratory [25]. This approach is a strategy whose importance is based on the need for a multidisciplinary team for performing tissue engineering, since it requires the physician or surgeon in charge of obtaining tissue samples by biopsy, the bioengineer, who usually participates in manipulating the tissues in bioreactors and prepares the means necessary for placing the cells obtained from biopsy samples, besides cell biologist, who will apply the principles of cell biology required for multiplication and maintenance of cells in the laboratory [1, 18, 26, 27].

Despite having different mechanisms, the three strategies for tissue formation have one characteristic in common: the use of polymeric materials. In conducting approaches, polymer is mainly used as a membrane barrier for exclusion of particular cells that can disturb the regenerative process. In the inductive approaches, these materials act as a carrier for delivery of proteins (e.g., BMP) or the DNA encoding the protein [24, 28]. With regard to approaches used to achieve control of the dose and bioavailability of biodegradable polymer carriers enable localized and sustained release of inductive molecules. The dose rate and the molecule to be delivered are controlled generally by gradual breakdown of the vehicle [24].

These delivery vehicles are often used in cell transplantation approaches. However, in this approach the vehicle serves as a carrier of intact cells and even partial tissues [1].

Besides acting as vehicles for the simple delivery of cells, the vehicles also serve as scaffolds to guide new tissue to grow in a predictable way from the interaction between cells or transplanted tissue and host cells. The collagen derived from animal sources, and synthetic polymers of lactic acid and glycolic acid are the main absorbable materials used for tissue repair in three types of approaches. The collagen is degraded by cells in the tissue during its development, whereas the synthetic polymers are degraded into natural metabolites of lactic acid and glycolic acid by the water action at the implant site. From the development and innovation of biotechnology in tissue engineering various new materials are also being developed for these applications, such as injectable materials that enable a minimally invasive delivery of inductive molecules or transplanted cells [1].

Below (Figure 1), a schematic view of the three types of approaches in tissue engineering:

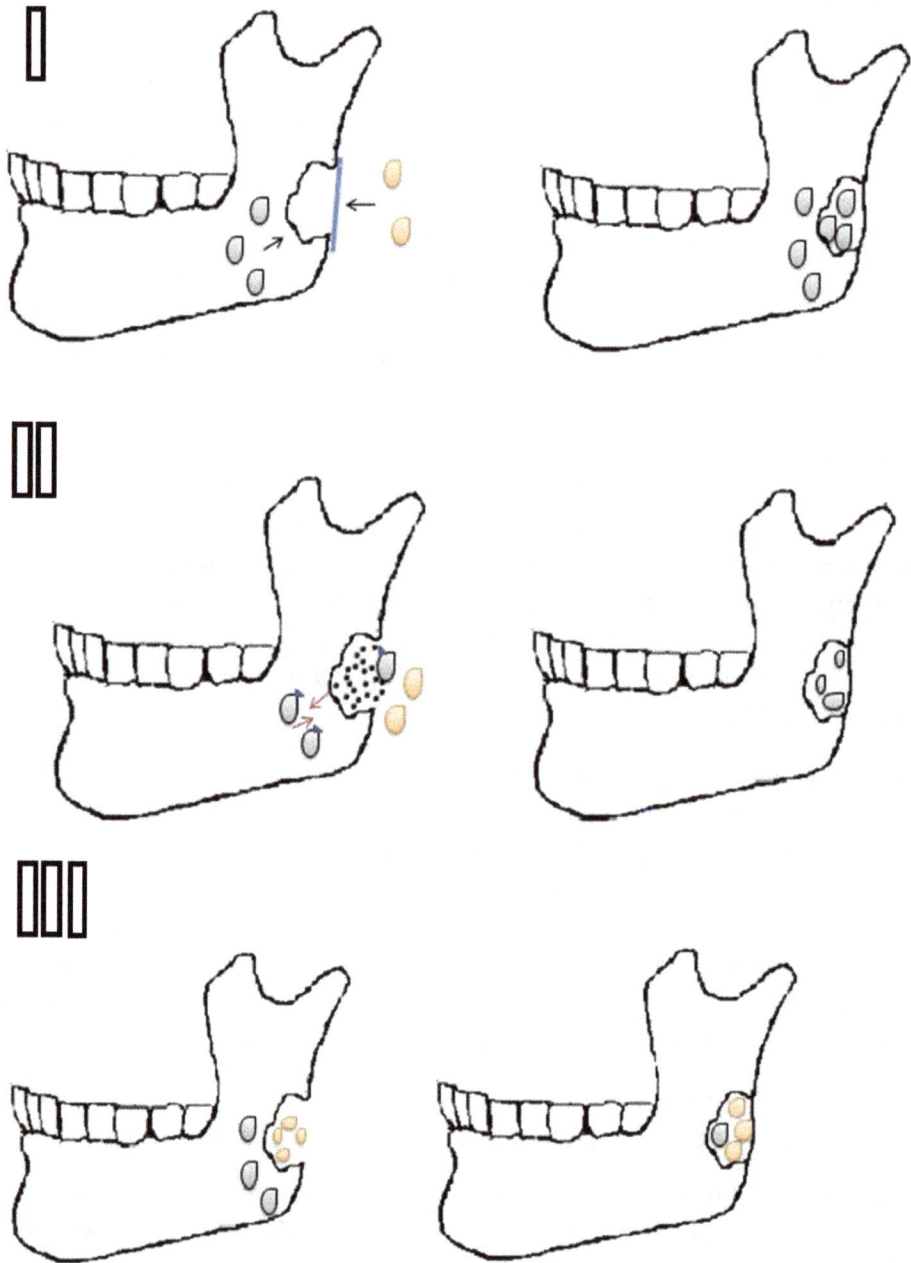

Figure 1. Schematic representation of the three main approaches for tissue rebuilding in tissue engineering in jaw: I) by the conductive method where use is made of a barrier that is able to exclude connective tissue cells that may interfere with the regeneration process and at the same time enables the desired host cells to populate the site to be regenerated. **II)** by the inductive method, in which a scaffold of the biodegradable polymer is used as a delivery vehicle for growth factors and / or genes encoding this factor in the desired location. As the polymer is being degraded, the growth factor is being released gradually. **III)** by the strategy of cell transplantation, which uses a delivery vehicle, similar to that used in an inductive approach, with the goal of transplanting cells and partial tissues to the place where we want to regenerate tissue. In this approach can be transplanted only tissues or cells previously formed in the laboratory from scaffolds.

Tissue engineering seeks solutions for the regeneration of various tissues associated with the oral cavity, such as, bones, cartilage, skin and oral mucosa, dentin and dental pulp, and salivary glands. But in fact, this science will probably have its most significant impact in dentistry through bone reconstruction and regeneration. The fact that cell transplantation approaches may offer the possibility of pre-formation of bone structures of large dimensions (for example, full jaw), which may not be possible to use the other two strategies, makes it the most important approach in the engineering scope for bone tissue formation [1] (Figure 2).

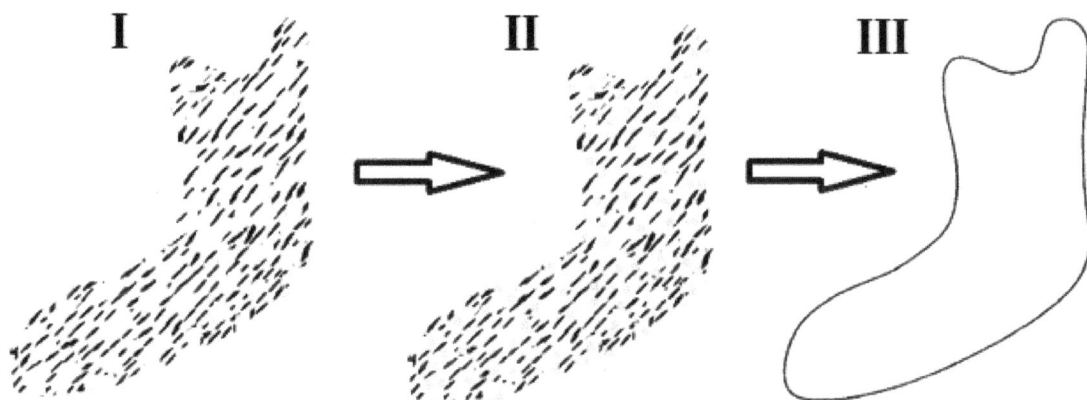

Figure 2. Schematic representation of the advances in tissue engineering to regenerate part of the jaw by means of cell transplantation. A scaffold consisting of biodegradable polymer in the shape of half of the jaw is built (I). Thereafter, bone precursor cells are seeded on the polymer (beige dots) and stimulated to grow in a bioreactor (II). The scaffold will then be gradually degraded, while facilitating growth of jaw-shaped bone (III) (Scheme adapted from [1].

Thus, the tissue repair from the in vitro tissue engineering requires the use of cells to completion and production of similar matrix to the native tissue. The main successful developments in this field have been using the transplant of primary cells taken from patient and used in combination with scaffolds to produce the required tissue to re-implant. However, this strategy has limitations due to the invasive nature of how the cells are removed. Thus, attention has turned to the use of stem cells, including embryonic stem cells and mesenchymal cells derived from bone marrow. In addition to being able to turn into all body tissues, these cells have the capability and advantage of being maintained in culture for long periods, thus having the potential to obtaining large amounts of cells to tissue. The extraordinary ability of these pluripotent cells is linked to their ability to form teratoma [29]. Besides the potential to differentiate into osteoblasts, the possibility of rejection of these cells is greatly reduced.

In cell transplantation, these units can be directly transplanted to the desired location or they may be cultured in the laboratory on scaffolding. In this case, those cells are stimulated to lay the groundwork matrix to produce a tissue for transplantation [29].

Currently, several products can be used to achieve tissue regeneration or reconstruction. These options are divided according to the approach to be used (Inducing, conductive or cell transplantation) as shown in the scheme below (Figure 3) adapted from [19].

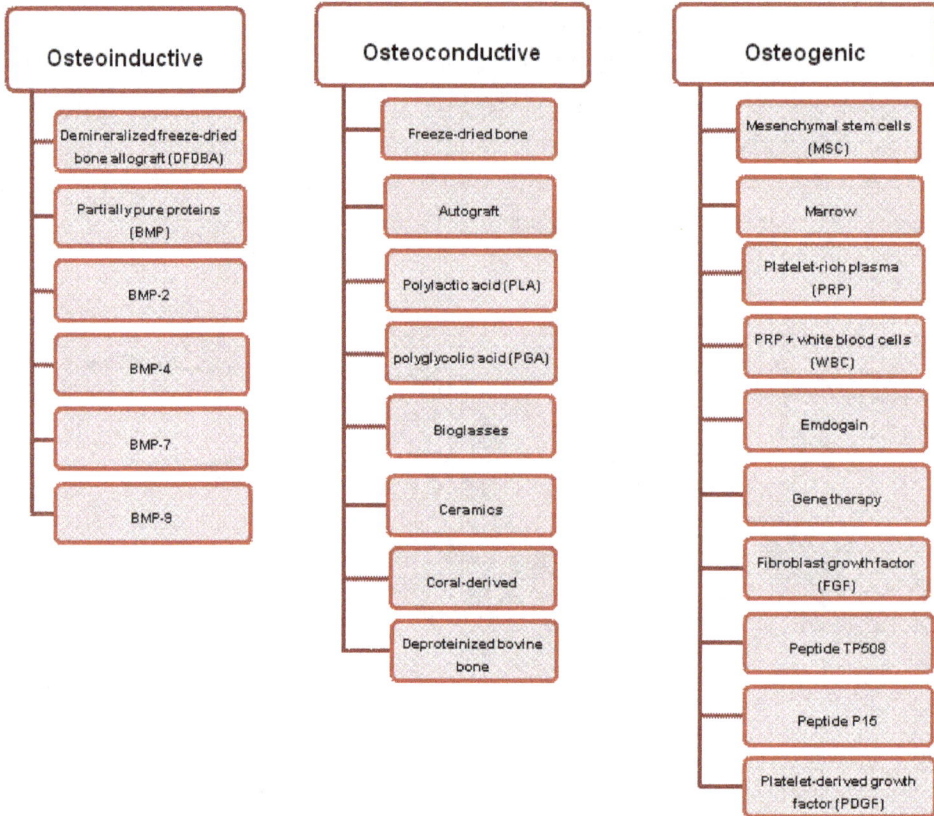

Osteoinductive
- Demineralized freeze-dried bone allograft (DFDBA)
- Partially pure proteins (BMP)
- BMP-2
- BMP-4
- BMP-7
- BMP-9

Osteoconductive
- Freeze-dried bone
- Autograft
- Polylactic acid (PLA)
- polyglycolic acid (PGA)
- Bioglasses
- Ceramics
- Coral-derived
- Deproteinized bovine bone

Osteogenic
- Mesenchymal stem cells (MSC)
- Marrow
- Platelet-rich plasma (PRP)
- PRP + white blood cells (WBC)
- Emdogain
- Gene therapy
- Fibroblast growth factor (FGF)
- Peptide TP508
- Peptide P15
- Platelet-derived growth factor (PDGF)

Figure 3. Products used for bone tissue repair in different types of approaches (Inducing, or conductive cell transplantation) (Adapted from de Kumar, Mukhtar-Un-Nisar and Zia, 2011) [19].

3. Importance of tissues for maxillofacial complex

The maxillofacial complex can be subjected to processes of physical, chemical and biological nature, which usually determine from minor tissue losses to the involvement of large areas of structures of this complex. In this context, dentistry has been explored new technologies in order to change this reality, adapting to new concepts, scientific innovations that include research on stem cells, tissue engineering, and molecular biology techniques, as tools to stimulate regeneration or replacement of damaged tissue by tissue engineering.

Considering the scenario of new technologies, however, still in 2001 it was asked: "What impact could have this engineering in dentistry?" And "What maxillofacial tissues have potential or are important for that engineering?" According to Kaigler and Mooney (2001) [1], at that time the answer to the first question was still being formulated, since the engineering probably would have a revolutionary effect on the field of Dentistry, once almost all types of tissues in the maxillofacial complex could have potential for engineering. Currently, reality has changed significantly due to which the tissue engineering has wide application to many different tissue types associated with the oral cavity, including bone, cartilage, skin, oral mucosa, dentin and dental pulp, and salivary glands.

As previously mentioned, inductive, conductive and cell transplantation strategies, which represent the most used techniques in tissue engineering, are of importance to typically use different material components in order to achieve the goal of regeneration and / or replacement of damaged tissues.

Absolutely, all tissues of the maxillofacial complex are important for its proper functioning, playing a crucial role also in facial aesthetics. Thus, some comments are required about the major oral tissues and their importance for tissue engineering.

With respect to bone, it can be said that tissue engineering has had a greater impact in dentistry, particularly with regard to bone regeneration. Bone loss associated with trauma, diseases or disorders can currently be handled through the use of biomaterials for auto-grafts, allografts or synthetic, morphogenetic proteins (BMPs) and growth factors. It is reported that even though these biomaterials stimulate, replace and / or restore the stability and function of tissues in a reasonably sufficient manner, there are still limitations in their use, which is of importance for research is increasingly carried out using the three main strategies of tissue engineering in order to optimize the mechanisms of regeneration in bone areas compromised by various damaging agents [1, 28, 30].

The importance of cartilage tissue to tissue engineering of structures of the maxillofacial complex lies in the possibility of reconstruction of craniofacial chondromatosous structures, the design of polymeric structures with defined mechanical and degradative properties that can serve as a support structures for cartilage cell proliferation of temporomandibular or intranasal joints if compromised by trauma or degenerative diseases. One of the limitations of the use of cartilage tissue in tissue engineering is due to its limited capacity for regeneration and lack of inductive molecules to the proliferation of their cells; thus it is one of the tissues of great interest among researchers to develop envisaging bioengineering techniques for transplanting of cartilage cells [1, 31, 32].

Researches have been and continue to be focused on the production of dentin and dental pulp by the use of tissue engineering strategies. The importance of these tissues for this engineering is associated with the possibility to replace material lost by carious processes. There is evidence that odontoblasts, even lost due to caries, it would be possible to induce the formation of new pulp tissue cells by tissue engineering based on the use of certain biomolecules stimulating or inducing odontoblast proliferation and / or nerve cells, and these new odontoblasts, in turn, could synthesize new dentin material. Furthermore, it is suggested that the tissue engineering of the dental pulp itself may be possible by using techniques of cultured fibroblasts in synthetic polymer matrices [33, 34, 35, 36, 37].

One of the most exploited tissues in research of tissue engineering in dentistry is the epithelial lining of the oral mucosa with significant advances in the use of these tissues in regeneration and / or replacement of structures of the oral mucosa damaged by various aggressors. Recently, the introduction of 3D reconstruction of the oral mucosa has significantly impacted the approaches to biocompatibility evaluation of tissues and materials to replace and / or regenerate oral soft tissues [2, 38, 39, 40].

One of the most challenging areas of genetic engineering applied to the structures of the maxillofacial complex is the replace of function of salivary glands, since these tissues play important roles in mastication, phonation and protection of hard and soft tissues of the mouth by saliva production. In this context, we study the possibility of salivary gland cells transplantation or creating a replacement for compromised glandular structures through the use of artificial salivary glands consisting of a polymer tube coated with salivary epithelial cells [41]. The success importance of future tissue engineering for these tissues might represent the possibility of new and more effective approaches to the treatment of conditions associated with loss of function of the salivary glands, including dysphagia, dysgeusia, rampant caries and mucosal infections [1].

Regarding the possibility of reproducing teeth, there are numerous growth factors involved in the development of dental organs and biological processes involved in odontogenesis are quite complex, reason why we still cannot form a complete tooth; however, some studies have shown the enamel and dentin formation from stem cells isolated from dental pulp [42, 43]. The replacement of missing teeth by tissue engineering in humans is still being researched, but with a real possibility of application in the future.

4. Biomaterials used in craniofacial tissue regeneration

Biomaterials play a crucial role in tissue engineering. They are used for the manufacture of supports or matrices which allow a suitable microenvironment for optimal cell regeneration.

Biomaterials for constructing scaffolds can be natural/synthetic and rigid/non rigid. Natural biomaterials offer good cellular compatibility i.e. ability to support cell survival and function thereby enhancing the cells' performance, and biocompatibility. Their disadvantages include source variability, immunogenicity, if not pure, limited range of mechanical properties and lack of control over pore size. Unlike natural biomaterials, synthetic biomaterials can be manufactured in unlimited supply under controlled conditions, are cheaper and can be tailored to obtain desired shape, cell differentiation properties and mechanical and chemical properties especially the strength, pore characteristics and degradation rate suited for intended applications. However, synthetic biomaterials lack cell adhesion sites and require chemical modifications to improve cell adhesion

During the last century, various natural or synthetic biomaterials have been used for the manufacture of supports for tissue engineering (fabrication of tissue engineering scaffolds) such as metals, ceramics and polymers. However, metals and ceramics are not biodegradable and its processing is limited, which prevents their application as effective supports (scaffolds) for tissue regeneration. Thus, the polymers has been the most commonly used because they have some important characteristics for tissue regeneration such as biodegradability, porosity, large surface area and ease of processing, among others [44, 45].

There are two types of polymers: natural and synthetic [46, 47]. The main biodegradable synthetic polymers include polyesters, polyanhydride, polyfumarate, polycaprolactone, polycarbonate and polyorthoester [7, 48]. The polyesters such as poly (glycolic acid) (PGA), poly (lactic acid) (PLA), and their copolymer of poly [lactic-co-(glycolic acid)] (PLGA) are most commonly used for tissue engineering. The natural polymers include proteins of natural extracellular matrices such as glycosaminoglycan, collagen, alginic acid and chitosan etc [49, 50]. These polymers of natural origin are biodegradable and possess known cell-binding sites. However, they have some disadvantages such as the level of immunogenicity and speed of degradation.

The tissue regeneration from cells transplanted into a polymer scaffold is summarized in Figure 4.

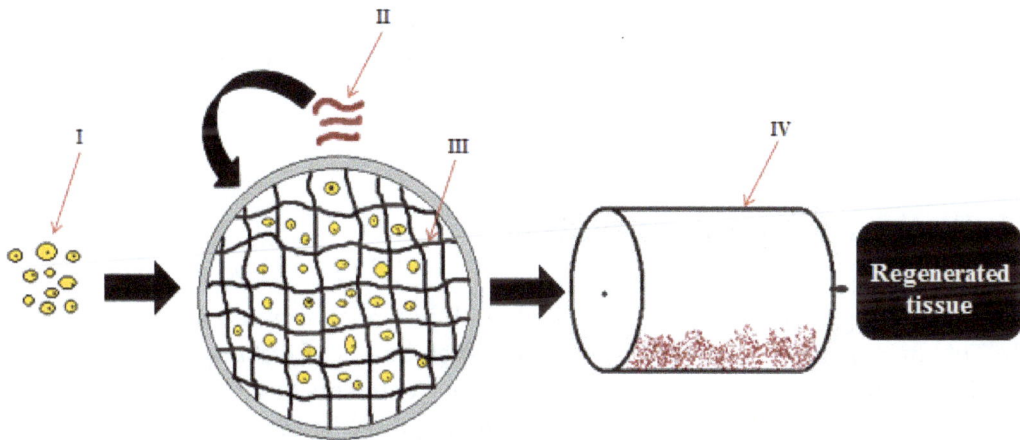

Figure 4. Schematic figure illustrating the steps performed in the laboratory for tissue regeneration from the use of transplanted cells stimulated to grow on biomaterials. It is necessary to understand the importance of biomaterial to perform this technique. It can be natural or synthetic and should meet the requirements of biocompatibility and other features already mentioned in this chapter. It is also important to realize the multidisciplinarity involved in this process. The physician is needed in order to perform the tissue biopsy to remove the cells **(I)**. This tissue/cell is then taken to the laboratory to be multiplied several times. Thereafter, the use of principles of cell biology, such as growth factors **(II)** to stimulate the cells to grow and maintain their functions will be necessary. It is also required the involvement of engineers for manufacturing matrices of biodegradable polymers **(III)** and the bioreactor **(IV).** When cells grow in appropriate number, they are seeded on the polymer scaffold. The tissue is then allowed to grow in the bioreactor until the time of transplantation by clinical surgeon. Biomaterials can be used to stimulate the growth of several types of tissues, e.g. bone, cartilage or skin. After the appropriate development, the tissue is transplanted and the area is regenerated.

Other extracellular matrices used as scaffolds include fibrin and fibrinogen. [51, 52, 53]. According to some studies, both can induce angiogenesis during tissue regeneration [54, 55, 56]. Chitosan is a derivative of chitin, a natural biopolymer which is biocompatible, biodegradable, antimicrobial and possesses tissue healing and osteoinductive effects. It has the ability to bind to growth factors, glycosaminoglycans and DNA and can be easily processed into membranes, gels, nanofibres, beads, scaffolds and sponges. Because of these properties, chitosan gel alone or in combination with demineralized bone matrix/collagenous membrane is quite promising in periodontal regeneration [57].

Considering the bone tissue engineering, porous scaffolds are designed to support the migration, proliferation, and differentiation of osteo-progenitor cells and aid in the organization of these cells in three dimensions. These scaffolds may be made from a wide variety of both natural and synthetic materials. The naturally derived materials include cornstarch-based polymers, [58] chitosan [59, 60] collagen, [61] and coral [62, 63]. Among these materials, the coral has been shown to be an effective clinical alternative to autogenous and allogenous bone grafts [64, 65].

Examples of synthetic materials include calcium phosphates [66, 67] and organic materials such as poly (phosphazenes), [68] poly (tyrosine carbonates), [69] poly (caprolactones) [70], poly (propylene fumarates) [71], and poly (α-hydroxy acids) [72, 73]. Composites of inorganic and organic materials have also been successfully used to create scaffolds for bone grafts [74, 75]. Poly (α-hydroxy acids) are the most commonly used polymeric materials for the creation of tissue-engineering scaffolds for bone. The most common of the poly (α-hydroxy acids) are poly (glycolic acid), poly (lactic acid) (PLA), and copolymers of poly (lactic-co-glycolic acid) (PLGA). These materials are readily metabolized and excreted when degraded by the body [44].

5. Challenges and future prospects

Tissue engineering is an emerging technology with potential application in various medical fields. The main focus of recent research is the development of techniques for manipulating stem cells, aiming at the achievement of restorative treatments of injured and/or lost tissues and organs. Apart from stem cells, bioengineering requires the presence of factors that allow their proliferation in a microenvironment closer to tissue reality, including the extracellular matrix and growth factors. The biomaterials, in turn, are necessary for serving as porous scaffold upon which tissue regeneration is set. As knowledge is acquired with respect to stem cells and biomaterials, the potential for treating diseases may extend beyond the craniofacial region of the body. However, the mechanisms of action of these biotechnologies are not yet fully understood and offer a promising future, so that research is needed to apply them clinically.

Author details

Andréa Cristina Barbosa da Silva*, Diego Romário da Silva, Rafael Grotta Grempel, Manuel Antonio Gordón-Núñez and Gustavo Gomes Agripino

*Address all correspondence to: andreacbsilva@gmail.com

Graduate Program in Dentistry, Center of Sciences, Technology and Health, State University of Paraiba, UEPB, Araruna, Paraíba, Brazil

References

[1] Kaigler D, Mooney D. Tissue engineering's impact on dentistry. J Dent Educ 2001;65(5) 456-462.

[2] Neel EAA, Chrzanowski W, Salih VM, Kim HW, Knowles JC. Tissue engineering in dentistry. Journal of Dentistry 2014;42(8) 915-928.

[3] Bonassar LJ, Vacanti CA. Tissue engineering: the first decade and beyond. Journal of Cellular Biochemistry Supplement 1998;30(31) 297–303.

[4] Griffith, L. G. & Naughton, G. Science, 295, p.1009 (2002).

[5] Langer, R. & Vacanti, J. P. Science, 260, p.920 (1993).

[6] Ikada Y. Challenges in tissue engineering. Journal of the Royal Society Interface 2006;3(10) 589-601.

[7] Hutmacher DW, Schantz T, Zein I, Ng KW, Teoh SH, Tan KC. Mechanical properties and cell cultural response of polycaprolactone scaffolds designed and fabricated via fused deposition modeling. J Biomed Mater Res 2001;55(2) 203-216

[8] Behravesh E, Yasko AW, Engel PS, Mikos AG. Synthetic biodegradable polymers for orthopaedic applications. Clin Orthop 1999;367 S118-129.

[9] Holmes TC. Novel peptide-based biomaterialscaffolds for tissue engineering. Trends Biotechnol 2002;20(1) 16-21.

[10] Yang S, Leong KF, Du Z, Chua CK. The design of scaffolds for use in tissue engineering. Part I. Traditional factors. Tissue Eng 2001;7(6) 679-689.

[11] Yang S, Leong KF, Du Z, Chua CK. The design of scaffolds for use in tissue engineering. Part II. Rapid prototyping techniques. Tissue Eng 2002;8(1) 1-11.

[12] Fishere Reddi 2003 (FALTOU).

[13] Sanborn TJ, Messersmith PB, Barron AE. In situ crosslinking of a biomimetic peptide-PEG hydrogel via thermally triggered activation of factor XIII. Biomaterials 2002;23(13) 2703-2710.

[14] Peter SJ, Miller MJ, Yasko AW, Yaszemski MJ, Mikos AG. Polymer concepts in tissue engineering. J Biomed Mater Res 1998;43(4) 422-427.

[15] Williams DF. On the mechanisms of biocompatibility. Biomaterials 2008;29(20) 2941-2953.

[16] Carvalho PSP, Rosa AL, Bassi APF, Pereira LAVD. Biomateriais aplicados a Implantodontia. Revista Implantnews 2010;7(3a-PBA) 56-65.

[17] Nyman S, Lindhe J, Karring T et al. New attachment following surgical treatment of human periodontal disease. J Clin Periodontol 1982;9(4) 290–296.

[18] Nakahara T, Nakamura T, Kobayashi E, Inoue M, Shigeno K, Tabata Y, Eto K, Shimi-zu Y. Novel approach to regeneration of periodontal tissues based on in situ tissue engineering: effects of controlled release of basic fibroblast growth factor from a sandwich membrane. Tissue Eng 2003; 9(1) 153-62.

[19] Kumar A, Mukhtar-Un-Nisar S, Zia A. Tissue engineering - the promise of regenerative dentistry. Biology and Medicine 2011;3(2) 108-113.

[20] Urist M.R. Bone: formation by autoinduction. Science 1965;150(698) 893-899.

[21] Cochran DL, Wozney JM, 1999. Biological mediators for periodontal regeneration. Periodontology 2000;19 40-58.

[22] Ripamonti U, Petit JC. Bone morphogenetic proteins, cementogenesis, myoblastic stem cells and the induction of periodontal tissue regeneration. Cytokine Growth Factor Rev 2009;20(5-6) 489-99.

[23] Heijl L, Heden G, Svardstrom G, Ostgren A. Enamel matrix derivative (EMDOGAIN) in the treatment of intrabony periodontal defects. J Clin Periodontol 1997;24(9 Pt 2) 705-714.

[24] Sheridan ME, Shea LD, Peters MC, Mooney DJ. Bioabsorbable polymer scaffolds for tissue engineering capable of sustained growth factor delivery. J Control Rel 2000;64(1-3) 91-102.

[25] Krebsbach PH, Kuznetsov SA, Bianco P, Gerhon Robey P. Bone marrow stromal cells: characterization and clinical application. Crit Rev in Oral Biol Med 1999;10(2) 165-81.

[26] Seo BM, Miura M, Gronthos S, et al. Investigation of multipotent postnatal stem cells from human periodontal ligament. Lancet 2004;364(9429) 149–155.

[27] Emily J, Arnsdorf MS, Luis M, Jones MS et al. The Periosteum as a Cellular Source for Functional Tissue Engineering. Tissue Eng part A 2009;15(9) 2637-2642.

[28] Nevins ML, Camelo M, Lynch SE, Schenk RK, Nevins M. Evaluation of periodontal regeneration following grafting intrabony defects with bio-oss collagen: a human histologic report. Int J Periodontics Restorative Dent 2003; 23(1) 9-17.

[29] Howard D, Buttery LD, Shakesheff KM, Roberts SJ. Tissue engineering: strategies, stem cells and scaffolds. J. Anat 2008; 213(1) 66–72.

[30] Alsberg E, Hill EE, Mooney DJ. Craniofacial tissue engineering. Crit Rev Oral Biol Med 2001;12(1) 64-75.

[31] Brittberg M, Lindahl A, Nilsson A, Ohlsson C, Isaksson O, Peterson L (1994) Treatment of deep cartilage defects in the knee with autologous chondrocyte transplantation. N Engl J Med 1994;331(14) 889–895.

[32] Puelacher WC, Wisser J, Vacanti CA, Ferraro NF, Jaramillo D, Vacanti JP. Temporo-mandibular joint disc replacement made by tissue-engineered growth of cartilage. J Oral Maxillofac Surg 1994;52(11) 1172-1177.

[33] Lianjia Y, Yuhao G, White F. Bovine bone morphogenetic protein induced dentino-genesis. Clin Orthop Relat Res 1993;295 305-312.

[34] Mooney D, Mazzoni CL, Breuer C, McNamara K, Hern D, Vacanti JP, Langer R. Stabilized polyglycolic acid fibre-based tubes for tissue engineering. Biomaterials 1996;17(2) 115-124.

[35] Gronthos S, Mankani M, Brahim J, Robey PG, Shi S. Postnatal human dental pulp stem cells (DPSCs) in vitro and in vivo. Proc Natl Acad Sci U S A. 2000;97(25) 13625-13630.

[36] Iohara K, Nakashima, M, Ito M, Ishikawa M, Nakasima A, Akamine A. Dentin regeneration by dental pulp stem cell therapy with recombinant human bone morphogenetic protein 2. J. Dent. Res 2004;83(8) 590-595.

[37] Nakashima M, Akamine A. The application of tissue engineering to regeneration of pulp and dentin in endodontics. J Endod, Baltimore 2005;31(10) 711-718.

[38] Kinikoglu B, Rodriguez-Cabello JC, Damour O, Hasirci V. The influence of elastin-like recombinant polymer on the self-renewing potential of a 3D tissue equivalent derived from human lamina propria fibroblasts and oral epithelial cells. Biomaterials 2011;32(25) 5756–5764.

[39] Moharamzadeh K, Colley H, Murdoch C, Hearnden V, Chai WL, Brook IM, et al. Tissue-engineered oral mucosa. Journal of Dental Research 2012;91(7) 642-650.

[40] Rastogi S, Modi M, Sathian B. The efficacy of collagen membrane as a biodegradable wound dressing material for surgical defects of oral mucosa: a prospective study. Journal of Oral and Maxillofacial Surgery 2009;67(8) 1600-1606.

[41] Baum BJ, O'Connell BC. In vivo gene transfer to salivary glands. Crit Rev Oral Biol Med 1999;10(3) 276-283.

[42] Duailibi SE, Duailibi MT, Zhang W, Asrican R, Vacanti JP, Yelick PC. Bioengineered dental tissues grown in the rat jaw. J Dent Res 2008;87(8) 745-750.

[43] Kim JY, Xin X, Moioli EK, Chung J, Lee CH, Chen M, Fu SY, Koch PD, Mao JJ. Regeneration of dental-pulp-like tissue by chemotaxis-induced cell homing. Tissue Eng Part A 2010;16(10) 3023–3031.

[44] Patil AS, Merchant Y, Nagarajan P. Tissue Engineering of Craniofacial Tissues – A Review. Journal of Regenerative Medicine & Tissue Engineering 2013;2 1-19.

[45] Sharma S, Srivastava D, Grover S, Sharma V. Biomaterials in Tooth Tissue Engineering: A Review. Journal of Clinical and Diagnostic Research 2014;8(1) 309-315.

[46] Kim BS, Mooney DJ. Development of biocompatible synthetic extracellular matrices for tissue engineering. Trends Biotechnol 1998;16(5) 224-30.

[47] Kim BS, Baez CE, Atala A. Biomaterials for tissue engineering. World J Urol 2000;18(1) 2-9.

[48] Burg KJ, Porter S, Kellam JF. Biomaterial developments for bone tissue engineering. Biomaterials 2000;21(23) 2347-59.

[49] Nehrer S, Breinan HA, Ramappa A, Young G, Shortkroff S, Louie LK, Sledge CB, Yannas IV and Spector M. Matrix collagen type and pore size influence behaviour of seeded canine chondrocytes. Biomaterials 1997;18(11) 769-776.

[50] Rowley JA, Madlambayan G and Mooney DJ. Alginate hydrogels as synthetic extracellular matrix materials. Biomaterials 1999;20(1) 45-53.

[51] Cassell OC, Morrison WA, Messina A, Penington AJ, Thompson EW, Stevens GW, Perera JM, Kleinman HK, Hurley JV, Romeo R and Knight KR. The influence of extracellular matrix on the generation of vascularized, engineered, transplantable tissue. Ann N Y Acad Sc 2001;944 429-442.

[52] Hofer SO, Mitchell GM, Penington AJ, Morrison WA, RomeoMeeuw R, Keramidaris E, Palmer J and Knight KR. The use of pimonidazole to characterise hypoxia in the internal environment of an in vivo tissue engineering chamber. Br J Plast Surg 2005;58(8) 1104-1114.

[53] Ye Q, Zund G, Benedikt P, Jockenhoevel S, Hoerstrup SP, Sakyama S, Hubbell JA and Turina M. Fibrin gel as a three dimensional matrix in cardiovascular tissue engineering. Eur J Cardiothorac Surg 2000;17(5) 587-591.

[54] Hall H, Baechi T and Hubbell JA. Molecular properties of fibrin-based matrices for promotion of angiogenesis in vitro. Microvasc Res 2001;62(3) 315-326.

[55] Bourdoulous S, Orend G, MacKenna DA, Pasqualini R and Ruoslahti E. Fibronectin matrix regulates activation of RHO and CDC42 GTPases and cell cycle progression. J Cell Biol 1998;143(1) 267-276.

[56] Vogel V, Baneyx G. The tissue engineeting puzzle: a molecular perspective. Annu Rev Biomed Eng 2003; 5 441-63.

[57] Boynuegri D, Ozcan G, Senel S, Uç D, Uraz A, Ogüs E, Cakilci B, Karaduman B. Clinical and radiographic evaluations of chitosan gel in periodontal intraosseous defects: a pilot study. J Biomed Mater Res B Appl Biomater 2009;90(1) 461-466.

[58] Gomes ME, Ribeiro AS, Malafaya PB, Reis RL and Cunha AM. A new approach based on injection moulding to produce biodegradable starch-based polymeric scaffolds: morphology, mechanical and degradation behaviour. Biomaterials 2001;22(9) 883-889.

[59] Madihally SV and Matthew HW. Porous chitosan scaffolds for tissue engineering. Biomaterials 1999;20(12) 1133-1142.

[60] Suh JK and Matthew HW. Application of chitosan-based polysaccharide biomaterials in cartilage tissue engineering: a review. Biomaterials 2000;21(24) 2589-2598.

[61] Rocha LB, Goissis G and Rossi MA. Biocompatibility of anionic collagen matrix as scaffold for bone healing. Biomaterials 2002;23(2) 449-456.

[62] Petite H, Viateau V, Bensaid W, Meunier A, Pollak C, Bourguignon M, Oudina K, Sedel L and Guillemin G. Tissue-engineered bone regeneration. Nat Biotechnol 2000;18(9) 959-963.

[63] Sartoris DJ, Gershuni DH, Akeson WH, Holmes RE and Resnick D. Coralline hydroxyapatite bone graft substitutes: preliminary report of radiographic evaluation. Radiology 1986;159(1) 133-137.

[64] Irwin RB, Bernhard M and Biddinger A. Coralline hydroxyapatite as bone substitute in orthopedic oncology. Am J Orthop (Belle Mead NJ) 2001;30(7) 544-550.

[65] Vacanti CA, Bonassar LJ, Vacanti MP and Shufflebarger J. Replacement of an avulsed phalanx with tissue-engineered bone. N Engl J Med 2001;344(20) 1511-1514.

[66] Flatley TJ, Lynch KL, Benson M. Recombined Xenograft of Cancellous Bone and Bone Morphogenetic Protein (BMP). Clin. Orthop 1983;11 55-58.

[67] Kon E, Muraglia A, Corsi A, Bianco P, Marcacci M, Martin I, Boyde A, Ruspantini I, Chistolini P, Rocca M, Giardino R, Cancedda R and Quarto R. Autologous bone marrow stromal cells loaded onto porous hydroxyapatite ceramic accelerate bone repair in critical-size defects of sheep long bones. J Biomed Mater Res 2000;49(3) 328-337.

[68] Laurencin CT, El-Amin SF, Ibim SE, Willoughby DA, Attawia M, Allcock HR and Ambrosio AA. A highly porous 3-dimensional polyphosphazene polymer matrix for skeletal tissue regeneration. J Biomed Mater Res 1996;30(2) 133-138.

[69] Lhommeau CL, Levene H, Abramson S, Kohn J. Preparation of highly interconnected porous, tyrosine-derived polycarbonate scaffolds. Tissue Eng 1998;4(4) 468.

[70] Zein I, Hutmacher DW, Tan KC and Teoh SH. Fused deposition modeling of novel scaffold architectures for tissue engineering applications. Biomaterials 2002; 23(4) 1169-1185.

[71] Fisher JP, Holland TA, Dean D, Engel PS and Mikos AG. Synthesis and properties of photocross-linked poly(propylene fumarate) scaffolds. J Biomater Sci Polym Ed 2001; 12(6) 673-687.

[72] Ishaug-Riley SL, Crane-Kruger GM, Yaszemski MJ and Mikos AG. Three-dimensional culture of rat calvarial osteoblasts in porous biodegradable polymers. Biomaterials 1998; 19(15) 1405-1412.

[73] Ma PX and Choi JW. Biodegradable polymer scaffolds with welldefined intercon-nected spherical pore network. Tissue Eng 2001;7(1) 23-33.

[74] Thomson RC, Yaszemski MJ, Powers JM and Mikos AG. Hydroxyapatite fiber rein-forced poly(alpha-hydroxy ester) foams for bone regeneration. Biomaterials 1998;19(21) 1935-1943.

[75] Ma PX, Zhang R, Xiao G and Franceschi R. Engineering new bone tissue in vitroon highly porous poly(alpha-hydroxyl acids)/hydroxyapatite composite scaffolds. J Bi-omed Mater Res 2001;54(2) 284-293.

Permissions

All chapters in this book were first published in CCDI, by InTech Open; hereby published with permission under the Creative Commons Attribution License or equivalent. Every chapter published in this book has been scrutinized by our experts. Their significance has been extensively debated. The topics covered herein carry significant findings which will fuel the growth of the discipline. They may even be implemented as practical applications or may be referred to as a beginning point for another development.

The contributors of this book come from diverse backgrounds, making this book a truly international effort. This book will bring forth new frontiers with its revolutionizing research information and detailed analysis of the nascent developments around the world.

We would like to thank all the contributing authors for lending their expertise to make the book truly unique. They have played a crucial role in the development of this book. Without their invaluable contributions this book wouldn't have been possible. They have made vital efforts to compile up to date information on the varied aspects of this subject to make this book a valuable addition to the collection of many professionals and students.

This book was conceptualized with the vision of imparting up-to-date information and advanced data in this field. To ensure the same, a matchless editorial board was set up. Every individual on the board went through rigorous rounds of assessment to prove their worth. After which they invested a large part of their time researching and compiling the most relevant data for our readers.

The editorial board has been involved in producing this book since its inception. They have spent rigorous hours researching and exploring the diverse topics which have resulted in the successful publishing of this book. They have passed on their knowledge of decades through this book. To expedite this challenging task, the publisher supported the team at every step. A small team of assistant editors was also appointed to further simplify the editing procedure and attain best results for the readers.

Apart from the editorial board, the designing team has also invested a significant amount of their time in understanding the subject and creating the most relevant covers. They scrutinized every image to scout for the most suitable representation of the subject and create an appropriate cover for the book.

The publishing team has been an ardent support to the editorial, designing and production team. Their endless efforts to recruit the best for this project, has resulted in the accomplishment of this book. They are a veteran in the field of academics and their pool of knowledge is as vast as their experience in printing. Their expertise and guidance has proved useful at every step. Their uncompromising quality standards have made this book an exceptional effort. Their encouragement from time to time has been an inspiration for everyone.

The publisher and the editorial board hope that this book will prove to be a valuable piece of knowledge for researchers, students, practitioners and scholars across the globe.

List of Contributors

Sukumaran Anil
Department of Periodontics and Community Dentistry, College of Dentistry, King Saud University, Riyadh, Saudi Arabia

Asala F. Al-Sulaimani
King Saud University, Riyadh, Saudi Arabia

Ansar E. Beeran and Harikrishna P. R. Varma
Biomedical Technology Wing, Sree Chitra Tirunal Institute for Medical Sciences & Technology, Poojappura, India

Elna P. Chalisserry
College of Dentistry, King Saud University, Riyadh, Saudi Arabia

Mohammad D. Al Amri
Department of Prosthetic Dental Sciences, College of Dentistry, King Saud University, Riyadh, Saudi Arabia

Ilser Turkyilmaz and Ashley Brooke Hoders
Department of Comprehensive Dentistry, University of Texas Health Science Center at San Antonio, Texas, USA

Fatma Deniz Uzuner and Belma Işık Aslan
Department of Orthodontics, Faculty of Dentistry, Gazi University, Emek Ankara, Turkey

Umit Karacayli
Department of Oral and Maxillofacial Surgery, Gulhane Military Medical Academy, Ankara, Turkey

Emre Dikicier
Department of Oral and Maxillofacial Surgery, Corlu Military Hospital, Tekirdag, Turkey

Sibel Dikicier
Department of Prosthodontics, Corlu Military Hospital, Tekirdag, Turkey

Sybele Saska and Larissa Souza Mendes
Institute of Chemistry, São Paulo State University-UNESP, Araraquara – SP, Brazil

Ana Maria Minarelli Gaspar and Ticiana Sidorenko de Oliveira Capote
Dental School at Araraquara, São Paulo State University-UNESP, Department of Morphology, Araraquara – SP, Brazil

Elena Preoteasa and Marina Imre
Department of Prosthodontics, Faculty of Dental Medicine, Carol Davila University of Medicine and Pharmacy, Bucharest, Romania

Laurentiu Iulian Florica
Private Practice, Bucharest, Romania

Florian Obadan
Private Practice, Alexandria, Romania

Cristina Teodora Preoteasa
Department of Oral Diagnosis, Ergonomics, Scientific Research Methodology, Faculty of Dental Medicine, Carol Davila University of Medicine and Pharmacy, Bucharest, Romania

Derek D'Souza
Consultant Prosthodontist, Pune, India

Ilser Turkyilmaz
Department of Comprehensive Dentistry, University of Texas Health Science Center at San Antonio, Texas, USA

Gokce Soganci
Department of Prosthodontics, Oral and Dental Health Center, Ankara, Turkey

Andréa Cristina Barbosa da Silva, Diego Romário da Silva, Rafael Grotta Grempel, Manuel Antonio Gordón-Núñez and Gustavo Gomes Agripino
Graduate Program in Dentistry, Center of Sciences, Technology and Health, State University of Paraiba, UEPB, Araruna, Paraíba, Brazil

Index

www.ingramcontent.com/pod-product-compliance
Lightning Source LLC
Chambersburg PA
CBHW061946190326
41458CB00009B/2800